I0165397

# THE
# HUNGER
# CRUSHING
# COMBO
## METHOD

Also by Abbey Sharp:

*The Mindful Glow Cookbook: Radiant Recipes*
*for Being the Healthiest, Happiest You*

# THE HUNGER CRUSHING COMBO METHOD

The Simple Secret to Eating Well
Without Ever Dieting Again

## ABBEY SHARP, RD

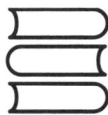

balance

New York   Boston

Neither this diet nor any other diet should be followed without first consulting a health-care professional. If you have any special conditions requiring attention, you should consult with your health-care professional regularly regarding possible modification of the program contained in this book.

Copyright © 2026 by Abbey Sharp Picov

Cover design by Terri Sirma
Cover images by Shutterstock
Cover copyright © 2026 by Hachette Book Group, Inc.

Hachette Book Group supports the right to free expression and the value of copyright. The purpose of copyright is to encourage writers and artists to produce the creative works that enrich our culture.

The scanning, uploading, and distribution of this book without permission is a theft of the author's intellectual property. If you would like permission to use material from the book (other than for review purposes), please contact permissions@hbgusa.com. Thank you for your support of the author's rights.

Balance
Hachette Book Group
1290 Avenue of the Americas
New York, NY 10104
GCP-Balance.com
@GCPBalance

First Edition: January 2026

Balance is an imprint of Grand Central Publishing. The Balance name and logo are registered trademarks of Hachette Book Group, Inc.

The publisher is not responsible for websites (or their content) that are not owned by the publisher.

The Hachette Speakers Bureau provides a wide range of authors for speaking events. To find out more, go to hachettespeakersbureau.com or email HachetteSpeakers@hbgusa.com.

Balance books may be purchased in bulk for business, educational, or promotional use. For information, please contact your local bookseller or the Hachette Book Group Special Markets Department at special.markets@hbgusa.com.

Print book interior design by Bart Dawson

Library of Congress Control Number: 2025034635

ISBNs: 9780306836794 (hardcover), 9780306836817 (ebook)

Printed in the United States of America

LSC-H

Printing 1, 2025

*To my boys, a.k.a. the real superstar combo of my life.*
*Thank you for the daily reminder that wellness,*
*self-care, and nourishment go well beyond*
*what we put on our plate (but sprinkles on yogurt*
*is always a good place to start).*

# CONTENTS

· · · · · · · · · · · · · · · · · · · · · · ·

# PART 3: PUTTING IT ON YOUR PLATE

# THE
# HUNGER CRUSHING COMBO
## METHOD

# INTRODUCTION

. . . . . . . . . . . . . . . . . . . . . .

# The Road to Abundance

It's a wild time to be alive, folks. And I'm not just talking about the political landscape, the acceleration of AI, the grim economy, or the superstardom that is Taylor Swift (basically, the only thing our generation seems to have going for us). The state of affairs when it comes to diet and nutrition information (or, should I say, misinformation) is enough to leave anyone aghast. Never before have we had so many competing ideas about what to eat. Gluten makes you fat. Seed oils are inflammatory. Eggs are good for you. No, wait, they're bad for you. No, actually we were right the first time, eat the damn eggs! Just make sure they're grass-fed, free-range omega-3–enriched eggs, or don't bother.

Every day, we're faced with hundreds of messages about food and our diet, the vast majority of which are contradictory and often just flat-out wrong. Between social media influencers, sensational-ized media headlines, and the notorious inconsistency of nutrition research, it seems the more we learn about nutrition, the less confident we become in our ability to eat intuitively. Man, for something as pri-mal as putting energy into our body, it's starting to feel like we need a PhD just to pack a basic lunch.

Not only is eating well now confusing and complicated, but it's also riddled with shame, morality, and judgment too. Chances are, you've felt the pressure to restrict what you're eating in some way, whether that's your total calories, sugar, or even the hours during which you're "allowed" to eat. Welcome to the modern world, my friend. Focusing on all the foods we can't have because they're bad is now so deeply ingrained into the fabric of our lives, it's largely invisible. But while diet dogma may help you at least temporarily control your body shape, size, or health markers, often it has a more permanent effect on your relationship with food and your body. The result is a longtime struggle with body dysmorphia, dissatisfaction, and disconnect from your own internal wisdom.

If you've been dieting your whole life, ask yourself this seemingly simple question: "What's the first thing I think of when I hear the word 'cake'?" My seven-year-old son who, hopefully, has years before he's made an acquaintance with diet culture, would probably say "birthday," "party," or "fun." But to so many of us who have been dieting our whole lives, just breathing in toxic messages about our bodies and food, "cake" isn't such a jolly word. It may conjure up words like "guilty," "cheat," "unhealthy," or "bad." And these words may even become absorbed into our own being. Suddenly, just the thought of red velvet makes us feel fearful and ashamed. This is the $300-billion-plus diet industry that feeds off our insecurities, forcing us (particularly women) to beg for another solution to our self-loathing and food fears. So, here we all are, indoctrinated to feel just as bad about having a mini biscotti at the office as we would about having an affair with *someone* at the office.

Let's change that, okay?

Food is not just a compilation of banal nutrients meant to sustain life; it's actually evolutionarily designed to be pleasurable. If it weren't, we'd be too distracted by other interesting earthly pleasures, like a bird in the sky or a new flower in the distance to get off our butts and find something to eat! Honestly, every time I see an influencer flex about spending $12 on a flavorless, 20-calorie bottle of celery juice, I imagine our caveman ancestors face-palming and rolling their eyes even more aggressively than I do. No matter how hard the diet industry pushes us to fight against our inherent love of food, it will always be one of life's great pleasures. Take it away, and the body sets off alarm bells that something is *very* wrong and that we need to rectify the uncomfortable situation stat. Cue the late-night pantry raid. The soul-gnawing guilt. The self-loathing and punishment all the weeks that follow. You're in the fiery depths of diet hell, and after just one or two kicks at the can, it can feel nearly impossible to climb out. I know, because I was shackled to this cycle for years, and it nearly cost me my life.

For most of my adult life, my motto has been, "If I'm not ahead, I'm behind," a mindset that I've embodied since I was young. Those who know me personally know that I'm a classic type A. And the constant battle of trying to keep up with the Joneses (and by Joneses, I mean my own unattainable high standards) has won me both praise and a lot of agony. At as early as six years old, I would cry in my bed, worrying myself sick over the next morning's dance competition. In high school, my focus shifted to my budding singing career and "winning" all the top theater parts. That success soon led me away from my supportive small rural community to try to "make it" in big-city Toronto, taking the year after high school to really sink my teeth into the music industry. Adults much older and wiser than I insisted I had the "it" factor; I just needed to get myself into the right rooms. Not surprisingly, my frenemy, anxiety, took full control. I had thrown everything away for this opportunity. I had moved away from my friends, I had put a pause on any higher education, and as a bona fide people-pleaser, I was paralyzed by the fear of letting everyone down. If I didn't make this happen for myself, who would I even be?

Meanwhile, I had always had a sensitive tummy. I almost thought it was just normal to constantly feel a little nauseated and bloated. But performance butterflies only amplified my daily discomfort. I didn't have a name for it at the time, but I know now that I had been suffering from irritable bowel syndrome (IBS). And thanks to a constant conversation between my deteriorating mental state and my perceptive gut, my digestion was perpetually on the fritz. It seemed that everything I ate caused some discomfort and pain, which, looking back, was likely more of a mirrored reflection of my tortured brain, than of any one triggering food or drink.

But, alas, I thought it was time to get some help with my tummy troubles. So, at the recommendation of a family friend, I enlisted the support of a local homeopathic naturopath. Her recommendation was simple and direct: Cut out all the sugar in my diet. According to her, sugar was toxic and it was poisoning my gut *and* my mental health. It needed to be eliminated.

Not surprisingly, once I started focusing all my energy on sugar elimination, I began losing weight. I also started receiving loads of praise from people around me. These compliments were pure ecstasy. And if cutting out sugar got me a round of applause, I figured that cutting out more "bad" foods might get me that standing ovation I so desperately craved.

I had already "mastered" the art of scanning every food product for words that end in -*ose* (shorthand for sugar in everything from bread to cereals to salad dressings to pasta sauce). I was ready for the gut-healing detox 2.0. Sugar may have been public enemy number one, but according to all the "health" magazines at the checkout, fat was also on the naughty list. It, too, had to go.

Very quickly, my list of safe foods got even smaller, and so, too, did my weak body. Compliments ceased and were replaced with whispers, looks, and words of concern. And just like that, my steady stream of people-pleasing dopamine was ripped away. The shame only drove me further into a state of depression and despair, and my only sense of satisfaction came from control.

Or at least the facade of control. After months of living off fat-free, sugar-free yogurt and massive bowls of lettuce sans dressing, my willpower self-imploded. I started to binge. But, of course, in the most "controlled" way possible. Every Sunday, I would spend the day fasting, pacifying my hunger with tea while running errands to distract myself. Then, at night, I would eat the equivalent of more than all my weekly meals combined, in the form of all the "forbidden foods" I had otherwise cut out. A multicourse smorgasbord of fries, pizza, pasta, cheesecake, doughnuts, and ice cream as soon as the clock struck five p.m. and the cheat meal began. Every waking moment between those feasts was spent drowning in food fantasies and planning my next "cheat," always with the sad knowledge that the life I was living in real time was so miserably gray. And despite the climax that was that end-of-week meal, I would spend the rest of the week in an even deeper depression. Each week, the binges got bigger, and the restrictions got tighter, and it became unimaginable to ever stop.

It became me.

And I hated that me. So, I retreated into my delicate shell, withdrawn, small, silenced. I had spent my whole life being the little girl with the big voice, and suddenly, I felt completely incapable of singing a single note. Symbolically and figuratively, I had fully lost touch with who I was. My quest for diet purity quite literally hijacked my brain, and my body was succumbing to its powerful control.

Eventually, the adults in my life woke up to the fact that this regimen was not serving me, and was quite possibly going to lead to my demise. I had to admit I had a problem, and it had a name: orthorexia.

Orthorexia is often described as "clean eating taken to an extreme." Unlike other eating disorders that focus primarily on restricting the quantity of food consumed, orthorexia involves an unhealthy obsession with the perceived quality, healthfulness, or purity of food. In my case, my orthorexia eventually evolved into a dangerous eating disorder cocktail that included both anorexia and binge-eating tendencies.

Recovery was not a simple linear journey. But after meeting with a dietitian (my first introduction to the profession), I was able to wake up to everything that diet culture had stolen from my life: the relationships, the experiences, the mental space to think, grow, and learn. Most people ease into recovery slowly and gently, but I knew I had to go all in. Seemingly overnight, I went from micromanaging every bite of food that grazed my lips, to attending nightly food events and restaurant launches where I had zero say in what I was eating. Yes, it was scary to fully relinquish control, but the freedom was so invigorating, so exhilarating, I knew I could never let myself go back. And it's this lived experience of mine that has guided me into my career as a registered dietitian specializing in helping people make peace with food for good.

As I've quickly learned as a professional, my experience is far from unique, and as such, I will sadly never be out of a job. Twenty years ago, I fell into disordered eating patterns likely due to my own personal comorbidities and circumstances, including preexisting anxiety, ADHD, perfectionism, and loneliness, all of which are major risk factors for eating disorders. Sure, I was also exposed to diet culture messaging in the media, but I wasn't fully immersed in it the way young people on social media are today. My eating disorder took hold long before the "What I Eat in a Day" videos, the social media echo chambers, the perfectly curated influencer feeds, and the nonstop proliferation of mis- and disinformation online. Today, you don't need any existing genetic or mental health comorbidities to be massively at risk. In fact, our collective obsession with "clean eating" is now so celebrated that orthorexia and general disordered eating are almost status quo. The message being: If you're not buying the sugar-free, gluten-free, dairy-free Paleo muffin, are you even trying?

I know that many reading this right now have struggled with their relationship with food in some way. It is estimated that 8 percent of the

US population[1] (nearly thirty million Americans across a variety of cultures, genders, and age groups) suffer from an eating disorder. And a 2008 survey with over four thousand American women found that 65 percent reported behaviors consistent with disordered eating.[2] So, even if your personal journey hasn't manifested as a full-blown eating disorder, worrying about food has still likely stolen years of life. The guilt you've felt when you swore you would only eat two fries, but polished off the whole plate. The shame of "cheating" on your diet with your kids' Halloween haul. The mental gymnastics of trying to calculate how many calories you can eat at breakfast if you plan to have a glass of wine at girls' night. You have been robbed of so many joyful life experiences by obsessing about food and your body, experiences that make you, *you*. And whether you've been trapped in this cycle for months or years, it's been too long.

You can't get that time back, but you're here today because, going forward, you want to do things differently. And by "differently," I'm not saying I'm going to convince you to not give a damn about your health, how you look, or what size of pants you're going to buy. We all have wellness goals! For one person, that may be to improve their daily blood sugars so they can reduce their medication dose. For others, it may be to lose 10 pounds so they can feel confident at the pool. It's not up to me (or anyone else) to judge whose goals are "valid" and whose are "vain." But when it comes specifically to numerical weight-loss targets, they're not always the most actionable goal. We can't *directly* control what our weight decides to do when we cut out sugar or integrate a daily run. And if the number on the scale is your sole indicator of success, it's nearly impossible to push through the discouragement when your progress doesn't move at a linear, predictable, or quick pace. We do, however, have control over behaviors that support our goals and health (assuming these behaviors are accessible to you). Although, in the past, you may have taken the *control* component into dangerous, extreme territory, I'm going to teach you a revolutionary approach to eating well without the common pitfalls and harm. No risk, all rewards. No scarcity, just abundance. No fear, just loads of delicious nourishing food.

Introducing the Hunger Crushing Combo, a revolutionary non-diet additive approach to eating and living well. You'll never look at a bag of potato chips in the same way again.

## PART 1

# WHAT IS THE HUNGER CRUSHING COMBO?

# CHAPTER 1

· · · · · · · · · · · · · · · · · ·

# The Nonrestrictive, Additive Approach
# to Eating and Living Well

You know the feeling. You reach into a bag of chips for what you swear is just a tiny taste. And somehow, someway, within minutes, you're fumbling with the crumbs at the bottom of the bag. Instant guilt. You blew it. You're weak. You're stupid. You royally F'ed up. And now you can never ever ever be trusted to bring chips into your house again. Chips are now a "fear food." Those Lay's marketers were right. You absolutely CAN'T eat just one.

What if I told you that the mere existence of these "fear foods" (that is, the belief that you can't trust yourself around something with a less-than-stellar nutrition CV) is what triggers these out-of-control binges in the first place? It wasn't until I was on my own journey of healing my relationship with food that I was able to unearth this pattern and nip the cycle right in the bud. That is, the restrictive scarcity mentality of fearing and avoiding foods I loved.

Once I cleared the mental distraction of obsessing over NOT eating my fear foods, I had space to listen to my body's true desires and needs.

That's when my Hunger Crushing Combo Method was born. This is an additive, gentle nutrition framework designed to serve as an evidence-based alternative to all the rigid rules that have failed you in the past. Rather than focusing on a laundry list of what you need to remove from your diet, it shifts the focus onto what you can add. Namely, your Hunger Crushing Compounds (HCCs): fiber, protein, and healthy fats.

The Hunger Crushing Combo will never tell you to swear off your favorite foods. In fact, it encourages you to work them into your diet every day. Sometimes, just as is, but often "dressed up" with the foods that keep you fuller longer. Adding one HCC, such as fiber, protein, or healthy fat, to a meal is great. Adding two or more offers even more perks! The key here is that you're *adding* foods to your meals and snacks that satisfy your physical and emotional needs, helping to quiet the "food noise" that robs you of a full life.

The Hunger Crushing Combo Method is a 180 shift that helps you escape the scarcity mentality that keeps you trapped in the binge–restrict cycle, and funnels you into a more sustainable mindset of abundance. Foods will never all be nutritionally equal, but we can make them morally equal by seeing them for what they are. Just different foods with various attributes, none of which defines us.

I've been using this framework for a decade now, and the results are pure magic. Cravings disappear. Hunger and fullness cues are restored. You have space in your life to think about things other than food. And you never have to diet again.

## Hunger 101

Despite all the unexpected and somewhat expected pains and trauma we put our body through, particularly as women (I'm going to file my eighteen-hour active labor under "unexpected trauma," thank you), our body still has our back. If we let it be heard, and trust the messages it sends, it holds the great power to help us manage our health, whether that's getting a mammogram after feeling a lump in our breast, or saving the rest of the carrot cake for the next day when we start to feel full. Our body can and should be our BFF.

The problem most of us face is that, at some point in our lives, we were conditioned to turn our back on our body. For a lot of us, the betrayal started with our first diet, with the tricks it taught us on how to purposefully ignore our innate body wisdom. Most "diets" require some form of restriction, triggering a wave of hunger to beg us to shut that diet down. And because hunger (physical and also emotional) is such an uncomfortable and gnawing state to live in, it's not long before we're washing down French fries with a triple-thick shake, thinking, "Eh, that just wasn't a good diet, I'll start a new one next week." It's easy to get frustrated by our hunger or see it as a marker of failure, but it's actually an important indicator that our body is alive and well! Back in our ancestors' days, if we didn't feel the discomfort of hunger, we might just lie around in our hut all day, making cave art until either something came to eat *us*, or we just starved and withered away. Hunger is a necessary survival cue, and when we stop seeing these sensations as the enemy, we can start to work *with* them to better reach our goals.

Working *with* our hunger doesn't mean never feeling hunger again. Let me say that again for the people in the back: The goal is not to suppress your hunger sensations so much that you get really good at ignoring what your body is telling you it needs. And it's certainly not to learn to "fear" or antagonize hunger and become anxious or worried you're doing something wrong if you feel stomach grumbles, blood sugar dips, headaches, or other indications that your body needs food.

Normal, regular hunger cues are imperative to helping us meet our nutrient needs and maintain our body's healthiest happiest weight.

However, if we've been stuck treading the toxic waters of diet culture for a while, perhaps restricting our food intake for many years, we have likely desensitized and dulled down our hunger and fullness cues. It's a bit of a *boy who cried wolf* scenario. Eventually, we habituate and the desperate cries for help just disappear into the background. This reduced sensitivity and interoceptive awareness makes it impossible to eventually find food freedom and get back in tune with our body's true needs.

Deprivation also results in emotional hunger, as well. That longing for something we don't or can't have. Incessant physical and emotional hunger takes up space, time, and energy in our lives that we could be investing in other responsibilities, things we enjoy doing, and important acts of self-care. And no one has time to make themselves a meal or snack only to be hit with hunger again an hour later, or to fantasize about the food they *wanted* but didn't eat. Thinking about food shouldn't be the predominant task of your day.

The goal with my Hunger Crushing Combo is for you to learn a wide variety of skills for doing the hunger-to-fullness line dance in a predictable, compassionate, and flexible way that fits your vibrant life.

## The Hunger Crushing Compounds

Let me introduce you to our MVPs, our Hunger Crushing Compounds (protein, fiber, and healthy fats).

Now, within this framework, a lot of foods will almost exclusively be made up of *one* of these Hunger Crushing Compounds. I like to call this their "primary residence." Something like egg whites, or fat-free yogurt, for example, would be pretty much exclusively protein. Broccoli or cauliflower live pretty exclusively in the fiber category.

But a lot of foods in nature have at least some kind of mix. In other words, they have "dual citizenship" with two or more Hunger Crushing Compound categories. Avocados, for example, are rich in fiber *and* fats. Full-fat yogurt contains protein *and* fat. Nuts, seeds, chia, and flax might be triple threats offering fiber, protein, *and* fat. If you're obsessing over where these dual-citizenship foods lie, you're overthinking the details. These foods are inherent Hunger Crushing Combos, and they're going to be amazing meal additions, no matter how you want to define them. More of those things, please!

Let's break down each category and where you can typically find these types of foods.

## Aren't the HCCs Just Macros by Another Name?

The Hunger Crushing Compounds are similar, but slightly different categories of the three main macronutrients we consume in food: protein, carbs, and fat. And that's because carbohydrates can be highly refined (what you'll soon know of as Naked Carbs) or they can already come somewhat "dressed" in fiber (or protein and fat), and these types of carbs behave dramatically differently in the body. Likewise, not all fats are created equal, hence the need for a little more direction, clarification, and education through the structure of the HCC.

## Protein

Protein can come from both animal and plant sources. Both offer really important health benefits,[1] including increasing satiety[2] after a meal, promoting a healthy body weight and composition,[3] helping build muscle and bone,[4] and supporting a healthy immune system. Here's a quick and dirty Protein 101.

Protein is made up of building blocks called amino acids, which our body utilizes in different proportions to help us grow and repair body tissue; make hormones and neurotransmitters; provide an energy source; maintain healthy skin, hair, and nails; build muscle; and sustain a healthy immune and digestive system (just to name a few of protein's main gigs).

There are twenty different amino acids that our body needs to thrive, nine of which must come from what we eat. We call these *essential* amino acids. Unlike the other eleven nonessential amino acids, our body cannot manufacture these in-house, so we need to get them from our diet.

The term "complete protein" is often used to describe a food that features all nine essential amino acids. All animal-based proteins are inherently complete proteins, so if you consume a few eggs postworkout, for example, you're getting all the amino acids your body needs to build and repair those worked muscles.

Soy, quinoa, buckwheat, amaranth, hemp, chia, nutritional yeast, and mycoprotein (found in Quorn products) are the only plant-based proteins that have all nine essential amino acids in sufficient quantities to build muscle or other protein-based tissues. This does not mean that if you're vegetarian or vegan, you're suddenly unable to build muscle. The cool thing about plant-based proteins is that what one source lacks, another makes up for. So, for example, legumes (e.g., peas) are rich in the essential amino acid lysine, but low in the amino acid methionine. Rice, on the other hand, is rich in methionine, but it's low in lysine. Serve them together (as so many cultures have been doing for centuries), and ta-da! A perfect little protein package is born. We also don't need to "combine" them perfectly at every meal, as we used to think. Our body keeps a little reservoir of amino acids on deck to be pieced together in different orientations as different protein jobs arise. So, as long as we're getting in a variety of plant-based proteins, we'll get in all of the essential amino acids we need to thrive. In other words, variety is key (and we'll go into a lot more detail on why in Chapter 4).

## Key Protein Sources

| Animal-based sources of protein | Plant-based sources of protein |
|---|---|
| Chicken | Beans, peas, lentils, and other legumes |
| Turkey | Soy (tofu, tempeh, and soy milk) |
| Beef and other red meats | Whole grains (including amaranth and quinoa) |
| Pork | |
| Fish | Nuts and seeds |
| Shellfish | Mycoprotein |
| Dairy | Nutritional yeast |
| Eggs | |

Dairy can be one of those foods that can lean toward a protein or fat "primary residence," depending on the variety. Greek yogurt, cottage cheese, and milk are considered protein primary residences because they're high in protein and generally low in fat. Yet soft cheese, like Brie and blue cheese, lean more toward the fat category (which we will get to shortly), as this macronutrient makes up the majority share. Don't overthink the framework; there will always be overlapping Hunger Crushing Compounds in food, and remember, dual citizens are our BFFs!

## Protein Dual Citizens

Fatty fish (salmon, trout, mackerel): Protein + Healthy Fats

Edamame: Protein + Healthy Fats + Fiber

Tempeh or tofu: Protein + Healthy Fats

Full-fat fermented dairy (yogurt, kefir, cheese): Protein + Healthy Fats

Whole eggs: Protein + Healthy Fats

Beans: Protein + Fiber

Legumes (lentils, peas, and chickpeas): Protein + Fiber

Quinoa: Protein + Fiber

Nuts (peanuts, almonds, pistachios): Protein + Fiber +
Healthy Fats

Seeds (pumpkin, sesame, sunflower): Protein + Fiber +
Healthy Fats

Hemp hearts: Protein + Healthy Fats

Chia seeds: Protein + Fiber + Healthy Fats

Flaxseeds: Protein + Fiber + Healthy Fats

## Fiber

Fiber is so much more than just the "poop" nutrient. It's actually one of our best tools for overcoming the restrict-binge-regret-repeat cycle, because it provides bulk to meals, helps slow digestion, makes us feel fuller longer, and is generally associated with maintaining a healthy body weight. Fiber is also important for managing blood sugar,[5] reducing our risk of heart disease[6] and certain cancers,[7] preventing digestive conditions like hemorrhoids[8] and diverticulitis, and supporting a healthy gut.[9]

Dietary fiber is derived exclusively from plants. Some of the best sources include fruits and vegetables; whole grains; beans, peas, lentils, and other legumes; and nuts and seeds.

There are two types of fiber: soluble and insoluble. Both types are super important. To my fellow Swifties, they're the Evermore and Folklore dynamic duo. You can't choose *just* one.

**Insoluble fiber** does not dissolve in water and remains intact as it moves through the digestive tract. Its main job is to add bulk to stool and prevent constipation, which in turn helps reduce the risk of digestive diseases. Foods that are rich in insoluble fiber include whole grains (e.g., wheat bran and barley), nuts and seeds, vegetables (e.g., broccoli, cauliflower, and kale), and the skins of fruits.

**Soluble fiber** dissolves in water to form a gummy or gelatinous substance in the digestive tract, helping make your poop smooth, soft, and easy to pass without needing to take a thirty-minute "poocation" in the loo. Its slow glacial velocity helps improve satiety, reduce blood sugar spikes, and lower "bad" LDL cholesterol. Plus, it serves as fuel (a.k.a. prebiotics) for the bacteria in our gut. Good sources of soluble fiber include oats, barley, legumes (e.g., beans, lentils, and peas), fruits (e.g., apples, pears, and berries), and some vegetables (e.g., carrots and sweet potatoes).

Most plants contain a mixture of insoluble and soluble fiber (and a lot of them are also dual citizens with other Hunger Crushing Compounds), so as long as you're getting a variety of plant-based foods, you're doing great.

## Fiber Dual Citizens

Avocado: Fiber + Healthy Fats

Beans: Fiber + Protein

Legumes (lentils, peas, and chickpeas): Fiber + Protein

Quinoa: Fiber + Protein

Edamame: Fiber + Healthy Fats + Protein

Nuts (almonds, hazelnuts, chestnuts): Fiber + Protein + Healthy Fats

Seeds (sunflower, sesame, pumpkin): Fiber + Protein + Healthy Fats

Chia seeds: Fiber + Protein + Healthy Fats

Flaxseeds: Fiber + Protein + Healthy Fats

## Healthy Fats

Fats help with vitamin absorption, provide a source of energy, contribute structure and function to cell membranes, and assist in cell signaling. Most important, they make food physically satiating and emotionally satisfying, because fat inherently tastes good. Food without fat will always leave you feeling a bit of longing, even if it's an otherwise good meal.

Like protein, dietary fats are made up of building blocks; these are called fatty acids. We categorize them based on their chemical structure and functions. This also helps play into how we classify our healthy fats. Here's a breakdown:

**Polyunsaturated Fats: Healthy Fats.** Polyunsaturated fatty acids, or PUFAs as we affectionately call them, are the omega-6 and omega-3 fatty acids. Omega-6s are found predominantly in vegetable oils, like corn and soybean oil, whereas omega-3s are found in fatty fish, like salmon; seeds, like flax, chia, and hemp; and plant oils, like walnut or flaxseed oil.

Omega-3 fats are legit fat superstars. We have ample research that they can help support the health of our heart, brain, cognition, mood, joints, and eyes. One large review[10] of the literature even found omega-3s were associated with a lower chance of early death from all causes!

Then, there are omega-6 fats. Despite what a lot of your social media feeds might suggest, these aren't inherently "bad." We will go into way more detail on debunking the seed oil slander, but in short, omega-3s and omega-6s work together in inflammation homeostasis. When the delicate balance of these two types of fatty acids get thrown off, there is concern that it can tip us into a pro-inflammatory state. But if we look at the greater body of research, including one large systematic review,[11] we see no strong link to suggest that omega-6s *in isolation* increased inflammation. That said, most of the omega-6s we get in our diet come from fried foods and highly processed snacks. So, though we don't want to denounce a naturally nutritious food just because it contains omega-6s, we do want us to try to reduce our reliance on highly processed foods and focus more on whole-food sources of omega-6s, like walnuts, Brazil nuts, almonds, and seeds.

**Monounsaturated Fats: Healthy Fats.** Research suggests that monounsaturated fats, or MUFAs (a.k.a. omega-9 fatty acids), can help us maintain a healthy weight,[12] while supporting heart health by reducing "bad" LDL cholesterol and improving[13] "good" HDL cholesterol. A diet rich in MUFAs is also associated with improvements in insulin sensitivity[14] and a reduced risk of certain cancers (e.g., breast cancer).[15] Some foods that are rich in monounsaturated fats include the following:

Avocado

Olives

Pistachios

Peanuts

Cashews

Macadamia nuts

Peanut butter

Pumpkin seeds

Pecans

Almonds

Sesame seeds

Hazelnuts

What about cooking oils from "healthy fat" sources, like olive oil? Since they're not in their "whole-food" state, does that mean they're bad? Absolutely not! In fact, as with Naked Carbs (more on these in just a minute), I encourage you to use oils in your meals, as they add nutrition, flavor, and texture to naturally nourishing foods. Extra-virgin olive oil is essential for making my signature Greek salad dressing. Coconut oil is delicious for cooking pancakes. And avocado oil is great for marinades and roasted veggies. But if you want to get the most out of this framework, you want to choose the fats that offer the greatest satiety bang for your calorie buck. We will be going into a lot more detail, with tips on how to do that, in the chapters that follow, but within this framework, our best healthy fat heroes are going to be those coming from whole foods that have dual citizenship with fiber and/or protein. A plate of olives will always be more satiating than a drizzle of oil.

**Saturated Fats: (Sometimes) Healthy Fats.** For most of the twentieth century, we were convinced that saturated fats were the devil, but recent reports are changing that tune. The argument for and against saturated fats could truly be its own book, but here's my attempt at CliffsNotes.

Decades ago,[16] a doctor named Ancel Keys hypothesized that saturated fat, or even just fat in general, caused heart disease. It was because of his theory and spotty research that dietary fats received their scarlet letter, and BAM! the "low-fat" and "fat-free" movement was born. Over the years, the research on saturated fats' impact on heart health has remained contradictory, with some studies finding fault, and others absolving them of culpability.

For example, in a controversial 2016 systematic review and meta-analysis,[17] researchers specifically looked at butter (which is high in saturated fat) and its relationship to cardiovascular disease. After careful review, the scientists found only a small or neutral effect of butter on cardiovascular disease, type 2 diabetes, and all-cause mortality.

Part of the reason for the inconsistent messaging may be the fact that saturated fats are not a homogenous group and their behaviors in the body may differ based on the length of their carbon chain. Most saturated fats in our diet are long-chain fatty acids (e.g., those found in beef and dark meat poultry). However, there is growing scientific interest in some of the unique properties of short- and medium-chain fatty acids. Short-chain fatty acids (SCFAs) like butyrate and acetate are found naturally in fermented foods like yogurt, sauerkraut, vinegar, and cheese, but they are also produced by our gut in response to eating fiber (more on this in Chapter 4). SCFAs are uniquely important for strengthening the intestinal barrier, supporting the immune system,[18] reducing the risk of chronic disease,[19] and even regulating appetite and metabolism.[20]

Medium-chain triglycerides (MCTs) offer other distinct metabolic benefits. Unlike long-chain fats, MCTs are transported directly to the liver, where they can be absorbed and metabolized as ketones for the brain and muscles to use as energy. For that reason, there is special interest in these fats for fat loss, appetite suppression,[21] and blood sugar regulation, plus the health of our brain, heart, and gut.[22] The greatest sources of MCTs in food are coconut oil, palm kernel oil, some dairy products, and pure MCT oil.

Whether a saturated fat is considered a "healthy fat" within this framework depends less on the minutiae of how many carbons its fatty acid chain has, and more on its dual-citizenship status. In other words, you want to choose *whole-food* sources of saturated fats that are bound up with protein and/or fiber.

Fermented dairy like cheese and yogurt are great sources of "healthy" saturated fats (including those beneficial SCFAs we just discussed), *plus* protein (along with a plethora of other important vitamins and minerals). Likewise, coconut is one of our best whole-food sources of those MCTs, plus fiber!

The bottom line on saturated fats is that they're not all created equal. Since we do have strong evidence that saturated fat may raise cardiovascular disease *risk factors* (even if it doesn't increase heart disease directly), it's not a bad idea to focus more intently on whole foods rich in unsaturated fats that we know have well-defined benefits. And when you do choose foods rich in saturated fats, to aim for those with dual citizenship status.

**Trans Fats: NOT Healthy Fats.** Trans fats are unsaturated fatty acids that exist naturally in minute amounts in some animal products, like beef and butter, but that are largely made artificially for ultraprocessed foods through a process called partial hydrogenation.

We used to think that they were better for us than saturated fats because they were naturally low in cholesterol and made of plants, but science has quickly confirmed that trans fats are one of the most concerning food components in our food system. Ironically, they're far worse for heart health than the saturated fats they were designed to replace, as they've been shown to increase the "bad" LDL cholesterol *and* decrease the "good" HDL cholesterol. The good news is that, as of December 23, 2023, the FDA has banned[23] the use of artificial trans fats in all processed foods, so our exposure today is greatly reduced.

## Healthy Fat Dual Citizens

Avocado: Healthy Fat + Fiber

Olives: Healthy Fat + Fiber

Fatty fish (salmon, trout, mackerel): Healthy Fat + Protein

Cheese: Healthy Fat + Protein

Eggs: Healthy Fat + Protein

Nuts (walnuts, pecans, brazil nuts): Healthy Fat + Fiber + Protein

Seeds (sunflower, sesame, pumpkin): Healthy Fat + Fiber + Protein

Flaxseeds: Healthy Fat + Fiber + Protein

Hemp hearts: Healthy Fat + Protein

Chia seeds: Healthy Fat + Fiber + Protein

Whole-milk dairy (yogurt, cottage cheese, milk): Healthy Fat + Protein

We are, however, still exposed to small amounts of trans fats in deep-fried foods, even if we're deep-frying in "healthier" unsaturated oils. I'm not suggesting you never eat a French fry again (skin-on chip truck spuds are a whole mood)! I'm just clarifying that we shouldn't be banking on deep-fried cooking oils as our "healthy fats" and that, when we can, we should aim to pair those foods with other Hunger Crushing Compounds.

## Naked Carbs

We've now established what Hunger Crushing Compounds are. Which leaves us to define the big category that ultimately does not make the cut: Naked Carbs. Don't skip this section, thinking that you just need to cut these foods out; they are actually an integral part of the framework. Let me explain.

Carbs are our bodies' preferred source of fuel, so we're biologically hardwired to seek them out! Our brain alone needs 130 grams per day just to function optimally, and this is just *one* of our many carb-loving organs! Those needs become much higher if you exercise. Most commercial diets, both the dodgy BS ones and the ones backed by research, generally have one thing in common: They limit or eliminate refined carbohydrates. And while there is some solid science to back this suggestion up, if you've struggled with your relationship with food all your life, "eliminating" anything can do more harm than good.

Humans seek pleasure-packed experiences, and eating carbs is an easy source. So, I want to be clear, I don't ever want you to cut out carbs if they bring you joy. Not to mention, some of the most nutritious foods and dietary patterns are rich in carbs. The Mediterranean diet, for example, is one of the most well-studied and celebrated dietary patterns for reducing the risk of chronic disease.[24] And it's the carbs, like those found in whole grains (e.g., brown rice and barley), legumes (e.g., chickpeas and lentils), fruits, and vegetables, that provide its disease-fighting foundation! That said, even though we can make all foods morally equal, not all carbs are created nutritionally equal, and health-promoting dietary patterns (e.g., the Mediterranean diet) emphasize higher-fiber carbs over refined.

- **High-fiber carbs** are those that have their energizing carbohydrates bound up with indigestible carbohydrates that only our gut microbiome can utilize as energy. It's a snack for us, and a snack for them!
- **Refined carbs**, on the other hand, are missing the protein, fiber, and dietary fat (yes, the HCCs!) that make carbohydrate-rich foods nutritious and satiating. Research[25] has consistently linked a diet rich in refined carbohydrates with an increased risk of heart disease, type 2 diabetes, and excess weight gain.[26]

Despite the clear difference in health outcomes between high-fiber carbs and heavily refined carbs, no one slice of white bread or bowl of Froot Loops is the problem. It's an excess of these heavily refined carbs, especially when they edge out other more nutrient-dense foods, that increases our risk of chronic disease.

I like to call refined carbohydrates Naked Carbs. Despite their name suggesting something exciting and racy, Naked Carbs are actually pretty basic. Generally, Naked Carbs are made from refined white flour, are rich in added sugar, and are not the best sources of vitamins, minerals, and antioxidants. Common examples of Naked Carbs are things like white bread, bagels, rice, and pasta, along with chips, pretzels, candy, pastries, soda, doughnuts, and cakes.

Naked Carbs are often associated with weight gain because they're just so damn easy to overeat. Consider how much easier it would be to down two cups of apple juice compared to eating six whole apples in one sitting. It might take six apples to make that 16-ounce glass of juice, but good luck getting past apple number three. Naked Carbs are stripped of all the beneficial compounds that satisfy our appetite and make us feel full, so naturally, we need to eat more of them to get our fill. And at the end of the day, overconsumption of calories from anything (whether apple juice or even something without any carbs at all, like a chicken breast) is the primary physiological factor in explaining weight gain. It's just a lot easier to pack the calories in from juice than whole apples, or chicken.

This is the part in most diet books where you'd see the list of foods you need to cut out, and at the top, it would probably say something like NO REFINED CARBS. Yeah, scratch that hot tip out of your notes. Despite everything I've told you about Naked Carbs' track record, I don't want you to cut them out. In fact, I want you to unapologetically work them into your diet whenever it suits you. Even every day, if you'd like. I sure do. When I was in the depths of diet culture, I had developed a real longing for sugary cereal. If it was in the house, I would think about it all day until I would give in and crush a whole box dry. Allowing myself to eat cereal, or any other Naked Carb sans judgment, helped neutralize the power that cereal had over me. Ultimately, when our choices aren't bound to a staunch sense of morality, we can actually listen to what feels best to our body each day.

And, honestly, what generally feels best to our body is balance. Sugary, crunchy things may bring the fun factor and emotional satisfaction, but protein (Greek yogurt), fiber (berries), and fats (hemp hearts) offer physical satiety. Suddenly, you have a formula where you can have your cake (or Froot Loops), and feel good eating it, too!

I get it. This might feel weird. Like, crazy AF. It's not easy to change your mindset about carbs. But, remember, the HCC framework was designed to help free us from the shackles of diet culture and our own self-induced scarcity mentality by shifting our focus from always taking foods away. By choosing foods that have at least one Hunger

Crushing Compound (protein, fat, and/or fiber), you'll feel more physically full and emotionally satisfied, and be better equipped to nourish yourself intuitively and pleasurably.

## The Benefits of the Hunger Crushing Combo

By now, you're starting to get a sense of what my Hunger Crushing Combo is all about. It has no calorie counting or off-limits foods, as we know all about the restriction to ice cream–binge pipeline. Instead, we have to ground our experience with food in an additive abundance mindset. Personally, I've never found joy in restriction or incessant hunger. But by "dressing up" the Naked Carbs we love with Hunger Crushing Compounds, we tend to naturally edge out some of the less nutritious, less satiating foods that are preventing us from maintaining our healthiest weight.

The benefits of my Hunger Crushing Combo go well beyond helping you stay full:

- The HCCs (protein, fiber, and fat) work together to slow the digestion of Naked Carbs, which helps flatten the blood sugar curve. This is not just of importance to folks with insulin resistance or type 2 diabetes, but rather, maintaining healthy balanced blood sugar levels just helps us *feel* our best. No one likes a midday meltdown or a three p.m. energy dip. And definitely, no one likes being around someone when they hit their wall. As my husband always says, *"Well-fed wife, happy life."*
- My Hunger Crushing Combo Method inherently provides you with all the nutrients your body needs to thrive. Planning a balanced diet shouldn't require a PhD, and nobody has time to be worrying about how many grams of folate they've

consumed each day. Focusing on integrating HCC categories into your diet helps you cover your macro- and micronutrient bases without thought.

- And, finally, and perhaps most important, this framework helps you redefine your relationship with food. Food is not "good" or "bad." It's not "clean" or "junk." It's just food. And by putting all foods on an equal playing field, and stripping them of their moral value, it encourages you to incorporate the foods you love in a way that *feels* good to your body, physically and emotionally.

Listen, I know this is not going to be an easy adjustment. Healing from years of diet culture takes work. A lot of work. But improving your relationship with food should be the first step in setting the stage for any other health goals. Add, don't restrict. It might seem radical, but it works.

## The How-To of the
## Hunger Crushing Combo Method

The Hunger Crushing Combo diverges from the usual restrictive route of every other diet in your little black book: There are NO hard-and-fast rules. I know, this can feel counterintuitive and a bit scary, but letting go of the rigidity and robotics of dieting is imperative to relearning your birthright body wisdom.

Obviously, we now know that it's advantageous to have balanced meals and snacks with fiber, protein, and healthy fats; however, not every meal or snack needs to be a "perfect" HCC package with fiber *and* protein *and* healthy fats. Not every meal or snack will have any HCCs at all. Sometimes, you will *just* have the fresh bakery croissant on its own. Sometimes, you will *just* want a handful of pretzels. Sometimes, you will *just* order the buttered pasta without any vegetables or protein in sight. Eating carbs in their birthday suit because that's what you want and crave at that moment is all part of normal healthy eating. Remember, this is a framework, not a diet. It may seem like just a word, but you've really got to embrace that nuanced distinction to make this work for you. This is a way of eating for the long haul; it's a gentle paradigm for real life. The goal is to neutralize the power of certain fear-provoking foods, overthrow them from their throne, and embrace the Naked Carbs that you love, without judgment or fear. Yes, most of the time, this will look like dressing them up in a way that feels good to your body while providing a balancing combo of nutrients to keep you satisfied and energized. Other times, it's just going to look like finger-forking a handful of chocolate chips while baking with your kids. And that, my friends, is all part of the beautiful, messy, unpredictable, delicious plan.

# CHAPTER 2

. . . . . . . . . . . . . . . . .

# Goodbye, Diets; Hello, Satiety— and Your Healthiest Weight

First up: a quick note about language as we get into discussing weight. As I will elucidate in more detail later on in the book (see "Why BMI Is Kinda BS," page 137), categories like "overweight" and "obese" are grounded in pretty poor science. A lot of folks in the body neutrality and positivity movement suggest these terms medicalize certain body sizes, and contribute to stigma and fat phobias, choosing descriptors like "fat" or "larger body" instead. I fully acknowledge and agree with these concerns. That said, I don't believe in censoring science, and since these are the official categories used in the literature, I will be occasionally using them throughout the book (along with more morally neutral descriptors) to describe the methods and outcomes of research studies.

## From Diet Culture to Wellness Culture

Diet culture is like an insidious force, almost omnipresent in our lives, dictating not only what we eat but how we should feel about our bodies.

Everywhere we turn, from social media and television, to even conversations with friends, the same message appears on loop: We will be happy *only* when we're thin. It perpetuates a cycle where our self-worth becomes intrinsically tied to the size of our bodies, and our ability to adhere to the diet du jour is a marker of moral value. We start to see ourselves as inherently "good" when we order the salad sans dressing, and we label ourselves as "bad," "lazy," or "incompetent" when we cave and polish off a friend's fries. Diet culture teaches us that we are nothing more than our bodies. Our achievements, relationships, and character are all second fiddle to how we look. And when this is the system we've all been groomed by, it becomes our truth. Research suggests that in the arena of public opinion, obesity serves as a proxy for low competence.[1] Fat people are consistently assumed to be less productive, less intelligent, and more prone to interpersonal problems than thin people. As a result, they are discriminated against in virtually every sector and service, including health care, education, media, public accommodations, and employment. In fact, every 64 extra pounds a woman carries is translated to a 9 percent decrease in wages.[2]

If this is our collective worldview of folks in larger bodies, it's really no wonder we're all desperate to be thin!

Unfortunately, this ideology is not without risk. Diet culture and our shared fear of fatness don't "motivate people to be healthier." Rather, they set people up for a lifetime of chronic dieting, self-loathing, obsessive food rules, and, ultimately, a disordered relationship with food and body. What may start as a thirty-day cleanse (post-all-you-can-eat holiday), can very quickly become a fatal disorder. Anorexia nervosa is the leading killer of all psychiatric conditions, taking the lives of 5 percent of all those diagnosed within four short years. And yes, it's possible to be both fat *and* have an eating disorder.[3] In fact, it's a rampant (yet undersupported) problem. Research suggests that, compared to normal-weight young adults, those with obesity are almost 2.5 times more likely to engage in disordered eating behaviors.[4]

Diet culture is also not a new phenomenon. In the 1920s, families were asked to trade their eggs for cornflakes as John Harvey Kellogg (yes, the cereal guy) convinced everyone to live off refined grains. The '60s emphasized the macrobiotic diet, the early seedlings of the so-called clean eating movement. The '70s brought us the low-carb Atkins diet, along with its distant cousin, the grapefruit diet. The '80s popularized our first "cleanse" with the cabbage soup diet (which sounds very . . . gassy . . .). And by the '90s and 2000s, we started to revitalize old diets with better PR campaigns, gamifying calorie counting with points systems and apps.

I would love to say we've emerged from these dark diet times as savvier, smarter consumers, but alas, diet culture has simply evolved into a slightly more sexy (and sneaky) new form: wellness culture.

To the uncritical eye, wellness culture appears to offer a holistic approach to health, prioritizing not just physical well-being but our mental, emotional, and spiritual needs as well. It offers an escape from the militant and deprivative nature of your grandma's steak and cigarette diet with a seemingly more gentle and aesthetic alternative. Instead of saying we want to be skinny, now we say we want to combat "bloating" to get that "snatched" flat tummy look. Instead of saying, "Sorry, I can't do dinner; I'm on a diet," we're now just doing a green juice cleanse to detox our liver.

Folks, do the duck test. If it quacks like a diet, swims like a diet, and looks like a diet, it's probably a diet. Wellness culture is simply diet culture with a new shiny coat of lipstick on. And even those who are vocally antidiet culture can be seduced by wellness culture's call.

Thanks to wellness culture, our diets have become deeply ingrained into our identity, leading us to defend our choices with zeal that mirrors religious or political fervor. This passionate advocacy can foster a sense of community and belonging, but can also create divisions or a feeling of superiority over those who choose different paths. The result is often that we shelter ourselves from any new information that contradicts our beliefs, and more problematically, from our own body's wisdom. When you've committed yourself to a bacon-and-egg lifestyle, eating, sleeping, and breathing keto for months, all while muscling through unpleasant side effects and cravings, it can feel really distressing to admit that it's not the diet for you.

Wellness culture also often propagates a new form of elitism and exclusion masked as investing in our well-being. It commodifies health as a status symbol reserved only for those who can afford the influencer-backed tinctures, fitness regimens, cleanses, and "clean" food. We are sold the narrative that without fulfilling a very specific set of wellness prescriptions, we will never be our healthiest selves, creating unrealistic exclusive benchmarks for living well.

And if you can't follow that influencer's program to a T because acai berries are too expensive or you can't make it to the gym five days a week? Wellness culture suggests that you just aren't investing in your health enough. Your health is *your* personal responsibility, and failing to live like a perky Peloton instructor is an epic moral fail.

Wellness culture just conveniently overlooks all of the cultural and systemic factors that negatively influence our health, like socioeconomic status, access to health care and nutritious food, health literacy, food skills, and more. Not to mention personal genetics and other nonmodifiable factors! And, listen, I'm a dietitian; obviously I want people to eat a generally balanced, mostly whole-food diet. But food is just one small piece of the wellness puzzle. And investing all of our energy in achieving diet purity in the name of better health often pushes us further away from our wellness goals. Not just because of the risk of disordered eating or eating disorders, but also because it can distract us from more important tools in our personal health toolbox. For example, telling a cancer patient to quit chemo and just do a juice fast could be deadly. But this is exactly the kind of advice we see in the shady grifter corners of online wellness culture. Wellness culture also often blurs the lines between evidence-based health practices and those rooted in pseudoscience and good marketing. And because it is so sneaky and persuasive, we need to be on extra high alert to sort through the noise. That is becoming increasingly more difficult in our digital era, when information moves across the world at an unprecedented speed. Everyone has a platform. Everyone is an "expert."

Listen, I get how overwhelmingly easy it is to fall into these traps. Our social feed is flush with stylized images of fit young women in sports bras, sharing what they (allegedly) ate that day. The unspoken message is that *if you eat like this, you can look like this*. What's more telling is what is absent from this content. The parties they might have had to skip out on. The meals they couldn't share. The full box of double-stacked Oreos they binged on after eating meal-prepped broccoli for five days straight. There is often a lot more going on behind the scenes that we don't see.

I can promise you this: Even if an influencer *is* being honest about their ultradisciplined diet, they are likely not being honest with you (or even themselves) about the emotional toll it takes. Diets like these (or cleanses, or detoxes, or whatever the wellness influencer wants to conveniently call them) will always fail you. And they fail not because they don't result in weight loss or temporary health outcomes (they might!). They fail because no one can stick to them in the long term.[5]

## Do You Have Orthorexia?

At the time of publishing, orthorexia nervosa is not yet considered an official mental health diagnosis that is classified in the *Diagnostic and Statistical Manual of Mental Disorders* (DSM-5) or the International Classification of Disease (ICD-10). That said, it is taken very seriously by mental health experts due to its associated physical and mental health complications. The following are some common signs and symptoms:

1.  Spending an excessive amount of time researching the "healthiness" of different foods, reading ingredient lists, health blogs, and other wellness media.
2.  Eliminating entire food groups or types of foods believed to be "unhealthy" or "impure."
3.  Severe distress or anxiety over food "violations" leading to guilt, shame, and even stricter rules.
4.  Social isolation as the individual withdraws from activities and people who do not align with their strict dietary regimen.
5.  Signs and symptoms of nutrition deficiencies, including extreme weight loss, weakness, fatigue, hair loss, and menstrual irregularities.
6.  Sense of superiority over others' eating habits, and viewing one's diet as the only correct way to eat.
7.  Increased rigidity over time with diet rules where breaking these self-imposed rules triggers severe emotional distress.
8.  An overwhelming and often unfounded fear of disease or illness from eating foods not on their safe list.
9.  Inability to allow others to prepare meals for them (leading to an avoidance of social eating experiences, restaurants, and events).
10. Extreme anxiety or fear when "healthy" or "safe" foods are not readily available, often resulting in skipping meals or undereating.

Only you and a trained eating disorder expert can determine whether your relationship with food is approaching or actively expressing itself as an eating disorder. If any of these attributes feel familiar, I recommend seeking advice from your health-care team or going to EatingDisorderHope.com to find support.

## Why Diets Have Failed You

If you're reading this book, you've likely tried, or at least have been tempted to try the whole lot of fad diet or wellness trends. From calorie counting to intermittent fasting to keto to raw vegan, they all promise they're "different" than every diet that came before. And sure, the "rules" you have to follow may help distinguish carnivore from juice cleansing, but if they're promising weight loss, they all have one very important attribute in common: Any diet can result in weight loss (at least temporarily) as long as it encourages a **calorie deficit**. This isn't my opinion; this is just science. A calorie deficit is a state of energy balance whereby the calories (energy) you consume undercut the energy your body expends (through exercise, digesting, moving, or just literally being alive).

It is often said that 1 pound of fat loss requires a calorie deficit of exactly 3,500 calories, which is why most commercial diets aim to reduce calories by 500 to 750 per day. Cutting 500 calories a day means eliminating 3,500 calories per week, and BAM! Like clockwork, you're down a pound by Monday. And in a year, you're 52 pounds lighter! A new person with just one go around the sun! Woot woot!

In reality, it's a lot more complicated than that. For one, the 3,500-calorie thing is kinda a farce.[6] I mean, you're (hopefully) not just going to continue to lose a pound a week until you disappear! But there are loads of metabolic adaptations that work to thwart your so-called summer body plans (side note: All bodies are summer bodies, but we'll get to that piece soon). See, our bodies like to keep us within a certain weight range, or what is generally called our set point weight. Set point theory suggests that our body weight is tightly regulated, like a thermostat that's been biologically set to have an upper and lower weight. Moving within these two numbers might be relatively easy (which is why the first 5 to 10 pounds tend to come off somewhat quickly). But if we try to push below our lower set point weight, we set off a cascade of metabolic adaptations to maintain homeostasis. And this is why losing a lot of weight (and keeping it off) is hard AF.

## Metabolic Adaptations to Weight Loss

The three main physiological adaptations involved in weight loss are metabolism, unconscious activity, and hunger.

When you lose weight, your metabolism slows down to maintain a smaller body size and conserve energy. It's estimated that within normal circumstances (that is, you're not losing 60% of your body weight on *The Biggest Loser*[7]), your metabolism might slow down by 5 percent.[8]

A bigger contributor to weight homeostasis is what we call NEAT: nonexercise activity thermogenesis (basically, the energy expended for everything we do that is not sleeping, eating, or sportslike exercise).[9] When we lose weight, our body naturally tries to slow down to conserve energy, and most of this results in subconsciously moving less. I'm not talking about skipping the gym one day; I'm talking about sitting down instead of standing, fidgeting less, taking the elevator instead of stairs, and so on. Believe it or not, when we are in a calorie deficit, our body burns 35 percent fewer calories from NEAT each day.[10] The decline in NEAT can absolutely make a difference in our ability to maintain weight loss over time.

Finally, in its desperate effort to squash that calorie deficit we expertly crafted, our body revs up its hunger hormones (ghrelin) and downregulates its satiety hormones (leptin, cholecystokinin, peptide YY, GLP-1, insulin, and adiponectin) to demand that we smarten up and just eat a damn burger. And that's just what's happening physiologically. Psychologically, deprivation cranks up the food noise, leaving no brain cell unoccupied by the thought of food. Cookies, cake, chips, pizza. If it's on the no-no list, it's all we want. Diet and wellness cultures set us up for a number of common traps, all of which leave us worse off than where we started. Chances are, you've experienced more than one.

**Binge–Restrict Cycle**

Let's be honest with ourselves. Restricting the foods we love almost always backfires. Let's say you love, love, love basic white bread. But your favorite clean-eating influencer says gluten is inflammatory junk (PS: that's BS). You think about bread all day and night until you find yourself sunbathing in the light of the fridge at two a.m., clearing out your kids' sandwiches in their lunch boxes. Cue the crushing guilt and negative self-talk. Now, you've got to pay for your indiscretions: no bread *or any other carbs* for a month! The harder you restrict, the harder your body fights back. Binge, restrict, repent, repeat. This depressing cycle is pretty much inevitable, because our bodies and minds don't like to be told no.

**Emotional and Comfort Eating**

Food is not just fuel. It's love, joy, and comfort. Our earliest interactions with food as babies are intrinsically linked to comfort and care. Our fondest memories of childhood and family are often associated with certain flavors or smells, such as a grandmother's pie or an uncle's game day dip. Sharing a meal helps foster community, unity, and cultural identity. As humans, we have also spent centuries celebrating and mourning with food as part of religious and spiritual rituals or traditions.

Food feels good, tastes good, and represents good in our lives; it is only natural and normal to eat for emotional reasons that have nothing to do with our physiological needs. Your tummy might be physically full, but you still need *something* to take the edge off. You don't *need* a Hunger Crushing Combo. That is okay. It's not realistic to never cry into a pint of ice cream ever again. But the goal is to get to a place where food isn't the only tool in your emotion regulation toolbox; it's not your only source of joy in life. And if you're struggling to find ways of managing big emotions outside of Sour Patch Kids and blue-box macaroni, which are beyond the scope of this book, I do recommend working with a therapist on some alternative ways to support yourself.

## The Satisfaction Hunt

How many times has diet culture taught us to eat X every time we're craving Y? Want chips? Eat carrot sticks. Craving candy? Get out the strawberries. Let's not kid ourselves, folks. Carrots and berries are both delicious, but they're *not* a replacement for your kids' Halloween haul. What typically ends up happening here is what I call the Satisfaction Hunt. You're craving ice cream, so you eat a bowl of frozen grapes. That doesn't cut it, so you bring out the low-fat Cool Whip from the freezer and start raw-dawging it. But you're still thinking of the real deal. So, now, you're breaking off pieces of dark chocolate *into* the Cool Whip, closing your eyes, hoping you can be duped, but you just can't shake this desire. Finally, you cave and plow through the fully loaded Rocky Road in the freezer. Had you just had a mindful bowl of ice cream you wanted in the first place, you would have consumed way fewer calories (and not felt so sick *or* ashamed by the end of it). When we eat around the craving with nonsensical "health swaps," the longing simply builds up into these wild unruly waves until we crash and break into a full-out binge.

## Last Supper Syndrome

If you've ever gone on a restrictive diet, you've definitely done this dance. Basically, you're about to start a diet where you *know* all of your favorite foods will be on the no-no list, so you clear out the pantry, fridge, and freezer in a full-on bender as you repeat in your head, *"Diet starts tomorrow."* Research suggests that even the thought of starting a new diet results in a binge.[11] We also tend to see this cycle on restrictive diets that allow "cheat days."

**Health Halos**

Wellness culture has created an entire dictionary of health qualifiers, making us less critical consumers of shady food marketing. Gluten-free, superfood, non-GMO, keto, Paleo, organic, all-natural. We've been conditioned to translate any one of these front-of-label claims to automatically mean it's a "good choice." These Health Halos make us hyperfocus on one specific "healthy" attribute of a food and extrapolate that to the food at large, encouraging us to basically miss the forest for the trees. An organic cookie automatically seems "healthier" than its traditional counterpart, driving us to conveniently overlook some of its less nutritious attributes, like the fact that it has just as many Naked Carbs as a regular old cookie. Folks, an organic cookie is still a cookie, regardless of what kind of pesticides were used to grow the crops. This tiny piece of marketing often also overshadows our body wisdom, and the data we've collected about how Naked Carbs like cookies, candies, and chocolates make us feel. The result? We often eat *more* of them. One study found that when M&M's were labeled as "low-fat," research participants ate significantly more than when they appeared as just regular candy.[12]

If you've fallen victim to these tricks, don't feel ashamed. Health Halos are manipulative by design. Fool me once, shame on diet culture. Fool me twice, shame on diet culture. You are not the problem to fix.

Is your diet history bingo card full yet? You're not alone. But just think back to all of your own past experiences with dieting and every bogus diet you've ever tried. Let me take a stab at the one thing they all have in common: They probably left you either physically hungry, emotionally deprived, or, most likely, both. And within days, weeks, and maybe months, you grew bored with the limited food options, tired of suppressing hunger with black coffee, and lonely skipping out on dinners with friends. And, then, you cracked. You ate all the "wrong" things, assumed you blew it, and threw in the towel. Give it a few days or weeks, and the weight comes right back.

And this is why most diets fail.

It's not because you're weak, or lazy, or have poor willpower. It's because the diet has pushed against everything that makes you human, and your body is fighting back. It's just doing its G-d–given job and we should actually be grateful for that.

This is why, whenever a pseudo-stranger at a dinner party finds out I'm a dietitian, and they ask me whether their "diet" is a good one to lose weight, I give the same answer, no matter what their plan. *Is this something you can do for life?* If the answer is no, it's a bad diet.

## Why My Hunger Crushing Combo Works

Eating is kinda, like, a big deal. It's a huge part of our lives and is so much more than just nutrients and fuel. It's emotional, social, and cultural, and if your diet doesn't align with all of these critical parts of your identity, you're not going to keep it up for long. Consistency and pleasure will always trump the minutiae of the plan.

With the HCCs, you're not giving up the foods you love (hello, emotional satisfaction) *and* you're absolutely not going to be hungry (I got you, physical satiety). By focusing on what we are adding to less-nutritious foods (e.g., dressing up Naked Carbs, to make them more satiating) we shift from a restrictive scarcity mindset to one of abundance. Yes, abundance and reaching your health goals, like weight loss, can finally coexist.

But, wait, doesn't weight loss require a calorie deficit? Love that you've been listening! Yes! Let me explain how this can happen without "dieting" the traditionally hyperrestrictive way.

When we retire from the crusty old restrictive mindset and give ourselves unconditional permission to eat the foods we love, we stop obsessing over the "bad" foods we can't have. We'll talk about this in more detail in Chapter 5, but letting go of this mindset is the first step to relearning our body's true needs.

> What feels good, and what doesn't?
> Which foods hold you until lunch, and which lead you back to the pantry an hour later?
> Are you "addicted to sugar," or are you just deeply deprived?

And when you *add* Hunger Crushing Compounds that are inherently filling and feel good, you naturally start to edge out the less-nutritious, less-satiating high-calorie foods that will leave you hungry for a snack again soon after. Without that *extra* snack, or *extra* serving of pasta, you create a calorie deficit. And you didn't even know it happened. This approach honors your emotional cravings, and your body's primal need to feel full, eliminating any need to throw in the towel with an epic "last supper" binge.

Let me give you an example of how this would work, with some hypothetical numbers to make a point. There's leftover birthday cake in the fridge, and you've got a hankering for something sweet. You might be "fasting" until noon, and when the clock strikes twelve, you face-plant into a girthy slice. Yes, you crushed the craving, *but also* acquired 500 unexpected calories in the process. The problem is that the cake isn't really that satiating. It's delicious and a lot of fun, sure, but it's mainly Naked Carbs without any Hunger Crushing Compounds to hold it up. So, naturally, an hour later, you're back in the pantry, looking for another pick-me-up. Maybe you crush a bag of chips (200 calories), a couple of rice cakes (100 calories), and a cup of juice (100 calories). And by three p.m., you're feeling your energy dip *again*. You can see how easy it is to pack in the calories without ever feeling truly *full*.

But let's try this scenario again, using my Hunger Crushing Combo framework. The cake craving hits, so you cut yourself a slice.

You know that cake tastes great, so you're not going to deny yourself a taste. But you've been practicing my Hunger Crushing Combo framework for a while now. You know that having *just* rich chocolate cake for lunch doesn't always feel so good. Your energy lags. You feel bloated and backed up. So, instead, you cut yourself a more mindful slice (200 calories), and serve it with a healthy portion of Greek yogurt (protein + fat; 75 calories), raspberries (fiber; 50 calories), and walnuts (protein + fats; 75 calories). *Adding* those supersatiating Hunger Crushing Compounds not only edge out 100 calories in the dessert, but they keep you satiated longer to *also* make obsolete the 400 calories in snacks that might follow. And that is how you create a calorie deficit without denial. You quite literally can have your cake, and feel good eating it, too. Now, obviously I'm not suggesting you have cake for lunch every day if your goal is to lose weight. But I used this as an extreme example; if you can create a calorie deficit by eating *cake*, then imagine the results when putting my framework fully into play.

## Powerful Protein:
## The Strength and Satiety Superstar

While all three of our Hunger Crushing Compounds help you feel full, protein is king of the satiety hierarchy, explaining why most, if not all, successful weight-loss diets are pro-protein. Research consistently shows that eating a protein-rich breakfast helps reduce appetite, increase feelings of fullness, reduce total daily calorie intake, and improve the quality of meal choices, compared to skipping breakfast or eating a meal that's higher in carbs.[13] In other words, simply making a protein-rich choice in the morning sets you up for a more nutrient-dense day of eating, *and* a calorie deficit without any additional effort at all. It also prevents you from slipping into the all-or-nothing last supper mentality that leads to a binge. You know, the whole *"Dammit, I'm so bad for eating pancakes for breakfast, my diet is ruined, so I might as well have a double cheeseburger and fries for lunch and finish off that jar of Nutella in the fridge. Diet starts again tomorrow!"*

There are a few reasons that protein is such a satiety superstar: how it's digested in the gut; the production of heat, a.k.a. thermogenesis; the support of metabolism-boosting muscle; and its impact on appetite hormones and cravings. Here's a snapshot of each:

### Digestion

Protein digestion starts in the stomach. The stomach releases gastric juices that combine with muscular contractions (a.k.a. peristalsis) to churn the protein into a substance called chyme. The protein structure is then broken down into individual amino acids (remember, those are the building blocks of protein) that enable them to be absorbed into the blood. This is actually a quite leisurely process, taking several hours to complete, and when it comes to satiety, slow and steady wins the race! A slower digestion process means a greater buildup of food volume in the gut to stretch and stimulate a bundle of our nervous system called the vagus nerve, to tell us we're full. The vagus nerve is crazy smart. It can sense the volume and type of nutrients (protein, carbohydrates, and/or fat) in the small intestine. If your diet is particularly high in sugar, your vagus nerve signaling can be disrupted, which can lead to overeating and, eventually, weight gain. This is one of the reasons that we tend to overeat when faced with a big bowl of Naked Carbs.

In contrast, a meal that is high in protein stimulates the vagus nerve to send a prompt message to your brain that you are, in fact, full. If you've been dieting most of your life, you've probably been taught to just "stop eating when you're full." But this advice is useless without an understanding of what helps you best achieve that fullness. As you can now understand, you're going to receive those messages to stop eating much clearer and faster if you choose to eat, say, eggs rather than white bread.

### Thermogenesis

In addition to protein's action on the vagus nerve, its digestion comes with another weight-management perk: thermogenesis. Thermogenesis is a measure of the heat produced in your body as a result of calories being burned during metabolic processes. Imagine your body as a little furnace, burning up energy from food and turning it into heat to help you maintain your body temperature. The more thermogenesis happening in the body, the more calories get burned.

There are several ways to rev up that internal furnace without sweating it out in the gym. There's NEAT, which, as we discussed in Chapter 2, is all of your unconscious and subconscious body movements, like fidgeting or shifting your weight while standing. Compared to intentional exercise (which contributes only 5% to 15% of the calories you expend in the day), NEAT makes up about 10 percent of calories burned in sedentary individuals (e.g., a receptionist who works a desk job) and up to 50 percent if you're highly active (e.g., a construction worker). I'm not knocking your boot camp class, but unplanned movement can make a huge difference.

Another contributor is the thermic effect of food (TEF), which contributes 8 to 10 percent of the total calories you burn each day from the energy expended in simply digesting what you eat. Protein has the highest TEF of all the macronutrients, with 20 to 30 percent of the calories from the protein you eat being expended during digestion (contrasted with 5% to 10% of calories from carbs, and 0% to 3% from fat).[14] This means that, if you ate 100 calories' worth of protein, your body would expend one-quarter of those in breaking it down, leaving you with net 75 calories. And this does add up! One study found that participants who ate around 40 percent of their daily calories from protein burned an additional 260 calories through TEF![15] That's literally the equivalent of doing an aerobics class!

**Lean Muscle and Metabolism**

The other really important role of protein is in maintaining calorie-torching muscle mass. Lean mass (specifically muscle) is the number one determinant of how many calories someone burns at rest (i.e., their resting metabolic rate).[16] Muscle cells have much higher energy demands than fat; the more muscle mass you have, the greater your metabolic rate, with each kilogram (2¼ pounds) of added muscle increasing your daily caloric expenditure by 20 to 30 calories per day.[17] And being that muscle is literally made up of amino acids (the building blocks of protein), it probably won't surprise you that eating enough protein is key to supporting your well-earned gains. Protein isn't just for hard-core bodybuilders; your needs are also quite high if you're trying to lose body fat. We will go into more detail in Chapter 6, but research consistently shows that a high-protein diet helps preserve lean body mass (muscle) while losing fat in a calorie deficit.[18] In the simplest terms, weight loss comes down to a straightforward equation:

$$\text{Calorie Input (How Much You Eat)} - \text{Calorie Output}$$
$$\text{(How Much You Burn)} = \text{Calorie Deficit}$$

You can create a calorie deficit a million ways till Sunday, but protein modifies both sides of the weight-loss formula. By boosting TEF and supporting healthy muscle mass, protein effortlessly increases your calorie expenditure, and that is a huge perk for supporting a healthy weight.[19] But it's actually protein's contribution to modifying caloric intake that really helps move the needle.[20]

**Appetite Hormones**

Part of protein's job description is in boosting satiety hormones, including the infamous blood sugar regulator, insulin. Insulin is more than just a messenger for sugar; it's actually an important satiety regulator as well.[21]

Protein stimulates insulin secretion, both directly, by activating amino acid nutrient receptors in the pancreas, and indirectly, by releasing hormones like glucagon-like peptide-1 (GLP-1).[22] If you think you've heard this acronym before, it's because GLP-1 is the hormone of interest in popular antidiabetes and weight-loss drugs like Ozempic, Wegovy, and Mounjaro (see sidebar "GLP-1 Weight-Loss Drugs," page 49). It's the hormone that enhances insulin secretion to help lower blood sugar levels, slow digestion, and reduce appetite and hunger. As protein travels through the digestive system, tiny receptors in the intestinal wall send signals to our neurons telling our brain, *"WOO HOO, protein is in the house!"* In response, GLP-1 gets activated to start to put that fuel to work. Research suggests that high-protein diets (with 30% of total calories from protein) boost this powerful appetite regulation hormone 50 percent higher than do diets low in protein.[23] Like insulin and GLP-1, leptin, cholecystokinin, and peptide YY also act as satiety hormones in the body. Leptin is actually our leading satiety hormone and is at the scene every time we eat. Interestingly, leptin is predominantly produced by our fat tissue, and how much of it is made is directly proportional to our body fat levels. This explains why, if you lose *too much* weight, you just can't seem to feel full. It's your body's way of trying to maintain enough body fat to keep you alive and well (and, yes, for most of us that means *not* having washboard abs).

Basically, this dream team of satiety hormones work together to help us get the message that we've had our fill. This is all-important body wisdom that diets often teach us to override. But focusing on protein can help us get the message more loudly and clearly. For example, one study found that when overweight men ate 138 grams of protein per day vs. 79 grams, spread out over three meals, they saw significant increases in peptide YY, and an enhanced sense of fullness.[24] Remember our set point weight? All of these hormones work together to help manage that! The more calories and protein in the meal, the more of these hormones get pumped out in our body's desperate attempt to help us maintain body weight homeostasis. Bottom line: Feeling full is not something to fear. Full feels good, and, particularly when it's driven by nutrient-dense Hunger Crushing Compounds like protein, it can serve as important interoceptive data that we're fueling our body well.

## GLP-1 Weight-Loss Drugs

Popular weight-loss drugs, including Ozempic, Wegovy, and Mounjaro, a.k.a. GLP-1 receptor *agonists*, work on the same GLP-1 hormone our body produces naturally in response to a meal. And much like protein, these drugs significantly suppress hunger and make a calorie deficit much easier to achieve. In fact, one study demonstrated that participants using semaglutide (the active ingredient in these GLP-1 agonist drugs) once per week managed to reduce calorie intake by 35 percent.[25] Study participants noted reduced hunger, appetite, and cravings, with increased feelings of fullness and satiety after meals. And there is no question, these drugs offer impressive results. Most studies have found that patients on GLP-1 agonists lose around 15 percent of their body weight.[26] But alas, it's not a free ride. There can be unpleasant side effects (mainly nausea, vomiting, and diarrhea), a high likelihood of weight regain when you come off, and the risk of a significant proportion of weight loss coming from metabolically active muscle (i.e., the type that burns calories). We will talk more about ways to avoid this in Chapter 6, but not surprisingly, protein will be key. Now, obviously a high-protein diet can't compete with a powerful pharmaceutical like Ozempic when it comes to how quickly you can lose weight. But, sometimes, slow and steady wins the race. And not only does protein act similarly on satiety, but it also supports healthy muscle mass, protecting our metabolism, body composition, and overall health as we age.

In the opposing ring to the satiety hormones is our lead hunger hormone, ghrelin. Ghrelin levels typically rise before meals and pipe down after you eat. But whenever you eat fewer calories than your body needs (as you've attempted to do on every diet you've ever been on), the stomach releases a mother lode of ghrelin to get you to maintain your set point weight. It literally is screaming at you to crush a cheeseburger, stat. Fortunately, protein significantly helps mitigate this effect by reducing the secretion of ghrelin after a meal. One study compared ghrelin concentrations after a high-protein breakfast and a high-carb breakfast.[27] Not surprisingly, the high-protein eaters had 40 percent lower ghrelin levels, along with slowed gastric emptying that helped the participants feel more full. This is one of many reasons that the more calories you cut trying to lose weight, the more protein you actually need.

### Cravings

Even when you're physically *full*, you can have cravings, emotional hunger, and "food noise" that stand in the way between you and your weight-loss goals. Once again, protein has your back.

One study compared a standard protein diet (14% of calories from protein) and a high-protein diet (25% of calories from protein) and found that the higher-protein group not only had greater fullness levels throughout the day, but had significantly less desire for late-night snacking and fewer preoccupying thoughts about food.[28] Managing cravings is important not only for supporting a healthy weight, but for your general relationship with food. Because if you're constantly thinking about what you want but *shouldn't* eat, it can quickly teeter into obsessive territory and leave little mental energy for what really matters in life. Thanks to its unique impact on fullness and hormones, protein absolutely helps quiet that noise. But giving yourself permission to eat the foods you love (judgment-free) is also key. In Part 2, we'll talk about how to put this into practice. But, generally, research suggests aiming to consume around 25 to 30 percent of our total daily calories from protein, or 1.2 to 1.8 grams of protein per kilogram (2¼ pounds) of our body weight each day, to help support a healthy body composition.[29]

## Fabulous Fiber:
## The Slow-Digesting Volumizer

There's a reason that fiber-rich foods like salads are also a mainstay across most popular diets: Research consistently shows that a diet rich in high-fiber fruits and vegetables improves weight loss and prevents weight gain.[30] According to one twenty-four-year study, each additional daily serving of fruit and veggies yielded a 0.53-pound and a 0.25-pound drop in body weight over four years, respectively.[31] None of that should come as a surprise. And yet, North Americans are notoriously slacking in their commitment to a produce-rich, fiber-full life. According to our dietary guidelines, we want to aim for around 14 grams of fiber per 1,000 calories we eat; so, on average, that's 25 grams of fiber per day for women, and 38 grams for men. In reality, most adults are consuming between 10 and 15 grams a day.[32] It's a miracle any of us poop!

But bathroom benefits aside, fiber is uniquely designed to help support a healthy weight in a number of important ways related to its affect on digestion, absorption, hormones, and the gut microbiome.

### Digestion

Unlike Naked Carbs, which are broken down into glucose and absorbed by your body quickly to provide energy (a.k.a. calories), fiber passes through the digestive system largely unaltered. Bacteria have the capacity to digest and utilize these fibers as their fuel, but humans lack the enzymes to break them down, so once our bacteria have had their fill, they end up excreted as waste. If you recall from Chapter 1, there are two types of fiber: insoluble fiber, which does not dissolve in water and therefore adds bulk to stool; and soluble fiber, which forms a gel-like substance as it moves through the gut. Both add volume and bulk (and typically a lot of water) that physically distend your stomach and move the food more slowly through the digestive tract.

Remember that vagus nerve? The vagus nerve *loves* fiber. Just think about the last time you ate a BAS (a.k.a. big-ass salad). Hopefully, there were some protein and fats in there for satiety and satisfaction, but the base of that bowl was probably greens and other vegetables. In other words, it was a mother lode of fiber bulk and fluid! And simply from volume alone, you probably felt *really* full.

### Absorption

Slow Sally fiber (along with the other HCCs—protein and fat) also creates a mini "traffic jam" in your gut, preventing the rapid absorption of sugars from the gut into your bloodstream. This means you don't get a blood sugar spike, *or* a subsequent blood sugar crash and hanger to follow, making it easier to maintain a calorie deficit.

### Appetite Hormones

Fiber takes between four and ten hours to finally reach the colon. And during its lengthy journey to the ivory throne, it triggers the cells in your gastrointestinal tract to release a cocktail of our BFF fullness hormones. Namely, it reduces the hunger hormone ghrelin, and pumps out the satiety hormones leptin, GLP-1, peptide YY, and cholecystokinin.

### Calorie Density

The indigestibility of fiber means you are not only eating a lot of bulk that makes you feel physically full for longer, but also that you're full on very few calories; for the most part, fiber-rich foods have the lowest calorie density of all the things we eat.

Calorie density refers to the amount of energy (calories) per unit of weight or volume in a food or beverage. Foods with high calorie density contain a large number of calories in a small package, whereas foods with low calorie density provide very few calories for a large volume of food. For example, a high-calorie-density food such as Ben & Jerry's Netflix & Chilll'd contains 200 calories for a pathetic ⅓-cup serving size (hilarious, right?). But if you tried to eat an equivalent amount of calories in spinach, your jaw would lock before you could finish the 30-cup serving. I'm absolutely *not* recommending anyone attempt that miserable feat, but this is one of the many reasons that it's much harder to overeat spinach than ice cream.

As world-renowned obesity researcher Kevin Hall points out, calorie density is the strongest factor associated with how many calories someone eats in a meal.[33] If your body needs 2,000 calories to thrive, it's going to be really hard to dupe it into thinking it's full on 1,000 calories because, at the end of the day, total calories still do matter. But at least in the transient short term, the volume and calorie density of the meal actually play a significant role in helping us feel full. Research suggests that the total weight of food we eat every day to feel "full" is generally consistent day to day.[34] In other words, if you have a big appetite, you might only feel satisfied if you fill a large dinner plate at every meal. However, even if the volume of food on the plate remains unchanged, you can manipulate the total calories you eat in a day by tweaking their calorie density. The fewer calories in each bite of food, the fewer calories you are likely to consume in a meal, across the day, and over time. This is what I mean when I say a specific food has the best satiety bang for its caloric buck.

This concept of calorie density helps explain a lot of scientific findings related to weight-loss success. For example, it explains why highly processed food consumption (a.k.a. Naked Carbs) is linked to weight gain, whereas a whole-food, unprocessed diet packed with fiber-rich fruits and vegetables is linked to weight loss. Research consistently shows that folks who eat low-calorie-density foods report greater fullness and weight loss on fewer calories, without ever needing to meticulously calculate or count.[35] That's the goal here, people! No counting. No obsessing. Just balance that *feels* good.

That said, calories still play a role in satiety, and eating a low-calorie-density diet can take you only so far. The premise of volume-eating large amounts of low-calorie foods can easily be misused, because a girl can't live on salad alone. While you might feel full in the moment, by the end of the day, or several days of this trickery, your brain will catch on that it's been bamboozled into believing lettuce is a good energizing meal. Thankfully, that's where fiber's sidekicks, protein and fat, will come into play. Sustainable weight loss isn't just about controlling hunger at one meal; it's about feeling satiated and satisfied for life.

The low calorie density of fiber-rich foods as it relates to its slow digestion, volume, and water content, all play an important role in promoting satiety. And researchers in Australia have actually attempted to categorize foods in terms of their fullness-promoting potential, by ranking them in their Satiety Index.[36] White bread (a Naked Carb) was considered the standard that everything else was judged against. Not surprisingly, an extra-sugary slice of cake was 33 percent less satiating than white bread, whereas a serving of boiled potatoes (which are rich in fiber and low in calorie density) was three times more satiating. In other words, you'd feel *at least* three times fuller by eating potatoes than a Naked Carb. Looks like it's time to rebrand the spud as a satiety superstar!

### Our Mighty Microbiome

There's another interesting perk to fiber that helps you manage your weight: its role in *feeding* the gut microbiome, the community of microorganisms living in the human gastrointestinal tract. It's been estimated that the average human gut harbors anywhere from 100 trillion to over 1,000 trillion diverse species of bacteria. As we've briefly established, humans lack the enzymes to effectively digest and absorb any calories from the fiber component of plant foods. But that BAS you had for lunch is like a Michelin-star meal to our friendly bugs!

To start, we need to clarify a few important (yet very confusing) terms that all sound the same, but are actually quite different.

**Pro**biotics are the beneficial bacteria in our gut. Common genera of probiotics you might find in foods and supplements include *Lactobacillus*, *Bifidobacterium*, *Streptococcus*, *Enterococcus*, *Escherichia*, *Bacillus*, and *Saccharomyces* (technically a yeast). These are further classified into specific species like *Lactobacillus rhamnosus*, a bacteria commonly found in yogurt, and even further into strains like *Lactobacillus rhamnosus* GG.

## Probiotics

If you're wondering how to get more beneficial probiotics to begin with, there are some key food sources you can add to your day, most notably fermented foods. Fermented foods include yogurt, kefir, kimchi, sauerkraut, kombucha, miso, tempeh, sourdough bread, and natto.

Obviously, I'm a dietitian, so food always comes first, and while incorporating more fermented foods into our diet has been shown to offer several health benefits (improved digestion, enhanced immunity, and greater weight loss[37]), for a clinical dose of probiotics, consider adding a high-quality probiotic supplement with at least 2 billion CFUs of bacteria.

**Pre**biotics are the fiber-packed fuel that feeds the good bacteria. Some of the best sources of prebiotics include most fruits, vegetables, and whole grains. A few that bacteria particularly like include green bananas, garlic, asparagus, and oats (but much more on that in Chapter 3).

**Post**biotics are the beneficial by-products from the fermentation (breaking down) of fiber by our gut bacteria. Common examples include vitamin $B_{12}$, folate, vitamin K, short-chain fatty acids (SCFAs), and certain amino acids.

The health of our microbiome is associated with the health of virtually every other organ and system in the body: digestion, immunity, brain health, mood, hormones, heart health, metabolism, and so much more. One of the more evolving areas of research is the link between our gut microbiome and our body weight. Research consistently shows that the gut microbiome of larger-bodied folks simply looks different from that of those who are thin.[38] Studies also suggest that losing excess body fat is associated with increased gut microbial diversity.[39]

Here's how fiber fits in. Let's say you had a simple meal of chickpea pasta with butter. The fat in the butter, and the starches and protein in the pasta, get broken down in your stomach, digested, and absorbed to be used as energy for your cells. But the fiber component (the prebiotics) in the pasta moves along to the intestines where your gut bacteria (the probiotics) await their feast. The more fuel for the probiotics, the more diverse and plentiful the microbiome, the lower the chances of dysbiosis (the disruption of a healthy diverse microbiome) and the fewer risk factors for obesity.

One of the potential mechanisms that explains the association between body weight and specific species of gut bacteria comes down to how different types of foods' calories are absorbed and utilized. Despite what common weight-loss dogma will have you believe, not all calories are processed the same. Our ability to manage our weight is not so much about how many calories a package says a food contains (a.k.a.

how many "available" calories are in a food), but rather, how many of those calories we can actually use and absorb. And that depends on the structure of the food and the vitality of our gut bacteria. In the simplest terms, imagine our body and our microbes are in a tug-of-war to "fight" over the calories in the food we eat. The more "simple" and processed the food is (as with Naked Carbs), the more easily *our* body can extract calories from it. In contrast, higher fiber foods are digested much more slowly, so they make their way to the large intestine, where our microbes await *their* feast, bypassing our ability to absorb all of their calories. If achieving a healthy weight is the goal, it's a fight we *want* to lose!

The effect of diet and microbiome quality was demonstrated in a very rigorous metabolic ward study where they gave one subject group a diet packed with prebiotic fiber (resistant starch, fruits, vegetables, beans, and whole grains), while the other group was given a diet rich in low-fiber, ultraprocessed foods and Naked Carbs (white bread, ground beef, American cheese, cheese puffs, cookies, and deli meats).[40] When the researchers looked at the participants' stool samples, they found that the high-fiber group "lost," on average, 217 calories per day, while the processed food group lost only about half of that. Some participants in the fiber group who assumedly had very active thriving microbiomes "lost" as much as 400 calories per day! That alone could create a big enough calorie deficit to result in almost a full pound of fat loss per week! The more "good" bacteria, and the more diverse the party down there, the more calories they can gobble up. And if you're thinking, well, wouldn't losing calories just make you hungrier for *more* calories, that is the beautiful thing about fiber. As we've established, fiber is super satiating, so despite "losing the fight" for some of those calories, our brains still register our guts as full.

And this is just part of fiber's healthy weight superpowers. This study also found that in addition to augmenting how many calories participants absorbed in their day, feeding the gut bacteria also produced short-chain fatty acids (a powerful postbiotic), which then increased the gut's release of the satiety hormone GLP-1. The more prebiotics there are for our probiotics to ferment, the more satiety-boosting postbiotics. I know, a lot of biotics in the house! In Chapter 4, we're going to get more into why eating a varied diet is important for our own overall nutrition status, but getting a wide range of plant foods into our diet rotation helps ensure *all* our gut critters are satisfied and well fed.

I probably didn't have to tell you that eating more salad would help support a healthy weight. But now you've got a mother lode of cool dinner party factoids to explain why! Bottom line: Eat more high-fiber plants.

## Hearty Healthy Fat:
## The Satisfaction Factor

Everything is better with butter. Unless you're vegan, allergic or intolerant to dairy, or just choose to avoid it, in which case I mean plant-based butter. And that's because butter is pretty much pure fat, and fat supplies food with its exceptional texture, flavor, appearance, quality, and satisfying characteristics. And while there's absolutely been a butter renaissance, you may recall the dark days of SnackWell's and other insipid fat-free foods lining the shelves. Thank goodness, the pendulum has swung back in its favor. Here's the skinny on fats and why we need them. Yes, even if losing *body* fat is desired.

### Digestion

Imagine the difference between a big bowl of lettuce, and a salad with avocado, nuts, and dressing. The former is rabbit food sure to drag you back to the pantry for a second lunch, and the latter is filling AF. Part of this satiety boost from rich sources of healthy fats comes down to their digestion. Fats are the last food component to leave the digestive tract, slowing down the digestion and absorption of everything in its tracks. The result is your meal remains in the stomach for longer, stimulating the vagus nerve and triggering our brain to tell us that we're full!

This explains why eating a few slices of Wonder Bread with jelly feels a bit like a bad Houdini trick: You remember chewing, but where the heck did it go after that? But if you were to add a thick slab of peanut butter, you actually *feel* the comfort of a meal in your gut.

## Appetite Hormones

Different types of fats stimulate different beneficial hormones in the gut. One of our star satiety hormones, cholecystokinin (CCK) is stimulated by long-chain fatty acids (think avocado, olives, fish, and full-fat dairy), while another fullness friend, peptide YY, is partial to medium-chain fats (e.g., coconut oil or pure MCT oils).[41] Then there's ghrelin, that pesky hunger hormone, nagging you to slip back into the staff room for your third doughnut of the day. Research suggests a diet rich in those beneficial long-chain fatty acids can help reduce the secretion of ghrelin.[42] The less ghrelin that is around, the less office tension over the last Boston cream doughnut (though I'm more of a cruller girl myself).

## Satisfaction

As humans, we are hardwired to derive satisfaction from fat. In fact, we naturally have unique fatty acid receptors in the mouth that detect and respond to the presence of fats in foods, helping to enhance the flavor, texture, satisfaction, and sensual experience of eating.[43] Not only are low-fat products not very satisfying, but even if they're lower in calories than the original, they are unlikely to offer major weight-loss perks. One study found that low- and nonfat foods contained up to 2½ times more sugar than did their full-fat counterparts (and sugar is far less satiating than fat![44]). So, even if you do slash a few calories by choosing the low-fat peanut butter over regular, you'll likely be hungry sooner and in need of another snack.

### Healthy Fats & Calories

There are 9 calories in every gram of dietary fat that you eat. This is more than twice as many calories as protein or carbs per gram, at 4 calories apiece. This largely explains why, for so long, low-fat diets reigned supreme. It only made logical sense that if you wanted to cut calories, you should do so from the most calorie-laden source: fat!

But this dismisses all of the metabolic and psychological adaptations that come with eating fat, not to mention all of its key health benefits. Most important, it doesn't consider the physical and emotional hunger that comes with livin' la fat-free loca.

This is where my unique approach to healthy fats comes into play. I want you to make most of your fat choices by focusing on those that hold dual citizenship in two or more HCC departments. Butter is amazing; butter is life. But think of butter as a bonus fat to be enjoyed in moderation. In just one paltry tablespoon of butter, you get 100 calories and 12 grams of fat. It's got a very high calorie density (lots of calories in a tiny package), doesn't offer volume or bulk, and doesn't have other Hunger Crushing Compounds to contribute better satiety bang for your calorie buck. In contrast, for 100 calories' worth of an all-star HCC, avocado, you'd be packing in an impressive 4 grams of fiber, 9 grams of healthy fats, and 1 gram of protein . . . and you're getting all that in four times the serving (¼ cup!). More volume, more HCCs, *way* more satiety bang for your caloric buck.

To summarize, any diet can technically "work" (at least in the short run) as long as it creates a calorie deficit. But creating a calorie deficit is easy. Staying in it is hard. The Hunger Crushing Combo helps you skip the punishment and learn how to build balanced meals that *actually* feel good. And who doesn't want that?

# CHAPTER 3

· · · · · · · · · · · · · · · · · ·

# Glucose, Insulin, and Managing Blood Sugars

If you have type 2 diabetes, prediabetes, insulin resistance, metabolic syndrome, or polycystic ovary syndrome (PCOS), this chapter is for you.

If you *don't* have type 2 diabetes, prediabetes, insulin resistance, metabolic syndrome, or PCOS, this chapter is for you.

Let me explain.

Even if you're an Olympic athlete or the "perfect" picture of health (whatever the heck that means), stabilizing your blood sugars just makes sense. Think back to the last time you grabbed a doughnut and pumpkin spice latte for breakfast on your way to work. You probably felt a surge of energy in your first meeting, but by round two, you were feeling the crash. You were fatigued, foggy, cranky, and hungry AF (probably not your company's MVP of the day). This is an example of blood sugar mismanagement, and while it's expected that healthy people will occasionally find themselves in a slump like this, it's just not a comfortable way to live routinely.

Managing "hanger" is an obvious priority for all (just ask my husband; this gal is not her best self when she hasn't been fed). But for a huge percentage of Americans, blood sugar management *absolutely* needs to be top of mind. According to the American Diabetes Association, 11.9 percent of US citizens have type 2 diabetes,[1] 40 percent of young adults (ages 18 to 44) have insulin resistance,[2] and almost one-third of people have prediabetes.[3] The problem with these conditions is that they rarely exist in a vacuum. In other words, poor blood sugar management can significantly increase your risk of obesity, cardiovascular disease, chronic kidney disease, liver disease, stroke, and so much more.[4] And while research does suggest that type 2 diabetes is about 50 percent hereditary,[5] learning how to balance your blood sugars (through diet and exercise) has been shown to reduce your risk of developing type 2 diabetes by 58 percent in adults, and by 71 percent for people ages sixty and older.[6]

Despite hearing statistics and risk factors surrounding diabetes *all* the time, most people don't fully understand what this common condition actually is.

## Blood Sugars 101

If you remember from Chapter 2, when we eat a meal (especially one high in carbohydrate-rich foods), our blood sugar rises, which then tells the pancreas to secrete a hormone called insulin. Insulin is like a key, and all of the cells that use glucose for energy (e.g., your muscles, brain, heart, red blood cells, liver, and kidneys) have locks that match that key. When sugar is detected in our blood, insulin says, *"Great, there's fuel, we don't need to eat more!"* It gives our brain a signal that we are full (at least, temporarily), while opening those locks to usher that sugar in. As glucose moves from the bloodstream into our cells, where it can be used as immediate energy or stored for the future, our blood sugar levels return back down to baseline. In an individual with a healthy working pancreas where this homeostatic process runs smoothly, their body is described as having strong **insulin sensitivity**.

But as we've just established, for a large proportion of Americans, this system has some kinks.

**Type 1 diabetes** is a chronic autoimmune condition whereby the immune system mistakenly attacks and destroys the insulin-producing beta cells in the pancreas. As a result, the pancreas produces little to no insulin. If not well managed with supplemental insulin therapy, folks with type 1 diabetes can experience dangerously high blood sugars (a.k.a. hyperglycemia), an increased risk of infections, unexplained weight loss (because sugar or energy isn't making it into the cells), and even coma or death. This is why those with type 1 diabetes have to track their carbohydrate intake and take insulin to keep their blood sugars safely within a normal range.

**Type 2 diabetes** is characterized primarily by **insulin resistance**, whereby the body's cells become less responsive to the insulin it *does* produce. Think of insulin resistance as a communication interference between our bloodstream (where the sugar is), our cells (what needs the sugar), and our pancreas and liver (the organs that help us maintain blood sugar homeostasis). Insulin resistance can be influenced by a wide range of variables, some of which are at least somewhat controllable, and some of which are not. Genetics, physical inactivity, age, hormonal dysfunction (e.g., PCOS), sleep disturbances, chronic stress, medications, non-alcoholic fatty liver disease, and more all play an important role. But most of the proposed theories to explain the development of type 2 diabetes, including the Twin Cycle Hypothesis, focus predominantly on the role of visceral fat.[7] Here's a quick and dirty explainer: When we eat more calories than our body needs, we start to gain fat, not just in our hips or butt, where we can see it, but around our internal organs as well (a.k.a. visceral fat). This fat blunts the communication among our pancreas, liver, and the glucose levels in our blood, so even when we've just eaten a bag of Haribo snacks, the liver doesn't get the memo, thinks we're running low, and dumps a boatload of glucose into the blood to compensate! And up our blood sugars go!

Visceral fat also secretes inflammatory substances called cytokines, which gum up the locks on our cells and block the insulin keys from getting in. The beta cells that produce insulin really don't do well rooming with a lot of cytokines, eventually leading these cells to dysfunction, burn out, and even die. Now we don't have enough insulin keys to open the locks on our hungry cells to let sugar inside, so we get a gnawing message to our brain to EAT. If this progressive system is not intercepted, we end up with surging blood sugars, inadequate insulin to manage it, insatiable hunger, and a propensity to gain more fat.

In addition to visceral fat's role in insulin resistance, physical inactivity is also a primary driver.[8] Not only does exercise help prevent and reduce visceral fat, but it also disrupts the inflammatory cytokine cycle that impairs insulin and glucose communication. So, inactivity can further accelerate the journey from insulin resistance to type 2 diabetes.

A formal diagnosis of diabetes is made when your fasting glucose (measured after not eating for 8 to 12 hours) reaches or exceeds 126 mg/dl (normal is 99 mg/dl or lower), or when your hemoglobin A1c level (a measure of average blood sugar levels over 3 months) is 6.5 percent or higher (normal for people without diabetes is 4% to 5.6%). The risks of unmanaged diabetes can range from weight gain in the early stages of insulin resistance, to poor wound healing, nerve damage, hypertension, Alzheimer's or other forms of dementia, and a lot of the same concerns that are also seen in unmanaged type 1 diabetes.

**Prediabetes** is essentially the early warning sign of type 2 diabetes, as blood sugar levels are recorded at higher than normal, but not high enough to warrant a type 2 diabetes diagnosis. If a normal fasting blood sugar is less than 100 mg/dl, prediabetes is diagnosed between 100 and 125 mg/dl. Without intervention, prediabetes can progress to type 2 diabetes over time.

Now, I want to make something very clear: Following a meal, even superhealthy folks without insulin resistance will see their blood sugars rise and fall, because that's how our body gains access to the nutrients (and energy) provided by what we eat. A balanced meal might make that curve less higgledy-piggledy than a once-a-year Thanksgiving-style carbo load, but even the latter on occasion isn't going to cause devastating or immediate harm. But that doesn't mean we should abuse our healthy pancreas privileges with nightly pizza parties either. Here's why. First of all, experiencing that "spike" in blood sugar after a meal full of Naked Carbs doesn't *feel* good. You might get a little shaky, thirsty, sweaty, or even anxious. As your pancreas pours in a flood of insulin to stabilize the situation, and your blood sugar abruptly declines, a new set of symptoms might arise. You might feel irritable, fatigued, weak, and hangry AF, leading you to instinctively seek out another hit for a high. This is the immediate hyperglycemia to reactive hypoglycemia roller coaster, and even healthy folks will get a dip in insulin sensitivity a few hours after a big carb-y meal.[9] The difference between a healthy individual and one with insulin resistance is that the former might feel like crap for an hour or two, but they recover fairly quickly, whereas someone with insulin resistance may be still flying high (*and* increasing their risk of nerve damage and other complications) for several hours.

The other reason that even healthy folks should focus on blood sugar–friendly choices is to reduce their risk of metabolic syndrome over time. **Metabolic syndrome** is a cluster of increased metabolic risk factors for developing cardiovascular disease, type 2 diabetes, and obesity.

Up to this point, we've painted insulin as this almighty satiety hormone swooping in and saving us from uncontrolled blood sugar. And while, yes, this is in fact insulin's job, it also helps us store anything extra in cells as fat for later use. You might have heard low-carb lifers calling out insulin as the "big bad fat storage hormone," claiming that if you eat anything with carbs, insulin will just bippity-boppity-boop it into fat. And, theoretically, this is *kinda sorta* true. But also sorta not. Your body secretes insulin when you eat, to signal that you're full, while simultaneously opening the doorways for glucose to be used as energy. But if you're struggling with high blood sugars, thanks to insulin resistance or type 2 diabetes, insulin will continue to be pumped out, telling your body that there is no need to dig into your fat reserves for fuel. Judging by the state of sugar in our blood, we clearly have got all the fuel we need! That said, in real life, insulin doesn't work like an on/off switch. It's more like a very sensitive dial that you need Barbie-size fingers to operate and fine-tune.

This is where an individual's insulin sensitivity and metabolic flexibility come into play. **Insulin sensitivity** is basically your body's ability to recognize and utilize small amounts of insulin, to prevent the need for more to be pumped out. There are a few ways we can improve our insulin sensitivity. One is related to body composition: Having a lot of excess fat, especially visceral belly fat, can hinder our liver and pancreas's ability to detect insulin and glucose.[10] Another is physical activity. Movement is one of the best ways to encourage glucose utilization and storage, especially in the muscle cells.[11] A third is sleep and stress management, as excess stress hormones like cortisol can decrease insulin sensitivity over time.[12] And finally, of course, is a balanced diet: Dressing up our Naked Carbs with Hunger Crushing Combos can reduce our need for frequent mega-dumps of insulin.

**Metabolic flexibility** is a related concept that depends on a combination of our insulin sensitivity, body fat percentage, and aerobic fitness level. Metabolic flexibility is our body's ability to adapt and switch back and forth between using carbs and fats as fuel. Imagine a professional runner for a minute. He's very fit; trains regularly; carb loads before a run; is tall, dark, handsome, my type (*okay, so those last few details don't matter here*). He might be using up glucose to fuel the first two legs of his triathlon, but once he's on the homestretch, his metabolic flexibility will allow him to tap into fat.

Improved insulin sensitivity and metabolic flexibility might *help* prevent insulin from turning into the "evil" fat-storing gremlin. But anticarb charlatans waxing poetic about carbs "spiking your insulin" and "storing fat" are missing the forest for the trees. And that forest is just excess calories. If carbs really were the enemy in transforming our body into a fat storage facility, we wouldn't see near-identical weight-loss outcomes in calorie-controlled studies comparing low-fat and low-carb diets.[13] In the end, weight loss will always come down to a calorie deficit. So while, yes, high insulin *can* encourage our body to store excess calories as fat, this only happens when we've eaten too many calories.

To summarize, sugar consumption (Naked Carbs), type 2 diabetes, and obesity are in a bit of a throuple love triangle. Naked Carbs, in and of themselves, don't *cause* diabetes, and they also don't *cause* obesity. But because Naked Carbs are so unsatisfying, they're hard not to overeat. This naturally creates a calorie surplus, which increases the risk of excess fat gain, which then interferes with our cells' insulin sensitivity, and sets the stage for insulin resistance and type 2 diabetes.

Now that we have a better understanding of how blood sugar regulation works (or fails to work optimally in many cases), let's discuss the different tools we often use for management.

## What About the Glycemic Index?

Since the 1980s, there's been a lot of talk about the glycemic index (GI), which is a method of classifying carbs based on how they affect our blood sugar levels. Most Naked Carbs are classified as high-GI carbs, meaning they result in a relatively high blood sugar spike equal to or greater than white bread (a GI of 70 or more). Rice crackers clock in at 87, cornflakes are 81, and pure glucose is represented at 100. In contrast, low-GI foods are those that cause a more gradual or modest increase in blood sugars after consumption, yielding a GI value of 55 or less. Apples have a GI of 36; lentils, 32, and barley offers an impressively low hit at 28. Research on people with prediabetes or diabetes suggests that a diet rich in low–glycemic index meals improves satiety, hemoglobin A1c (markers of high blood sugar over three months), fasting glucose, body mass index (BMI), total cholesterol, LDL cholesterol, and triglycerides, especially over the long term (at least 12 weeks).[14]

Despite the glycemic index being one of the most widely used methods of classifying carbs as "good" or "bad" for blood sugars, it doesn't actually make a whole lot of sense in the real world.

For one, GI values are just based on average responses observed in research studies; they are not meant to be able to accurately predict how a food affects us. Second, we don't usually just eat a single carbohydrate-containing food in isolation. Like, when was the last time you just shoved a piece of Wonder Bread by itself into your mouth, or ate a bowl of dry cornflakes, or a spoonful of table sugar? Portion size also matters (did you have a cup of cornflakes, or half a box)?

Finally, reducing the value of a food to one single data point is useless at best, and dangerous at worst. For example, if you were following a low–glycemic index diet and avoiding all high GI foods, you might be choosing ice cream (GI of 51) over watermelon (GI of

76). The glycemic index fails to identify the source of sugars in a food (naturally occurring vs added), along with beneficial antioxidants, micronutrients, and calorie density. Remember, you can eat ⅓ cup of Ben & Jerry's Netflix & Chill'd or 4½ cups of watermelon for the same amount of calories. And while watermelon is never a replacement for a creamy dreamy brownie- and cookie-packed ice cream dessert, you can probably imagine which is a more nutritious and satiating choice.

The glycemic load is a related concept, developed to try to standardize the serving size discrepancy. Using the glycemic load definitely aligns better with the satiety level of that food, but it still fails to recognize the myriad of factors that make a food a nutritious choice. It also requires that you spend your precious brain space and energy doing math equations all day. And that's a hard pass for most folks (including me).

The glycemic index is just one of many tools in the blood sugar management toolbox. It gives some valuable information, and can be a good start for helping people preempt a difference in blood sugars. But in the real world, it sorely misses the mark.

## Low-Carb Diets & Diabetes

Before we had nutrition education tools like the glycemic index, folks with type 2 diabetes were simply told to just remove carbs and sugar from their diet.[15] Forget about a celebratory birthday cake; you're celebrating with sugar-free Jell-O with a candle on top. Womp womp. The thought process was sound, albeit juvenile: If sugar spikes blood sugar, stop eating it! Fortunately, science has evolved and dietitians have led the pack. On the one hand, there is no question that a lot of research supports the use of low-carb diets for the management of unruly blood sugars.[16] But this research is not without its flaws. Namely, that there's typically a huge variation in what "low carb" even means, study designs don't often assess weight loss over the long term, and dropout rates are notoriously high because, let's be real, for most of us, the low-carb life kinda sucks. We don't live in a science lab where all of our meals are carefully prepared for us every day. We live vibrant, complex, messy lives in the real world where carbohydrates are abundant and delicious. We need to learn how to live and work *with* them in a way that helps us feel good physically (by managing our blood sugars appropriately) and emotionally (by enjoying the birthday cake on our special day). My Hunger Crushing Combo helps you dress up high-GI Naked Carbs to prevent wild fluctuations in blood sugar and insulin secretion, helping you effectively manage, prevent, or reverse existing insulin resistance.

### Tracking Your Blood Sugars

Technology for people with diabetes is continually improving, with most folks who depend on supplemental insulin now wearing a continuous glucose monitor (CGM). A CGM works via a sensor under the skin that can take and record continuous measurements of your blood sugars in real time. CGM technology is often combined with insulin pumps for folks with diabetes, to deliver the most accurate doses of medication without having to count every carb or be subject to human calculation errors.[17] We also have research on patients with prediabetes and type 2 diabetes, for whom CGM use can help encourage healthy blood sugar management behaviors.[18] For example, if you were always getting a notification that your blood sugar was spiking after you eat pizza, it may encourage you to try having a salad first, to flatten out the curve. For this reason, I do think that the benefits of CGMs for the population for whom they've been studied and validated (folks with insulin resistance and diabetes) likely outweigh the risks we will soon discuss.

But in an age of information overload, it's almost become "cool" to wear a CGM, with wellness influencers (who do not have insulin resistance) constantly sharing the results of their meals. Often, when these content creators see any kind of increase in blood sugar, they make a whole video outlining why that food is now "bad." In one video, an influencer noticed that a peach increased his blood sugars, concluding that he will be "careful" not to have peaches as a regular snack. And just like that, a single metric in the hands of someone who doesn't need that information (or know how to use it) can turn a whole population off eating a nutritious peach. What a tragedy! And this is despite the fact that we have ample evidence that a diet rich in fruits and vegetables helps reduce the risk of diabetes, insulin resistance, and obesity.[19]

What these influencers neglect to tell their disciples is that seeing an increase in blood sugar after you eat basically anything is *normal*. They also like to just ignore the fact that their blood sugars promptly go right back down because that is what a healthy working body is designed to do. As a dietitian, I don't recommend wearing a CGM if you *don't* have diabetes. At this point, there is very little data to suggest improved health outcomes with CGM use in folks without diabetes, and I can think of a lot of risks of using it.[20]

When a single transient metric informs what, when, and how much we eat, we quickly lose trust and connection with our innate wisdom. This is no different than hopping on the scale daily: It's an *okay* data point to check on occasion (to be used only in conjunction with many others), but I would never recommend that a healthy person weigh themselves that often. So, why would you need to be checking any other external metric multiple times a day? When you turn a single reading into a rule that you can never eat a Naked Carb again, or you can only eat foods that basically flatline your blood glucose all day, you distort the data into another potentially disordered obsession. I'm not saying that every healthy individual who uses a CGM will end up with an eating disorder, but it can be a slippery slope. Internal information, related to energy levels, hunger, alertness, mood, stress, attention span, and stamina, offers a much more robust and accurate database of metrics for helping you improve your health and well-being.

### Diabetes & Weight Loss

So, does losing weight improve blood sugar levels? Or does managing blood sugar help us lose weight? It's likely a bit of a chicken-or-the-egg situation, as these two goals have reciprocal benefits for each other in folks with insulin resistance or for those at risk of developing it. Let's take a closer look:

**Losing Weight Improves Blood Sugar Levels.** As we've established, excess fat, especially around the midsection, can make it difficult for insulin to make its way to cells to let energy in, while releasing hormones that interfere with normal insulin signaling. This is insulin resistance in a nutshell. The less excess body fat, the better insulin sensitivity, and the greater our chance of preventing type 2 diabetes or putting our existing diabetes into remission. Studies suggest that we can reduce our hemoglobin A1c by 0.1 percent for every percentage of total body weight loss.[21] So, if you are considered overweight or obese, even very modest weight-loss outcomes could stop type 2 diabetes in its tracks.

**Managing Blood Sugar Levels Helps Support Weight Loss.** These benefits work in reverse as well. Making a meal out of six-month-old Halloween candy can send our blood sugars flying higher than a Gen Zer at Coachella. In the case of insulin resistance or diabetes, our insulin signaling just isn't up to snuff, so we don't get the satiety cues our body needs. Our muscles also aren't effectively getting the fuel they need. Cue the "hunger hormones" to get us to eat more, increasing our total calorie intake and risk of gaining fat.

In contrast, when our blood sugars are stable, our body can use up the steady stream of glucose for energy without getting the message that we need to eat more. Also, without a stark blood sugar spike, we don't get a crash, which reduces the inescapable cravings for another high-sugar hit. Ultimately, when our blood sugars are controlled (from either diet or medication, or a combination of both), we're just better equipped to manage our appetite and hunger, making a calorie deficit easier to maintain.

**Improving Blood Sugars Without Weight Loss.** Despite the documented benefits of weight reduction on blood sugar management, the number on the scale doesn't tell us everything about our metabolic health. And pouring all of our energy into our weight can have both emotional and physical risks when our progress doesn't perfectly align with our goal. So, if you've struggled with your relationship with food and body, it's often helpful to think about weight loss more as a (potential) side effect of some other actionable behavior that you *can* directly control. What our body decides to do when we cut out sugar, begin a new exercise program, or even start to build Hunger Crushing Combos into our day, is highly individual. And despite all of our best efforts, sometimes we just kinda have to accept that the outcome is what it is. We *might* lose 10 pounds, we might not! But setting aside one's access to nutritious foods, socioeconomic status, physical ability, medical conditions, and other roadblocks to health-promoting behaviors, we can more readily control what we eat and how we move our body.

Focusing solely on weight loss also misses the mark on improving our 360 wellness. Shrinking our body at *any or all* costs risks disrupting other important elements of our health. What about social connections, mental health, diet quality, and stress reduction? All of these can be put in jeopardy when we measure our health solely by the number on the scale. This is why a lot of folks will benefit from a weight-neutral approach that allows their body to find its happiest healthiest weight when it's given the gentle tools and supportive environment to do so.

The good news is that, even if our weight doesn't budge, blood sugar–stabilizing behaviors still provide massive perks. For example, in one study, researchers tested different protein, carb, and fat ratios to see how they affected blood sugars in folks with uncontrolled type 2 diabetes.[22] Compared to a diet with only 15 percent of calories from protein, participants who bumped their calories from protein up to 30 percent saw significant improvements in glucose response (38%) and a reduction in fasting glucose to near normal levels. And this was all without any change in weight, at all!

And it's not just dietary changes; movement is another amazing tool in our blood sugar–balancing toolbox that we can actively control. Research suggests that getting in around 150 minutes of exercise per week helps improve insulin sensitivity and metabolic flexibility, while reducing one's chance of developing type 2 diabetes by 40 to 70 percent.[23] No time for a full-out sweat sesh? No problem! Try an "exercise snack." Researchers have found that taking just a three-minute movement break every half hour can improve postmeal blood sugar, insulin, and triglyceride levels.[24] Yes, please!

I know the world loves to focus on the size and shape of our body as visible evidence of our "health" status, but we know that it's actually much better to be overweight and fit, than thin and unfit. Loads of data demonstrates that having a higher fitness level (specifically, a high $VO_2$ max (the maximum amount of oxygen our body uses during intense exercise) puts us at lower risk of insulin resistance and disease as compared to people who are leaner but unfit.[25] So, while body fat does play an important role in insulin sensitivity, we can absolutely override this by focusing on fitness! This is known as the "fat but fit paradox" and it serves as further proof that health doesn't always have a specific look.

Sleep and stress management are also important blood sugar–regulating supports that are somewhat within our control (okay, maybe not so much if you have a newborn baby or scared preschooler in your bed). Poor sleep and mismanaged stress increase our cortisol levels, which can disrupt our hunger hormones (including insulin), raise our blood glucose, and reduce our insulin sensitivity.[26] Research suggests that aiming for seven to eight hours of restorative sleep, and taking on a stress-reducing activity like yoga or meditation can help lower blood sugar levels by 10 percent.[27] Even just a few minutes of finding your Zen can prove beneficial!

### Blood Sugars & Well-Being

Purposeful blood sugar management, through all the strategies we just discussed, may be a very meaningful act of self-care, because it *can* and *does* actually *improve* how we feel on the inside.

The roller coaster of uncontrolled blood sugars takes a toll on every system in our body, including our mental health. Even if you don't have diabetes, you can probably relate to a scenario like this: You rush out the door and skip breakfast, grabbing a sweetened coffee and Danish at the office cafeteria. An hour later, you're feeling the crash, but you're in back-to-back Zoom calls. You get a little more sassy and snippy with your manager in the staff meeting, and get hit with a wave of anxiety that your boss is unamused. So, you skip lunch and stay late in the office, trying to get back into their good graces. Working on fumes, by four p.m., you dive headfirst into the communal candy dish, giving you just enough energy to get home and take out your frustration on your spouse and kids. You feel like garbage (physically and emotionally), face-plant into a box of Nutter Butters to self-medicate from the trauma of the day, and spend the rest of the night replaying the day like a Swiftie with a new album. I'm not saying that a random morning pastry is going to get you fired from your job or served with divorce papers. Sometimes, that cream cheese blueberry bun is the *best* start of the day. But when this pattern becomes your every day, it can grind you right down.

We also know that stress specifically is a major contributor to unruly blood sugars, insulin resistance, and type 2 diabetes.[28] And bidirectionally, research shows that high-sugar diets increase the risk of anxiety, depression, and other mood disorders.[29] In fact, one review of the NHANES survey found that consuming 100 grams of sugar per day correlated with a 28 percent higher prevalence of depression.[30] To put this amount of sugar into perspective, that could potentially look like a 12-ounce can of soda, a venti flavored coffee drink, and a cup of sweetened yogurt, so it's really not an outrageous amount to consume.

But what if we look at this from a different point of view? If you are already struggling with your mental state, are you soothing yourself with baby carrots and broccoli? Probably not. Although mental health issues may cause some people to lose their appetite, others may be dealing with their emotions by eating more, especially foods high in sugar and other Naked Carbs. To me, this is another chicken-or-egg situation. Do you eat more sugar because you are depressed or are you depressed because you are eating more sugar? If we want to break this cycle and improve our overall sense of well-being, we need a gentler, nonrestrictive sugar strategy. When you feel your best, physically and mentally, you can be your best self: in your job, at home with your family, and for your own sense of self-purpose and joy. This is the real value of my Hunger Crushing Combo: to help you evolve and improve yourself from the inside out.

Let's break down how each of our Hunger Crushing Compounds comes into play when blood sugar management is our primary goal.

## Powerful Protein:
## The Steady-State Superstar

Not just a satiety superstar, protein is also a winner when it comes to stabilizing blood sugars. Here's how it works:

**Digestion.** Protein digests significantly more slowly than carbs: The digestion of protein happens at an average rate of 2 to 10 grams per hour, so it takes *at least* two hours for 20 grams of protein to completely absorb (compared to 30 grams per hour for Naked Carbs like white bread).[31] Casein in dairy products (e.g., cottage cheese) is one of the slowest-digesting proteins, taking almost seven hours to fully digest![32] So, what happens if we were to throw a little honey on that cottage cheese or eat it alongside a couple of Oreos (pro tip: Crush the Oreos *into* the cottage cheese! Game changer, I swear). Good news: Protein helps slow down the digestion of that sugar, too. It's as if the Naked Carbs are moving their turbocharged legs toward the finish line, while protein is pulling them back with their muscled Popeye arms. Even if carbs still make it there first, their finish time will be impaired. And despite being supercompetitive, I know that this is one race we actually don't want to win!

The result is that the impending blood sugar spike and crash just don't happen. Instead, a steadier stream of nutrients and glucose is delivered to your cells, where they can supply energy much longer over time.[33]

**Blood Sugar–Stabilizing Hormones.** Protein also can help stabilize blood sugar levels by stimulating insulin. This is really one of the unique hallmark superpowers of protein. If you recall from Chapter 2, a high-protein diet can result in a 20 percent boost in our hunger and blood sugar–stabilizing hormone, GLP-1, and GLP-1 signals insulin to get to work.[34] By increasing insulin secretion (without also increasing blood sugars as carbs would), we have *extra* insulin to deal with the sugars in our blood. It's like having two parents to manage one unruly toddler, rather than a solo parent trying to wrangle a whole brood.

Now, if we zoom out for a minute and bring this back to food, we can clearly see that *adding* protein to Naked Carbs significantly helps flatten the postmeal blood sugar response. For example, one study showed that adding 20 grams of whey protein reduced the peak blood glucose reading by 27 percent, and the total-meal blood sugar response by 40 percent.[35] It turns out that the more protein consumed before a carb-rich meal, the more profound the glucose-lowering effects.[36] So, this study (and many others) prove that you don't have to *eliminate* carbs to improve your blood sugars; you just have to *add* protein!

**Satiety.** Here's an all-too-common scenario: Your kids have back-to-back sports tournaments, and you're going to spend all day on the field. It took all of your effort and patience just to get everyone else well fed, dressed, packed, and out the door, so you skipped breakfast and forgot to pack yourself anything to eat. You're starving, so you hit the concession stand for a bag of chips and a warm pretzel that is *literally* the size of your head. A full meal of delicious, salty Naked Carbs. Not surprisingly, you're starving by the time the team heads out to grab pizza to celebrate. So, you crush a few slices of cheese pizza, four garlic knots (and a cold one, because *what a day*). You feel stuffed in the moment, but fatigued once the kids go to bed, setting yourself up for a midnight crash that disturbs your sleep. This tumultuous blood sugar roller-coaster ride not only feels chaotic, but it can be really hard to get off if you don't intervene with a more balanced meal.

But as we've uncovered, protein is filling AF because it is slow to digest and triggers high returns on key satiating hormones. Starting our day with higher-protein meals can significantly reduce excess hunger, cravings, food noise, and total calorie consumption as the day goes on.[37] I'm not saying you wouldn't have taken part in the pizza party if you had just eaten a cup of Greek yogurt at seven a.m. (you absolutely should get in on that 'za!). But when we fuel our body regularly and take panicked hanger out of the equation, our brain has the calmness to make more mindful blood sugar–balancing choices.

**Muscle Health.** Protein is the building block of muscle. But despite what some gym bros might believe, maximizing muscle isn't just about looking ripped in your gym selfies. Muscle mass *also* plays a role in glucose metabolism.[38]

Remember the analogy: Insulin is the key that unlocks our cells to let glucose (energy) into our cells, and 80 percent of the glucose we consume is used by our muscle cells.[39] The more muscle mass we have built (which requires protein and progressive overload to build and maintain), the more muscle cells to sop up the sugar in our blood. So, *just* having muscle mass on board can significantly reduce your risk of type 2 diabetes!

And it's not just a muscle cell numbers game. The improved blood flow and muscle contraction helps expedite the movement of sugars out of our bloodstream and into our cells. Exercise is actually such a powerful contributor to glucose metabolism that some research has demonstrated that it may even be able to fully reverse insulin resistance and diabetes![40]

## Fabulous Fiber: The Sugar Shield

Fiber and sugar are like brothers that look alike, but whose personalities clash (and as a mom of two boys, I could write a whole book about that). Sugar is a bit of a boisterous party crasher: It makes its presence known, it sings karaoke (badly, I might add), and it passes out on the lawn an hour later. Fiber is a lot more chill. It has a few quiet conversations, hangs around until last call, all while carrying its brother around on its back. In most cases, foods with carbs are a combination of sugars and fiber; fruits and vegetables, for example, have both. And while there are so many benefits of those sugars in whole-food form, being bound up by their supportive partner, fiber, helps us reap those benefits without the blood sugar spike. This is why an apple (which contains natural sugars *and* fiber) helps stabilize blood sugars *and* satiety better than a box of refined strained juice. A lot of these benefits relate back to how fiber is broken down and digested in the gut.

**Digestion.** As you'll recall from Chapter 2, fiber doesn't break down nearly as easily as carbs, protein, and fat. In fact, part of its superpower is that it resists digestion until it makes its way to the intestines, where our microbes get to work.

This long, slow, and largely unsuccessful process of trying to break down fiber in the gut doesn't just keep us full longer; it also means that any other components of a meal (specifically the sugars that often come packaged up with fiber) get dragged at a snail's pace, too. The result is that those sugars get digested and absorbed more slowly, preventing the dramatic blood sugar spike and drop.

**The Gut Microbiome.** Many types of fiber are prebiotics, which, as you know from your microbiome 101 on pages 54–58, are essential fuel for the bacteria in our gut. Inulin, oligosaccharides, pectin, and resistant starches are four of our gut microbes' favorite treats. And each of these prebiotic fibers has unique benefits and roles:

- **Inulin** (found in green bananas, asparagus, sunchokes, and chicory) stimulates the growth of some of the noblest strains of probiotics, including *Lactobacillus, Bifidobacterium,* and *Bacteroides*, while also edging out potentially harmful bacteria.[41] This at least partially explains why research has found that supplementing with inulin fiber helps improve blood sugars in folks with insulin resistance.[42]

- **Oligosaccharides** (found in legumes, garlic, and onions) have been shown to enhance the effects of a-glucosidase inhibitors (which prevent the absorption of carbohydrates), improve leptin and insulin resistance, and provide other powerful anti-inflammatory effects.[43]

- **Pectin** (found naturally in apples, okra, and potatoes) swells and thickens in the gut to help improve satiety and flatten the glucose curve.[44]

- **Resistant starches** are found naturally in green bananas, legumes, and grains. These microbe delicacies have a superpower so cool, you're going to swear it's TikTok lore! By simply cooking and cooling the starch, you can transform some of the absorbable carbs in the food into nonabsorbable resistant starch, effectively reducing that food's blood sugar impact, and its calorie content. I know, wild! See the box "The Magic of Resistant Starch" for more details and tips.

## The Magic of Resistant Starch

Increasing the resistant starch in your favorite carbs is really as easy as *not* throwing away your leftovers. Through a scientific phenomenon called retrogradation, cooling a starch that's been previously cooked traps the starch molecules in a matrix of hydrogen bonds that prevent our enzymes from accessing the carbohydrates to use them as energy. Researchers in the highly publicized preliminary Sri Lanka experiment found that a straightforward rice cooking hack could increase resistant starch levels tenfold and reduce the absorbable calories by 10 to 15 percent.[45] They simply added 1 teaspoon of coconut oil to boiling water, added ½ cup of white rice, cooked the rice for 40 minutes, then cooled it in the fridge for 12 hours before reheating it the next day. It is very important that, if you are planning to use leftover rice, you should refrigerate leftovers immediately after cooking. Due to how rice is grown, it is uniquely at risk of contamination with a dangerous bacteria called *Bacillus cereus*. It's therefore really important to refrigerate your rice within an hour after cooking, reheat it until steaming (reaching 165°F or higher, and only once), and to eat your leftovers within a day or two, to reduce your risk.

You can use this same cooking, cooling, and reheating technique to increase the resistant starch in pasta, potatoes, bread, and more. All the more reason to keep that leftover takeout rice and turn it into a Hunger Crushing Combo fried rice the next day!

You may be thinking, "Okay, Abbey, I get it, fiber is great! But all those fiber farts? Not so much!" Amen to that! So despite all the health perks of our gut's working hard to break down those indigestible fibers, there can definitely be too much of a good thing. This is why it's important that, when adding some fiber to your routine, you go slowly. A massive fiber feast is going to feel like napalm for your bowels, and nobody's got time for that. Rather than maxing out on as much fiber as you can possibly eat, try adding one extra serving of fiber at a time. Another pro-fiber tip is to add an extra 2 to 3 ounces of water for each gram of fiber you add to your stack, or around 2 liters (8⅓ cups) of water total when reaching your 25-gram goal. Fiber without water is just asking to get backed up.

## Low FODMAP and IBS?

Most prebiotic fibers in our diet can also be classified as FOD-MAPs, which is a much cuter name than its long-form moniker, fermentable oligosaccharides, disaccharides, monosaccharides, and polyols. If you already have irritable bowel syndrome (IBS) or a sensitive gut, you might have been told you need to cut out FODMAPs or go on a "low FODMAP diet" for a period of time, to manage your symptoms. But the low FODMAP diet is designed to be used as a step-by-step trial to identify triggers, not a long-term way to eat. Working alongside a health professional like a registered dietitian, you would temporarily eliminate all major sources of FODMAPs to get a symptom-free baseline, and then strategically challenge your gut by adding back a food from each category in different preparations and graduating amounts. The goal is to identify exactly *which* FODMAPs are uniquely triggering for you and how much you can tolerate. If you suspect you may be sensitive to some FODMAPS, seek professional help before swearing off all of them. Your gut microbiome (and blood sugars) will thank you!

### Fiber & Meal Order

One of the most popular concepts making the rounds in low-carb circles is this idea of the "correct" order in which to eat your meal. That is, if you want to flatten the blood sugar curve and reduce the insulin spike, you need to eat your nonstarchy low-carb fiber foods first, then protein and fat, and *then* your carbs. Normally I would let out one of my big ol' signature eye rolls on a hard-and-fast rule like this. But there is at least some decent evidence to support this approach. In a 2023 review of eleven studies, researchers concluded that people who saved their carbohydrate-rich foods for the end of the meal, after they ate their veggies and proteins, had significantly lower blood sugar levels than when they consumed them first.[46]

All of this makes sense for a few reasons. First, high-fiber foods like veggies help slow gastric emptying, which prevents dramatic spikes in your blood sugar levels. And then protein stimulates the hormone GLP-1, which further slows digestion and tells your pancreas to secrete insulin to start moving glucose from your blood into your cells. Still, most research on "food order" has been very small-scale or pilot studies, and largely done on folks with insulin resistance and diabetes.[47] They also typically give these Hunger Crushing Compound "preloads" a good thirty minutes before they offer participants their carbs. Um . . . are we really expecting people to take apart their sandwich, eat the lettuce first, then wait thirty minutes, then eat the turkey, then wait, and *then* eat the bread? This is the difference between understanding what data says may be helpful, and understanding how it applies in real life.

Yes, there may be some benefits to starting your meal with a little green salad, if it makes sense. But parsing out your meal like a picky toddler is no way to live. Nor do the potential benefits significantly outshine those of simply combining these HCCs into a satiating and satisfying meal you actually want to eat. In fact, the research on simply *adding* these components in a mixed meal as opposed to the minutiae of *timing* or *order* is far more robust. Adding some vegetables, chicken, and olives to your pasta is something you can commit to, because balance feels good and just makes sense. Freaking out if you accidentally swallow a piece of penne before your bell pepper does not.

## Hearty Healthy Fats: The Blood Sugar Breaks

Every macronutrient plays a part on the blood sugar management team. You might be surprised to see *fat* and *blood glucose* together in the same sentence, but thousands of people are bringing butter back in the hopes of better blood sugar control. So, how does dietary fat affect our blood sugar? Well, it doesn't, at least not directly. And that comes back around to how fats are digested.

**Digestion.** Compared to protein and carbs, fats tend to take the longest time to digest: six to eight hours or longer, depending on how much of them was in the meal.[48] But this is actually part of fats' superpowers when it comes to blood sugar management.

As we discussed in Chapter 2, adding fats to our meal slows down digestion and absorption, not just of the fat itself, but of everything else in that meal. It's as if a roadrunner (Naked Carbs) got stuck behind a geriatric horse and buggy, forcing the roadrunner to take a breather. Everything consumed with that fat gets absorbed at a slower, more stable pace, which is then mirrored in a more sustained blood sugar release.

One 2020 study, for example, compared small sugar-based, fat-free 250-calorie meals with meals that were almost double the calories (450 calories), each with 30 grams of fat and carbs.[49] Even though the meals containing fat were significantly larger, they had less of an impact on blood glucose and insulin levels, thanks to the digestion-slowing superpowers of fat. That's pretty powerful stuff!

### Healthy Fats & Insulin Resistance

The general role of dietary fat in improving metabolic health is actually not that well understood. Some studies have found no association between how much fat we eat and our blood sugar control, whereas others suggest that a high-fat diet is associated with worsened HbA1c.[50] This is where critical analysis of the literature is key. Because it's not just any sources of fat that appear to increase the risk; it's specifically a diet rich in animal-based saturated fats like those found in red meat, butter, cream, and bacon.[51]

Not only are the animal fats associated with diabetes risk, but saturated fats from plants may alter glucose metabolism, as well.[52]

So, what's the deal with saturated fat? Saturated fat seems to make it harder for insulin to attach to its receptors to effectively lower blood sugar. Saturated fat, compared to unsaturated fats, is also more likely to be stored as visceral fat.[53] This means, if someone gains weight and they are consuming a high–saturated fat diet, more of it is likely to be stored around their organs, including the critical ones for blood glucose management, such as the liver and pancreas.

In contrast, while research is admittedly mixed thanks to the heterogeneity of studies, unsaturated fats don't seem to carry the same set of risks. There may even be some clear benefits for improving insulin resistance and reducing the risk of comorbidities like heart disease.[54] In one randomized controlled study on folks with prehypertension or early-stage hypertension without diabetes, researchers concluded that "a diet that partially replaces carbohydrates with unsaturated fat may improve insulin sensitivity in a population at risk for cardiovascular disease."[55] In other words, lone wolf carbs (a.k.a. Naked Carbs) are best dressed up with healthy fats, to better manage blood sugar control in at-risk populations.

Monounsaturated fats (found in olives, avocados, nuts, and seeds) and polyunsaturated omega-3 fatty acids (from fatty fish, walnuts, and hemp hearts) may be particularly beneficial in helping lower "bad" cholesterol levels and improving insulin sensitivity.[56]

To sum it up, protein, fiber, and healthy fats all have unique roles to play in blood sugar management, insulin sensitivity, and risk of type 2 diabetes, with some playing a greater role than others. One 2019 study found adding sprouts (fiber), oil (fat), and egg (protein) to white rice

(Naked Carb) lowered blood sugar significantly more than any one Hunger Crushing Compound alone.[57] This was also concluded by another set of researchers when they combined white rice (Naked Carb) with bok choy (fiber), oil (fat), and chicken (protein).[58] In other words, when we combine our Hunger Crushing Compounds, we get the synergistic blood sugar–balancing magic of the Hunger Crushing Combo!

# CHAPTER 4

· · · · · · · · · · · · · · · · · ·

# Effortless Nutrition for Vitality and Immunity

A t this point, we've been fangirling over protein, fat, and fiber's physiological capacity to keep our blood sugars stabilized and our tummy full. But we don't eat just macronutrients, such as the amino acids in protein. We eat food. And food is so much more than the sum of its parts. When we look at the types of foods that our Hunger Crushing Compounds are typically found in, we find a bounty of important micronutrients and antioxidants that help us live our lives to the fullest. We call this the whole-food matrix, and it's a huge part of the benefits package of starting to focus on building Hunger Crushing Combos. No counting. No tracking. Just inherently balanced nutrition for health that *feels* good.

## Diet Variety and Quality for Health

You know that popular adage "Variety is the spice of life"? That applies to our diet, too. The more variety we include in our daily menu, and more important, over a period of weeks and months, the more tools we're giving our body to thrive.

Research consistently shows that diets offering a wide variety of foods in rotation, rather than just a handful of "healthy" staples, are associated with a lower risk of all-cause mortality (a.k.a. death from any cause).[1] The diverse diets of those living in many Blue Zones are another testament of that.[2] You might think that a vegetable is a vegetable. They're all healthy, so just pick one you like and stick to it! But each has their own unique fingerprint of nutrients consisting of phytonutrients, polyphenols, and other antioxidants; even green grapes offer different nutrients than do red!

Diet quality and food variety might even be more important than how *much* we eat. One 2023 study looked at fruit and vegetable consumption and all-cause mortality among nearly twenty thousand older Chinese adults.[3] Interestingly, the authors found that the subjects' consumption of a wider variety of fruits and vegetables was actually more important than the total amount they consumed.

In an ideal world, we're adding an array of different colors, textures, and flavors to our routine. But that doesn't mean you're going to die early if you meal-prep a big batch of bean salad for a week's worth of lunches, or if you eat oatmeal three days in a row. Most of us aren't living on a cruise ship with endless daily options, nor should we be expected to muster up the mental energy to plan hundreds of new recipes a year. A lot of us also derive comfort from the familiar, and that's okay! But even just a little rotation or tweaking throughout the weeks, months, and year can make a big difference in our overall health. One study following fifty-nine thousand women found that those who rotated sixteen or seventeen "healthy" foods in their diet had a 42 percent lower risk of all-cause mortality than did those who included fewer than eight "healthy" foods in their meals.[4] The researchers of this study concluded that encouraging *more diversity in "healthy" foods* was actually more important than limiting or focusing on eating *less "unhealthy" food*. Adding, not restricting.

The importance of *adding* more variety and healthy options at meals is also supported by fascinating research on a phenomenon called sensory-specific satiety (SSS).[5] If you've ever felt stuffed to the brim after your Thanksgiving turkey dinner, but suddenly had an appetite for pie, that is sensory-specific satiety at its finest. You're satiated, or full, on one flavor, texture, or type of food, but if presented with other options, you suddenly have more room. The opposite is true as well. When you've been served the same food over and over again, your hedonic interest in that food quickly declines. You get bored. You maybe even get the ick. This is one of the reasons that weight-loss diets that severely limit the number of foods you're allowed to eat can "work" (at least in the short run, before you binge on all the forbidden foods). When we're bored and no longer derive pleasure from the specific flavors and textures put in front of us, we just tend to eat less.

The science of SSS has traditionally been used to encourage kids to eat more vegetables and fruit, but it applies here, too. By using the psychology of SSS and a nonrestrictive additive approach to nutrition, we effortlessly achieve two big benefits in one behavioral shift: (1) We increase important nutrients in the diet, and (2) we subconsciously edge out the less-nutrient-dense foods, all without falling into a scarcity mindset.

## How to Incorporate More Variety
## (Without Going Crazy)

There are a lot of reasons that we tend to eat the same rotation of foods: for example, budget or time restraints, mental energy limitations, picky eating, and neurodivergence. And even if you don't identify with any of these specific reasons, most of us have a go-to Rolodex of maybe half a dozen dinners we're making over and over again during any given week. I'm not suggesting you become an inspired chef overnight, but let's go over some practical ways to overcome the most common barriers to gently switch things up.

**Budget Restraints.** If you're cooking for one or two, it can feel wasteful and financially inaccessible to try to buy four different vegetables in an effort to reap the benefits we've just discussed. This is where frozen produce really comes into play. Frozen produce is picked at the peak of ripeness, then flash frozen to lock in those nutrients. These days, there are plenty of innovative and delicious fruit and vegetable medleys that allow you to get a combination of fruits and vegetables in every meal (without spending an hour slicing and dicing). Think tropical fruit or berry blends for your smoothies and oats; Asian-inspired vegetable blends for your stir-fry night; and a classic corn, carrot, and pea medley for your go-to casserole recipe. Variety doesn't have to cost an arm and a leg.

**Time Restraints.** When time is tight, maximizing variety in your meals can require strategic planning and more efficiency in your decision-making. Start by diversifying your pantry and freezer staples to include versatile ingredients that can be used in a variety of ways (e.g., whole grains, herbs and spices, canned goods, and legumes). If you have even a short window of unassigned time on the weekend, try batch-prepping a few ingredients to be used in more than one dish in the week ahead. For example, you might whip out your Instant Pot for a big batch of rice that you could use to make stir-fry, protein bowls, and salads, and add to homemade veggie burger patties. Grill a big batch of chicken breasts for adding to salads, sandwiches, pasta dishes, and stir-fries. And prechop a head of lettuce or a few bell peppers for nutritious bowls, salads, and taco night. With a few main players already prepared, you can then fill in the gaps and add variety with convenience staples. Today, there are plenty of great prechopped, preseasoned raw veggie medleys and salad kits in the produce section, and premarinated proteins near the butcher section that combine a number of ingredients into a single meal. Fresh and frozen meal kits can also help you sneak a few new or unexpected vegetables, proteins, or grains into your routine, for minimal time or work.

**Mental Energy Limitations & Decision Paralysis.** If you've ever found yourself oscillating between opening the fridge and freezer doors and walking to your pantry, but being completely unable to take meal-time action, you've probably experienced decision paralysis. This is when simplification, structure, and a little inspiration are key. Start by scheduling themed-meal nights during the week, to help guide your meal-making decisions: for instance, Meatless Monday, Taco Tuesday, World-Cuisine Wednesday, Leftovers Thursday, Pizza Friday, Soup Saturday, and Spaghetti Sunday. This helps provide an easy meal structure that you can switch up on the regular without the overwhelm of endless options. For example, week one's pizza dinner could be made with BBQ sauce, Cheddar cheese, jalapeños, onions, and leftover chicken, whereas week two's could be mushrooms, peppers, and olives. One theme, endless opportunities for variety!

**Picky Eating and Neurodivergence.** Folks who are neurodivergent or are exhibiting signs of extreme picky eating or eating disorders like avoidant restrictive food intake disorder (ARFID), often have a limited number of "safe foods," due to sensory sensitivities, the need for routine, or the comfort of predictability. In cases of neurodivergence, folks often get stuck in "food fixation" loops, whereby they want to eat the same food every day until they eventually grow tired of it and that extreme preference shifts.

A good place to start is to identify textures, flavors, and colors that are preferred or disliked, and then make yourself a list of all the acceptable options within those parameters. Experiment with different cooking methods, encourage participation in meal planning and prep, and celebrate small victories in a supportive and nonjudgmental environment. So, for example, if French fries are a safe food because you (or your kiddo) likes the soft middle and crispy texture, see whether you can get the same fry-like experience using another vegetable like carrots or parsnips. A favorite dip is also a great way to "bridge" one familiar safe food to a related but different food: for example, switching from chicken nuggets to fish nuggets. If you or your child is dealing with a limited diet due to picky eating or neurodivergence, I strongly recommend working with a registered dietitian who specializes in eating and feeding disorders for one-on-one support.

We now know that variety is not only an effortless way to help us subconsciously (and enjoyably) work more nutritious foods into our day. It's also a well-established dietary pattern for longevity and good health. And while nutrient synergy yields a food that is much more than the sum of its parts, the parts are worth appreciating, too. Namely, the unique nutrients in each of our Hunger Crushing Compounds beyond just fiber, protein, and fat.

## Health Benefits of Protein-Rich Foods

Obviously, protein's hunger crushing capacity and role in supporting a healthy body composition are important drivers in why we love it so much. But the benefits of building protein into your Hunger Crushing Combos go well beyond just bro science or aesthetics.

For one, protein serves as the building blocks of immune fighting and messaging compounds (e.g., T cells, B cells, macrophages, antibodies, and cytokines) that spring into action when daycare virus number 59,205 is staring you down. Protein deficiency is rare in industrialized nations, but it can result in immune organ atrophy, increased susceptibility to infections, slowed immune response, and impaired healing.

Protein is also an essential structural component of cells and tissues. Our skin, hair, joints, cartilage, bones, neural tissue, enzymes, hormones, and even blood contain different types of protein! Skin, for example, is made up of collagen and elastin proteins, which provide structure and elasticity. Our epidermis (outermost layer of skin), hair, and nails, on the other hand, also contain collagen but are predominantly made up of keratin protein, which helps provide protection and resistance to mechanical damage. And as I just alluded to, proteins are also critical for repairing damaged tissues from a physical injury like a cut, scrape, or burn, while also employing immune defenses to prevent infections.

## Do You Need Collagen Protein Supplements?

Thanks to its unique triple helical structure and amino acid composition, some studies suggest that collagen supplements may help reduce the signs of skin aging by improving skin hydration and elasticity, and reducing wrinkles.[6] Many (but not all) studies also suggest that collagen supplementation may help improve joint stiffness, and mobility pain in folks with osteoarthritis.[7] It's very promising stuff! That said, collagen protein on its own is not a great source of dietary protein. Unlike whole-food sources of protein, or other protein supplements like whey or pea, which contain all of the amino acids needed for muscle protein synthesis, collagen's job is highly specialized. So, if you are choosing to supplement with collagen, see it as an addition, not a replacement for more high-quality, protein-rich foods. When choosing a collagen supplement, look for one that contains the type of collagen most specific to your needs (type I: skin, bones, and tendons; type II: cartilage and joints; type III: skin and blood vessels), that is hydrolyzed (predigested to improve bioavailability), and that is third-party tested for quality and purity.

Protein's role is evident in a lot of ways we can physically see and appreciate, but there's even more going on behind the scenes. One of protein's many roles is to act as enzymes that help make digestion, energy production, and other metabolic processes possible. Without adequate protein on board, all of these biochemical reactions would happen just too slowly to sustain life.

Likewise, some proteins also function as hormones. Remember insulin (our blood sugar regulator) and glucagon (our energy storer)? Both of these are made of protein! Our bodies may be 70 percent water, but protein makes up more than half of the other 30 percent! So, when I say protein is important, you now know it's not just because it helps get you from lunch to dinner without stopping for gas station snacks on the way home.

### Key Nutrients in Protein-Rich Foods

Foods that are typically rich in protein also offer a bounty of other essential micronutrients that support immunity, sleep, heart health, and everything in between. While every different protein source offers its own unique cocktail of nutrients, there are some major players that naturally come with the package deal. Here are some of the heavyweights.

| Nutrient | What it does | Key sources |
|---|---|---|
| Iron | Supports muscle and brain function, energy levels, and our immune system by helping our body respond to infection. Fatigue, weakness, frequent illness, and impaired cognition are all common symptoms of iron-deficiency anemia, which is one of the most common nutrient deficiencies in the first world.[8] | Heme iron is found in animal protein like liver, red meats, pork, dark meat poultry, and fish. Non-heme iron can be found in plants like legumes, lentils, seeds, nuts, whole grains, leafy greens, and fortified cereals. Non-heme iron is not absorbed as efficiently as heme iron, so pair it with a source of vitamin C for a boost! |

| | | |
|---|---|---|
| Zinc | Plays an important role in our immune system, skin integrity and wound healing, fetal growth throughout pregnancy, growth throughout childhood and adolescence, hormone regulation, and enzymatic pathways. | Oysters, beef, pork, dark meat chicken, eggs, Cheddar cheese, pumpkin seeds, chickpeas, lentils, firm tofu, and oats. |

## B Vitamins

| | | |
|---|---|---|
| Vitamin B$_1$ (Thiamine) | Helps metabolize carbs, and support nerve, muscle, and heart function. | Pork, beef liver, eggs, fatty fish, fortified breakfast cereal, whole grains, legumes, sunflower seeds, and edamame. |
| Vitamin B$_2$ (Riboflavin) | Plays a key role in metabolizing fats, while also maintaining healthy skin, eyes, and nerves. | Beef liver, eggs, dairy, lean meats, fish, fortified grains, almonds, mushrooms, spinach, quinoa, and avocados. |
| Vitamin B$_3$ (Niacin) | Reduces skin inflammation, improves cholesterol levels, supports cognition and mood, and protects cells from stress and aging. | Poultry, tuna, lean beef, pork, fatty fish, eggs, dairy, fortified cereals, peanuts, brown rice, whole-grain bread, and legumes. |
| Vitamin B$_5$ (Pantothenic acid) | Essential in the production of neurotransmitters and hormones (e.g., estrogen and cortisol), supports skin barrier function and tissue repair, and synthesizes energy from food. | Beef liver, dark meat poultry, egg yolks, fatty fish, dairy, avocados, sunflower seeds, mushrooms, sweet potatoes, and legumes. |
| Vitamin B$_6$ (Pyridoxine) | Critical for normal brain development, maintaining a healthy immune system, and metabolizing amino acids from protein. | Poultry, beef, liver, fatty fish, eggs, dairy, bananas, avocados, potatoes, chickpeas, and cooked spinach. |

| | | |
|---|---|---|
| Vitamin B$_7$ (Biotin) | Supports strong hair, skin, nails, and energy metabolism. | Egg yolks, liver, fatty fish, pork, dairy, sunflower seeds, sweet potatoes, almonds, cooked spinach, broccoli, and oats. |
| Vitamin B$_9$ (Folate) | An essential nutrient for healthy brain function and development, particularly during pregnancy when it supports the production of DNA, RNA, and rapid cell division and growth.<br><br>Inadequate folate in pregnancy can increase the risk of neural tube defects, which is why pregnant people are told to take at least 400–600 mcg DFE of folic acid per day. | Cooked spinach, asparagus, Brussels sprouts, romaine lettuce, beets, avocados, lentils, legumes, fortified cereals, eggs, liver, seafood, and dairy. |
| Vitamin B$_{12}$ (Cobalamin) | Critical for red blood cell formation, energy production, and the health of our brain and nervous system. Approximately 38% of older adults, and up to 86% of vegetarian adults, do not get enough B$_{12}$ without fortified foods or supplements, leading to fatigue, weakness, brain fog, irritability, and "pins and needles" in the extremities.[9]<br><br>People with certain gastrointestinal disorders, like Crohn's disease, celiac disease, and gastritis, and those on certain medications that affect stomach acid production, may also be at increased risk. | In animal protein like liver, beef, eggs, fish, salmon, plus some fortified plant-based foods like cereals, nondairy milks, tofu, and nutritional yeasts.<br><br>Vegetarians and vegans should look for fortified products and should speak to their doctor or dietitian about supplementation. |

| | | |
|---|---|---|
| Calcium | Provides the structure and strength of bones and teeth while playing a key role in muscle contractions, nerve impulse transmission, blood clotting, and hormone and enzyme regulation. Calcium deficiency is associated with an increased risk of low bone mineral density and fractures. | Dairy milk, yogurt, and cheese along with fortified plant milks, tofu with calcium sulfate, chia seeds, cooked dark leafy greens, almonds, and fish with edible bones (e.g., canned salmon). Vegans should look for fortified products and should speak to their doctor or dietitian about supplementation. |
| Phosphorus | Provides strength and structure to bones and teeth, assists in energy production and cellular function, acts as a buffer to maintain your body's acid-base balance, and helps the kidneys' natural detox mechanisms by filtering waste in our urine. | Poultry, pork, fish, beef, eggs, dairy, lentils, nuts and seeds, whole grains, and firm tofu. |
| Vitamin D | Helps the gut absorb calcium and phosphorus to regulate bone mineralization and prevent such conditions as osteoporosis and rickets. It also modulates the immune response, regulates inflammatory cytokine production, and plays a role in serotonin regulation. Low levels of vitamin D have been associated with increased risk of depression, heart disease, frequent infections, cancer, type 1 diabetes, multiple sclerosis, rheumatoid arthritis, and cognitive decline.[10] | Our skin produces vitamin $D_3$ when exposed to UVB rays (it takes only 10 to 30 minutes, a few times per week!). Food sources include fatty fish (salmon, trout, sardines, and tuna), cod liver oil, UV-exposed mushrooms, and fortified milks, plant milks, and cereals. Most adults who are not consistently exposed to sunlight year-round should consider a supplement with at least 1,000 to 2,000 IU of vitamin $D_3$.[11] |

| | | |
|---|---|---|
| Vitamin A | Supports vision (especially at night), promotes cell turnover in the skin, strengthens immune function by maintaining mucosal barriers, and produces white blood cells to prevent and fight infection. In pregnancy and infancy, vitamin A also plays a critical role in embryonic development and cell differentiation.<br>    Deficiency is associated with night blindness, dry eyes, frequent infections, dry skin or keratosis pilaris, and growth retardation in children. | Preformed vitamin A is found in beef liver, fatty fish, butter, cheese, and eggs.<br>    Provitamin A (beta-carotene) is converted to active vitamin A and is found in orange and yellow vegetables and fruit, along with dark greens. |
| Probiotics | Live microorganisms that improve digestion and nutrient absorption; strengthen our immune function; support glucose metabolism, the gut-brain axis (affecting mood, anxiety, and brain function), periodontal and vaginal health; and may help reduce inflammatory skin conditions (e.g., eczema, psoriasis, and acne). And that's honestly just scratching the surface. | Fermented foods (e.g., yogurt, kefir, miso, tempeh, kombucha, and pickles) naturally contain some probiotics.<br>    For a clinical dose, consider adding a probiotic supplement with at least 2 billion CFUs of active bacteria. |

## Animal vs. Plant-Based Protein

If you compare animal protein to plant-based protein on paper, it will often seem that you're getting the better nutrient bang for your protein buck when you go with meat, poultry, or fish. Typically, animal-based proteins contain more protein per gram, plus greater concentrations of such essential nutrients as zinc, iron, calcium, and vitamin $B_{12}$ (among others). But the healthfulness of a food depends on much more than a few micro- and macronutrients, and we have ample evidence that a diet rich in plant-based proteins offers some unique rewards.

For example, one large meta-analysis examined the relationship between total protein, animal protein, and plant protein and the risk of all-cause death, heart disease, and cancer.[12] It found that a higher intake of total protein was associated with an overall lower risk of death. However, a high-plant-protein diet was associated with a lower risk of all-cause death and death from cardiovascular disease. In fact, for every 3 percent increase in calories from plant proteins in a day, there was an associated 5 percent lower risk of death from all causes. Translation? All protein is protective, but loading up on plant-based options offers a few additional perks.

Other research has come to similar conclusions. For example, one 2020 prospective study looked at data from four hundred thousand men and women and found that swapping in just 3 percent of their daily calories to plant-based protein from animal protein slashed their overall mortality risk by 10 percent and reduced the risk of death from cardiovascular disease by 11 to 12 percent.[13]

So, does that mean that the occasional burger or barbecued steak is now on the no-no list? Absolutely not. We don't *do* off-limits over here! If you or your family are meat eaters, forcing yourself to go full vegan in the name of "health" is likely only going to backfire. As a dietitian and an omnivore myself, who enjoys an occasional cheeseburger (with extra pickles, ketchup, and mustard on top), I believe in meeting people where they are. And encouraging folks to work in one or two meat-less meals a week is an amazing start!

## Health Benefits of Fiber-Rich Foods

As we briefly discussed in Chapter 2, the very basic recommendation for fiber is to aim for at least 25 grams daily for women, and 38 grams for men. While this is the standard minimum recommendation (and honestly, this is a C+ to B–, max), these numbers are good goalposts to help reduce the risk of chronic disease, especially since 95 percent of American adults are currently flunking in fiber 101 and consuming nowhere close to these recommended amounts.[14] We've already covered fiber's role in helping promote regular complete bowel movements, keeping us fuller longer, and reducing blood sugars, but it also offers a wide range of remarkable disease-fighting perks.

**Reduces the Risk of Chronic Disease.** Soluble fiber acts like a sponge to soak up cholesterol-derived bile acids, which forces the liver to pull cholesterol out of the blood to replace the bile acids that were lost. This sneaky Houdini move effectively reduces our "bad" LDL cholesterol and improves our heart health markers. Research suggests that for each 5 to 10 grams of soluble fiber you consume, you can expect a 5- to 11-point reduction in total cholesterol and LDL cholesterol.[15] That's the amount of soluble fiber in just a cup of black beans! We got this! Other great sources of soluble fiber include oats and oat bran, barley, apples, pears, carrots, Brussels sprouts, psyllium, and other legumes.

**Insoluble** fiber doesn't dissolve in water, acting a bit like a massive wrecking ball (*cue our girl, Miley Cyrus*) that forces everything in its path to move. This doesn't just make for a good bowel movement, but it also helps reduce the amount of time that potentially harmful substances are in contact with your intestinal lining, helping prevent such digestive disorders as diverticular disease and possibly even colon cancer. Research suggests that for every 10 grams of daily total fiber, your risk of colon cancer decreases by 10 percent.[16] Some of the best sources of the insoluble variety, specifically, are hiding right under your nose, so load up on whole grains, nuts, seeds, wheat bran, and such veggies as carrots, celery, and tomatoes.

Another way that fiber can reduce cancer and digestive disorders is through the release of short-chain fatty acids during digestion (the *post*biotics of fiber fermentation). If you remember from Chapter 2, we talked briefly about the benefits of short-chain fatty acids (SCFAs) like butyrate. And while there are some food sources of these unique fats (namely, dairy fat: e.g., butter, ghee, and cheese), our body almost exclusively derives these from our microbes breaking down dietary fiber.

Butyrate is a preferred energy source for the cells lining your colon (called colonocytes) that help maintain the integrity of your gut barrier. Emerging research on colon cancer suggests that butyrate specifically may help inhibit the growth of cancer cells, kill existing cancer cells, and promote healthy cell turnover in the colon.[17] (And remember, we get this stuff for *free* every time we whip up something delicious like avocado toast on whole-grain bread!)

## Too Much of a Good Thing?

Fiber is a fickle thing: Too little can back you up, but also, too much can back you up (or at the very least, it can create some major GI warfare if you hit it hard out the gate). If you're experiencing bloating, gas, abdominal cramping, or other GI symptoms when you increase your fiber intake, try making these simple adjustments:

- Up your fluids. Remember to drink an extra 2 to 3 ounces for every gram of fiber you add.
- Aim for a balance of fibers. While insoluble fiber helps add bulk to stool, this can make constipation worse if it's not balanced with soluble fiber and enough fluids.
- Slow down, Sally! If you're new to a plant-rich life, start with a small portion of fiber-rich foods (e.g., a single serving of produce or grains) and allow your gut to adjust before adding more.

**Microbial Diversity.** Fiber is our gut microbiome's BFF. Simply put, fiber (the *prebiotic*) is our microbes' (*probiotics*) fuel of choice. But just as one of your kids prefers rice and the other wants pasta, different types of bacteria feed on different types of fiber.[18] For example, *Bifidobacterium* species (which support our immune system and improve regularity) prefer the inulin fiber in onions, garlic, and sunchokes, whereas *Lactobacillus* (great for preventing urinary tract infections, a.k.a. UTIs; yeast infections; and eczema in infants) has a penchant for the oligosaccharides in legumes.

You don't need to memorize the tongue-twister names or functions of all these microbes (unless you want to bust out some *very* specific facts at your next staff lunch). But by simply consuming a variety of fiber-rich foods, you promote a more diverse and vibrant microbiome, which positively affects every other aspect of physical and mental health. Bad mood? Blame it on the microbes. Breaking out before a big event? Those damn bacteria. Picked up your hundredth daycare sickness?? The good bugs are sleeping on the job again! No, but seriously, a healthy gut microbiome plays a role in the health of virtually every other bodily process.

### Fiber-Food Matrix Magic

As we've established, fiber is only found in plants: fruits, vegetables, whole grains, nuts, seeds, and legumes. So, if you think you fall within the 95 percent of Westerners who are not eating enough fiber, it's a pretty safe bet that you could use some more green things in your life (in addition to cash, obviously, which could surely come in handy for most of us in an economy like this). The cool thing about plant foods is that they're the best damn packaged deal you'll ever get, with loads of disease-fighting vitamins, minerals, and antioxidants in every bite. And when you look at data on a diet rich in plant-foods, particularly fruits and vegetables, you can quickly understand that the benefits of these foods are more than the sum of their parts.

Despite what the fringe carnivore dieters might try to make you believe, the benefits of a diet rich in fruits and vegetables make it a truly open-and-shut case. The evidence is basically indisputable that adding more fruits and vegetables helps reduce the risk of heart disease, certain cancers, obesity, and all-cause mortality.[19] Research like this is largely responsible for the nearly worldwide nutrition guideline consensus to aim for five to ten servings of fruits and vegetables per day.

## How to Get Your Five-a-Day

We hear it all the time: "Aim for at least five servings of fruits and vegetables per day." But what the heck is a "serving" anyway? In the context of the Dietary Guidelines for Americans, a serving size isn't a suggestion of how much we "should" eat in one sitting; it simply allows us to visualize how many pieces of any given food we should aim to consume, to meet the average adult's nutrition needs.

### 1 serving of fruit:
- 1 cup of fresh, frozen, or canned
- ½ cup of dried fruit
- 1 whole fruit the size of your fist
- 1 small banana

### 1 serving of vegetables:
- 1 cup of fresh, frozen, or canned vegetables
- 1 large whole vegetable (e.g., bell pepper, tomato)
- 2 cups (two large fistfuls) of raw leafy vegetables

If five servings seems like a big number, let's put it into practice with an example meal plan.

**Breakfast:** Latte with protein smoothie made with **1 banana, ¼ cup cherries**, protein powder, and peanut butter.

**Snack:** Greek yogurt with ¼ cup blueberries

**Lunch:** Grilled chicken salad with 2 cups spinach, ½ cup tomatoes, ½ cup bell peppers, quinoa, feta cheese, pistachios, and vinaigrette

**Dinner:** Tofu stir-fry with 1 cup bok choy, ½ cup carrots, rice, and cashews

Still a bit overwhelmed? Baby steps are key. Finding little ways to add a little color to your day can yield huge rewards. And we're going to have loads more examples to help you do just that in Part 3.

## Key Nutrients in Fiber-Rich Foods

So, what is it exactly about plant-based foods that keep the old engine running? In addition to being rich in fiber and water, they're packed with essential disease-fighting chemicals. Most notably, antioxidants. Antioxidants are compounds that help protect the health of your cells by "neutralizing" the erratic disease-promoting compounds called free radicals.[20] Imagine antioxidants as little handcuffs that keep the free radicals from doing harm. And fiber-rich foods are full of them!

| Antioxidant | What it does | Key sources |
|---|---|---|
| Vitamin C (ascorbic acid) | Stimulates immune cells (e.g., leukocytes) to fight infection, improves the absorption of non-heme iron, and supports the synthesis of collagen (a vital protein in skin, bones, tendons, ligaments, and blood vessels). | Citrus fruit, guava, papaya, strawberries, kiwi, red bell peppers, broccoli, Brussels sprouts, and kale. |

| | | |
|---|---|---|
| Vitamin E (tocopherols and tocotrienols) | Protects skin from harmful UV rays while promoting skin healing, reduces the risk of heart disease by preventing the oxidation of LDL cholesterol, reduces the risk of age-related macular degeneration and cataracts, and may help protect against such neurological conditions as Alzheimer's.[21] | Sunflower seeds, almonds, nut butter, wheat germ oil, avocados, and dark leafy greens. |
| Vitamin K phylloquinone (K1) & menaquinone (K2) | Vitamin $K_1$ promotes essential blood clotting, so you don't die of blood loss every time you nick yourself shaving. Vitamin $K_2$ supports bone and heart health by improving bone mineral density, and preventing atherosclerosis. | $K_1$ is found in cooked dark green vegetables: e.g., Swiss chard, spinach, and collard greens. $K_2$ is found in aged cheeses, natto, egg yolks, liver, and dark meat poultry. |
| Carotenoids (beta-carotene, lutein, zeaxanthin, lycopene) | Reduces the risk of heart disease, cognitive decline, and certain cancers (e.g., lung, breast, and skin).[22] Lutein and zeaxanthin specifically help prevent macular degeneration and cataracts.[23] Beta-carotene supports immunity (as a precursor to vitamin A) and protects against sunburns and UV damage.[24] And lycopene reduces the oxidation of "bad" LDL cholesterol and protects against prostate cancer. | Beta-carotene is in carrots, sweet potatoes, and dark leafy greens. Lutein is in kale, spinach, and broccoli. Zeaxanthin is in corn, oranges, red bell peppers, and cooked kale. Lycopene is in tomatoes, watermelon, and grapefruit. |

| Polyphenols (flavonoids, phenolic acids, stilbenes, lignans) | A large diverse group of plant-based compounds shown to protect against signs of premature aging, heart disease, cancers, and such neurodegenerative disorders as Alzheimer's and Parkinson's disease. Some polyphenols (e.g., flavonoids, catechins, isoflavones, and flavanols) may also improve insulin sensitivity and metabolic health.[25] | Flavonoids: Berries, green vegetables, soy, cocoa, tea, and wine.<br>    Phenolic acids: Berries, apples, nuts, and tea.<br>    Stilbenes: Red grapes, berries, wine, and peanuts.<br>    Lignans: Flax, whole grains, legumes, and sesame. |
| --- | --- | --- |
| Glutathione | Supports detoxification to eliminate harmful substances and heavy metals, enhances the activity of immune-supporting natural killer cells and lymphocytes, and supports healthy brain aging. | Avocados, asparagus, dark leafy greens, garlic, onions, and cruciferous vegetables. |

## Other Fiber Food Perks + Additional Nutrients

| Nutrient | What it does | Key sources |
| --- | --- | --- |
| Potassium | Key electrolyte responsible for normal fluid regulation, muscle contractions (including those of our heart), and communication between your nerves. Works to counterbalance sodium intake to reduce the risk of heart disease.[26] | Potatoes, squash, spinach, avocados, legumes, tomatoes, and bananas. |
| Water | Consuming adequate fruits and vegetables offers around 25% of your total daily fluid needs.[27] | Cucumbers, leafy greens, tomatoes, strawberries, celery, and citrus. |

In addition to some of their unique selling features, many fiber-rich plant-foods also contain a lot of the nutrients we covered in previous chapters, such as

- Magnesium (avocados, spinach, Swiss chard, and quinoa)
- Iron (dried apricots, legumes, beet greens, and spinach)
- Calcium (collard greens, broccoli, kale, and dried figs)
- Iodine (seaweed, cranberries, and leafy greens)
- Zinc (legumes, oats, green peas, asparagus, and fortified whole grains)
- Phosphorus (oats, potatoes, avocado, and lentils)
- Selenium (brown rice, barley, and oats)
- B vitamins (leafy greens, fortified whole grains, broccoli, bananas, and mushrooms)

Listen, you don't need another dietitian to tell you to eat more fruits and vegetables. You probably had a mother who's done plenty of that. But if you take anything away from this section, let it be an appreciation of the remarkable bundle offer you get when you *add* more fiber-rich foods to your diet. It's more than just a good poop, or better appetite management during the three p.m. slump. It's the all-inclusive package deal of antioxidants, hydration, and gut-friendly prebiotics that unequivocally supports our health. Focus on fiber. Every system in your body will thank you.

## Fat-Rich Foods Are Good for You

Dietary fat has ridden quite the roller coaster over the years: One day, we're told to load up on sugary rainbow sorbet and Twizzlers because they're fat-free; the next, we're watching influencers mow down on a brick of butter.

Not surprisingly, the secret to good health lies somewhere in the middle. Fat is an essential nutrient for good health, but as I established in Chapter 1, not all fats get classified as healthy fats in my Hunger Crushing Combo framework. That doesn't mean that fat sources without an HCC badge should be cut out or eliminated. It simply means that we want to put emphasis on the fats we know offer a nutritional edge. Let's go over our VIPs.

### Omega-3 Fatty Acids

Omega-3s are the Bruce Banner of the healthy fat team. It's the fat that has the greatest power and strongest potential to make the most significant changes in the body, which range from lowering blood pressure, to reducing joint stiffness, to improving mental health.

As briefly introduced in Chapter 1, omega-3s are a type of polyunsaturated fatty acid (PUFA) that helps support heart health, brain function, and inflammation reduction in the body.[28] They're considered *essential* fats because our body isn't able to manufacture omega-3s on our own, so we must get them through the foods (or supplements) we consume. This is why every healthy lifestyle magazine you have probably ever picked up features some kind of omega-3–rich salmon recipe on the front. We all should probably be making an effort to eat more. But there are actually three main types of omega-3 fatty acids to consider:

- **Alpha-linolenic acid (ALA)** is a short-chain omega-3 fatty acid predominantly found in such plant-based foods as flaxseeds, chia seeds, hemp seeds, walnuts, and soybeans. ALA is a precursor to the two long-chain omega-3s (EPA and DHA) we'll discuss next, meaning that your body can convert some ALA into these two. Unfortunately, the conversion rate is kinda meh (just 3 to 6 percent).[29] Still, that doesn't make ALA omega-3s total deadbeats! You can boost their conversion and bioavailability by reducing sources of omega-6s in your diet (from such foods as vegetable oils) that compete with conversion enzymes; increase foods rich in enzyme cofactors like zinc, magnesium, and vitamin E; and choose whole-food sources of ALA (e.g., flaxseeds) over oils (which are more prone to oxidation).

- **Eicosapentaenoic acid (EPA)** is one of the long-chain omega-3 fatty acids and is primarily found in fatty fish like herring, mackerel, salmon, tuna, sardines, and trout. EPA is a critical player in reducing chronic disease, largely through its conversion to molecules called eicosanoids, which have powerful anti-inflammatory effects. As a result, research has found that EPA can help lower triglyceride levels for better heart health, reduce the risk of dangerous blood clots, promote better brain function, and improve mental health.[30]

   While our most impressive research has been done using supplemental omega-3s (which are easier to control than whole foods), it is always ideal to get most of our nutrients from food. A 3-ounce serving of farmed salmon, for example, has 600 mg of EPA, 1,240 mg of DHA, and a combined omega-3 content of 1,830 mg; that is more than three times the daily recommended minimum of 500 mg in a very small protein package![31]

- **Docosahexaenoic acid (DHA)** is another long-chain omega-3 fatty acid found in fatty fish and seafood. DHA makes up about 8 percent of our brain's total weight, which is why it is extremely important for normal brain growth and cognitive function. Research has linked DHA supplementation during pregnancy and lactation to improved cellular immune health in infancy, and DHA intake in early life is associated with improved eyesight, higher IQ, better social skills, fewer behavioral problems, and reduced risk of developmental delay.[32]

DHA is also highly concentrated in our retinas, which explains why research has found that eating fatty fish just once per week could reduce the risk of macular degeneration by 50 percent![33] In addition to serving our brain and eyes, DHA helps reduce inflammation in our body and supports our cardiovascular wellness by lowering triglyceride levels, helping boost HDL cholesterol, and preventing atherosclerosis.[34] Atlantic herring is one of the best dietary sources of DHA, with an impressive 940 mg DHA (and 1,700 mg total omega-3) per 3-ounce serving.[35]

## Microalgae: Omega-3s for Vegans and Vegetarians

Seeing as DHA and EPA are only found in fish, and our plant-based version, ALA, offers a far less potent health punch, the question becomes, What if you don't eat seafood?

Such fish as salmon and sardines aren't inherently omega-3 factories. They, too, need to get their nutrients from the food *they* eat. And fish get *their* EPA and DHA largely from eating microalgae. And great news! There are now lots of algae-derived omega-3 supplements that have been shown to increase EPA and DHA levels comparably to fish oils.[36] Currently, there is no established RDA for DHA and EPA, only for ALA, but the Global Organization of EPA and DHA Omega-3s (GOED) recommends 500 mg per day for healthy adults, to help lower the risk of heart disease (but no more than 3,000 mg per day from supplements.[37]) The ideal ratio of EPA to DHA will largely depend on your goals and existing health conditions, so always work with a registered dietitian to determine the best option for you.

## Omega-6 Fats

As we discussed in Chapter 1, omega-6s have had a bit of a tough go lately, largely thanks to a whole lot of "seed oil" slander on social media. But despite their current PR crisis, omega-6 fats are essential for good health, and we can obtain them *only* from our diet. The main source of omega-6 in our diet is linoleic acid, which is found most abundantly in vegetable and seed oils (largely from highly processed food). If you recall, omega-3 fats offer anti-inflammatory benefits through their conversion to molecules called eicosanoids. Eicosanoids are like tiny chemical messengers that play various roles in the body, including helping regulate inflammation, blood pressure, and our immune system. And like omega-3s, omega-6s like linoleic acid can also be converted to eicosanoids. Sounds great, right?

Well, here's where the 3 and 6 lines get crossed. The eicosanoids that omega-3s produce are anti-inflammatory, whereas the ones produced by omega-6s can be more pro-inflammatory (which we also need as our first line of immune defense). A lot of "seed oil demonizers" point to this *mechanistic theory* that, when we have an imbalance of pro-inflammatory molecules (omega-6) and anti-inflammatory molecules (omega-3), we disrupt healthy physiological homeostasis. And while it's often been suggested that the optimal omega-6 to omega-3 ratio is around 4:1, on average, Americans are consuming closer to 20:1. In other words, we may be tipping the unsaturated fats scale in favor of more pro-inflammatory processes. And, yes, this all does make sense when we zone in on the biochemical pathways.

BUT (and she's a big but), this theory doesn't seem to hold up to testing in the real world. The consensus of human research shows that varying the amount of omega-6 in the diet doesn't actually have much impact on pro-inflammatory eicosanoids in the body.[38] And varying omega-6 levels in the body doesn't actually seem to increase inflammation.[39] In fact, a huge meta-analysis and systematic review on over three hundred thousand people found an association between omega-6 intake and *improved* health.[40] There are very few things in nutrition research that have been as profoundly and robustly debunked as the seed oil slander game.[41] So, omega-6 in isolation isn't the problem, and *just* reducing it won't necessarily be the fix. But increasing our intake of omega-3 may be. This is why, again, we add, not subtract.

However, it is important to consider the foods where omega-6 fats are typically found. In the standard American diet, most of our omega-6 fats are coming from fried foods and highly processed snack foods, most of which are generally low in Hunger Crushing Compounds and overall nutrition. So, obsessing over the omega-6 content in your deep-fried chicken tenders is really missing the forest for the trees. Alternatively, avoiding a bountiful salad just because the vinaigrette is made with sunflower oil is a bit like not buying a mutual fund that has one low-hanging stock when the overall portfolio is way up. It's just not a good life hack. What constitutes a "healthy" choice is always going to come down to context and the big picture. So, continue to enjoy vegetable oils to enhance naturally nourishing foods and other Hunger Crushing Compounds, such as on roasted vegetables, colorful salads, and marinated seafood and poultry. And then focus on adding more whole-food sources of omega-6 fats that offer dual-citizenship status with fiber, protein, and/or other healthy fatty acids. Walnuts, Brazil nuts, almonds, and seeds are some of our favorite sources.

**Monounsaturated Fats**

We've covered the PUFAs (omega-3s and omega-6s); now, let's talk about the omega-9 monounsaturated fats (MUFAs). Ninety percent of all MUFAs exist as oleic acid, which not only can be made by the body, but is most famously found in olive oil. Like omega-3 fats, MUFAs are amazing for your heart. In fact, research suggests that extra-virgin olive oil is one of the leading drivers in a reduction in cardiovascular disease risk associated with the Mediterranean diet, likely through its role in lowering "bad" LDL, blood pressure, and such inflammatory markers as CRP.[42]

Monounsaturated fats may also help support a healthy weight. One study measured changes in body fat, cholesterol, blood pressure, energy burned, and insulin concentrations, and after four weeks of replacing saturated fats with monounsaturated fats, it found that the participants had reduced their fat mass and total body weight with an average weight loss of about 4 pounds![43] The mechanism isn't fully understood, but it appears that MUFAs can boost feelings of fullness after eating, improve insulin sensitivity (which can curb appetite), promote fat burning, and may even be associated with a lower risk of abdominal fat accumulation (a risk factor for heart disease).[44]

Finally, MUFAs are fabulous fuel for our brain. The general trend we're seeing in the research suggests that diets high in saturated and trans fats, and low in MUFAs and PUFAs, are more likely to create an environment for dementia to develop.[45] Does this all mean we should be drinking olive oil by the gallon, for our health? Please don't do that. Since fluid oils lack dual citizenship with other Hunger Crushing Compounds, they're low volume, calorie dense, and just don't offer a great satiety ROI. This is why I recommend using added oils with purpose as part of this framework: enough to improve cooking, flavor, and texture (plus add some nutritional perks), without unexpectedly adding hundreds of (less satiating) calories per meal. So, enjoy your favorite PUFA and MUFA cooking oils in moderation, and load up most often on the whole-food sources of healthy fats like nuts and nut butters, seeds, avocados, olives, and fatty fish.

### Nutrients in Fat-Packed Foods

One of the key reasons the Hunger Crushing Combo defines "healthy fats" as those that come predominantly from whole-food unsaturated sources is all the extra nutrient benefits you get packed into fat-rich foods that go beyond their fatty acid components. Here are a few of those perks.

| Nutrient | What it does | Key sources |
| --- | --- | --- |
| Selenium | A trace mineral and antioxidant that helps regulate thyroid function, support immunity, and reduce the risk of some cancers. | Brazil nuts, sunflower seeds, organ meats, and seafood. |
| Magnesium | A key electrolyte involved in normal muscle and nerve function, blood pressure, and bone health. It's also been shown to help lower risk of heart disease, anxiety, insomnia, and depression, and can help prevent constipation. | Nuts and seeds, fish, avocados, dairy, and dark chocolate. |

Many fat-containing foods also provide other healthy nutrients that we've already covered, which help round out their benefits:

- Folate (avocados, peanuts, sunflower seeds, and eggs)
- Zinc (shellfish, pumpkin seeds, cashews, almonds, and Cheddar cheese)
- Calcium (Greek yogurt, Cheddar cheese, sesame seeds, canned sardines, and salmon)
- Iron (meat, fatty fish, dark meat poultry, almonds, and cashews)
- Copper (organ meats and avocados)
- Antioxidants (walnuts, flaxseeds, fatty fish, and avocado)

**Fat-Soluble Vitamins**

Fat-soluble vitamins A, D, E, and K (see pages 97–98 and page 105 for a full rundown of their functions) need dietary fats to be properly absorbed, utilized, and stored in your body. While you can always pair your vitamin A, D, E, and K with a source of fat to boost absorption (a drizzle of olive oil on your sweet potatoes will do the trick), a lot of fat-rich foods already offer a packaged deal:

Beef liver, fatty fish, butter, cheese, and eggs: vitamin A

Fatty fish, eggs, fortified full-fat dairy: vitamin D

Nuts and seeds: vitamin E

Aged cheeses, natto, egg yolks, liver, and dark meat poultry: vitamin K

When we focus on foods that naturally combine fiber, protein, and healthy fats, we're not just checking off boxes for individual nutrients. We're getting the benefit of the whole-food matrix, where nutrient synergy helps fuel, nourish, and satisfy. By embracing these foods as part of your everyday meals, healthy eating becomes less about micromanaging nutrients and more about effortlessly and intuitively enjoying the simplicity of whole, balanced choices. Start thinking about some new hobbies. You're about to free up a *ton* of mental space.

# CHAPTER 5

. . . . . . . . . . . . . . . . .

# Healing Your Relationship
# with Food

So, you now have the nutritional *what* of the HCC method, you know the science-based *why* of the combos, and are starting to get a hang of the *how*. But there's one more thing I want to address head-on before we dive deeper into the particulars. For so many of us who have lived and breathed diet culture since childhood, it might seem hopelessly implausible that we'll ever escape. The erratic nonsensical diet rules and food fears, the constant weight cycling, and the body image and self-esteem struggles feel so familiar, it's hard to imagine a life where they're all left behind. But repeat after me: Your diet and your body are the least interesting things about you. And rejecting diet culture and healing your relationship with food may be the first step in rediscovering what lights you up.

## Antidiet Culture

In response to the mounting evidence of the damage of diet culture and wellness culture, we've seen a strong counterculture emerge. One that explicitly rejects the diet mentality, advocates for weight inclusivity, and focuses on achieving food freedom. While there are many important movements that one could argue fit under the "antidiet culture" umbrella, a few of the notable ones include body positivity, health at every size (HAES), and intuitive eating. Understanding a bit of their backstory is imperative to understanding why a gentle additive approach like my Hunger Crushing Combo is so important for long-term happiness and health.

### Body Positivity & Neutrality

The body positivity movement was designed to challenge traditional beauty standards while advocating for the acceptance of all bodies, regardless of their size, shape, color, gender, and physical abilities. Rooted in fat liberation, body positivity aims to affirm that all bodies are worthy of dignity and respect, to challenge discrimination and fatphobia, and to advocate for more inclusive body representation in fashion, media, and society at large. But body positivity has faced increasing criticism in recent years for becoming overly commercialized, exclusionary, and, at times, performative, leaving many people feeling duped (especially those in larger bodies or with visible differences whom the movement was designed to support). In response to this pushback, a gentler but growing movement toward body neutrality has emerged. Body neutrality suggests that you can respect and care for your body, even if you're not vibing with it every day. So, to many, it offers a more sustainable and realistic mindset that emphasizes respect, functionality, and detachment from appearance-based self-worth.

### Health at Every Size

In the 1990s, the term "health at every size" (HAES) was adopted by health-care providers, researchers, and fat-acceptance activists looking to shift the definition of health away from a sole focus on body size and weight. In 2008, Dr. Lindo Bacon, a researcher and author, formalized the now popular HAES principles through his groundbreaking best-selling book *Health at Every Size: The Surprising Truth About Your Weight*. The HAES movement was designed to challenge standard health metrics that depend primarily on weight and BMI, while focusing on health behaviors over weight loss, challenging societal weight stigma, and advocating for more inclusive, respectful care. But HAES is also not without its criticism. Many argue that it's often misinterpreted as "You can be healthy at any and every size," downplaying the risks of obesity and potentially discouraging behavior change in populations at risk. Critics also argue that it invalidates the real health and social struggles of living in a larger body, doesn't address their systemic inequalities or unique barriers to nonstigmatizing care, and paints a desire for weight loss as a moral failure. Finally, many folks in marginalized bodies (e.g., people of color, disabled, trans, or "superfat") point out that mainstream HAES messages still seem to come from predominantly smaller or midsize, white, able-bodied persons, which seems counter to its original intentions.

## Intuitive Eating & Food Freedom

One of the most powerful attributes of my Hunger Crushing Combo is its role in supporting food freedom and relearning how to eat more intuitively. The official "intuitive eating" framework is considered an antidiet mind-body philosophy that encourages individuals to tune into their body's cues rather than adhere to external diet rules that reject body wisdom.[1] Developed by fellow dietitians Evelyn Tribole and Elyse Resch in the 1990s, intuitive eating is based on ten core principles, including rejecting the diet mentality, honoring hunger and fullness, respecting our body regardless of its size, and incorporating joyful movement and gentle nutrition strategies into our day.[2] This is where my Hunger Crushing Combo can be utilized, since at its core it is an additive framework for gentle nutrition.

Intuitive eating is also an evidence-based framework, with over 125 studies to support its use in practice. One 2021 meta-analysis summarized a number of its important health benefits suggesting that intuitive eaters were significantly *less likely* to[3]

- Restrict their intake by following rigid rules
- Eat emotionally or in response to external, rather than internal, cues
- Engage in disordered eating, binge eating, and purging
- Become preoccupied with the size or shape of their body or concern themselves with society's "ideal" body
- Report experiencing mental health challenges like anxiety or depression

In contrast, intuitive eaters were significantly *more likely* to

- Appreciate all of the amazing things their body does
- Have a strong sense of self-esteem
- Exercise flexibility in their body image while experiencing body acceptance from others
- Have a strong social support system
- Have a greater sense of well-being

Despite the data in support of intuitive eating, it, too, is not without criticism and pushback. Intuitive eating assumes a high level of body awareness and privilege that not everyone has clear access to, especially when it comes to folks navigating chronic illness, neurodivergence, food insecurity, or a history of trauma or disordered eating. It's also been criticized as being rooted in Western, white, individualistic values, which doesn't leave room for cultural practices like spiritual fasting, meal rituals, or communal eating. All of these are absolutely valid criticisms, and I am very much aware of my own privilege in benefiting from the intuitive eating model in my own life.

The other issue is that as intuitive eating has become commodified, watered down, and co-opted by wellness and diet culture, its tenets are often misrepresented or distorted.

For one, intuitive eating is not just the "eat when you're hungry, stop when you're full" diet. No different than with my Hunger Crushing Combo, there are no hard-and-fast rules. So, while we want to offer tools to teach interoception (like the Hunger–Fullness Scale that we'll unpack shortly), it doesn't mean you're "doing intuitive eating wrong" if you don't always listen to them. Remember, it's normal to eat past the point of fullness because your aunt makes the best pumpkin pie (and you've already had two servings of stuffing and mashed potatoes). It's also normal to sometimes let yourself get so busy that you skip lunch. Don't turn intuitive eating into another big dirty D!

Intuitive eating is also *not* a weight-loss diet. If any "food freedom coach" on Instagram is trying to sell you an "intuitive eating 30-day weight-loss challenge," they are absolutely co-opting the movement to sell you antidiet culture *and* diet culture at the same time! As we've already well established, what your weight decides to do when you change your diet (or start exercising more often) is ultimately not directly within your control. When you're honoring your hunger and satiety cues (as I teach you to do with my Hunger Crushing Combo), your weight might stay the same, you might gain weight (especially if you've been severely restricting yourself), or you might lose weight (particularly if you've been chronically dieting and rebounding for years). This likely explains why weight loss is a common "side effect" of intuitive eating in studies on folks who are classified as overweight or obese.[4] When you stop with the overt restriction, break out of the scarcity mindset, and quit obsessing over food, you're just better equipped to hear and respond to your body's true needs.

Part of this process is learning to exercise self-compassion and body respect, and rejecting the status quo assumption that your weight is a reflection of your worth. This is particularly important for those of us who have struggled with our relationship with food and body. If you just jump into thinking about adding protein to your meals, but you're still trapped in the diet culture mentality of "all carbs are bad," you're likely to turn the Hunger Crushing Combo into another hard-line obsession. Suddenly, a gentle recommendation like "Make a fully stacked sandwich with your white bread" will quickly become "If I don't have four layers of vegetables in that sandwich, I'm not allowed to eat it." Remember, I want you to eat the Naked Carbs. I even want you to be able to eat the Naked Carbs *alone*, if that's what brings you joy. When we shed our rule-binding skin, we're able to collect data on how all of the different foods make us feel, listen to our body's true needs, and, ultimately, eat in a way that serves us: mind, body, and soul.

## HCC: A Framework That Works for You

Intuitive eating (IE) is a framework distinct from my Hunger Crushing Combo, with some unique intersections and synergies. Most notably, these are both *additive* approaches to eating that encourage you to reject external indicators of when and what to eat, and instead to focus on foods that satisfy and satiate *your* body.

Both IE and the HCC are also both *not inherently* weight-loss diets. *Wait, what?! Haven't you spent a bunch of chapters talking about the different Hunger Crushing Compounds and their role in maintaining a healthy weight, and there's a whole upcoming chapter on using the HCC if you're hoping to reduce your weight?* This is where the nuance of nutrition comes into play. Ultimately, the HCC framework can be adapted to suit everyone's health desires, whether they want to lose weight, gain weight, manage their blood sugar, run faster, or just stop obsessing over food. In its core definition, it's simply a gentle guideline for building balance into our day and increasing the chances of better health. And as much as I subscribe to the antidiet culture, as a dietitian I am also patient- and client-centered. I believe in body autonomy and I am all about meeting people where they are. For some people, they're just going to want to lose weight, and whether that is for health or aesthetic reasons, there is nothing wrong with that! We don't judge or shame anyone's desires or goals over here. But how we approach that goal helps determine how sustainable that weight loss is, and I would much rather people navigate their weight-loss journey from a place of abundance rather than scarcity. The HCC can therefore be tweaked to respectfully guide you toward a pattern of eating that is consistent with the research on best practices, without the restrictive mindset. In the next section, we're going to go through all of these little adjustments, but regardless of what health "side effects" you're hoping come of the HCC, the core outcome is the same: You're learning to make choices from a place of self-care that *feels* good.

For some people, the HCC may offer an amazing tool for bringing all ten intuitive eating principles together, whereas other people (especially those who are still desiring weight loss) may only be able to relate to a few. This is why I prefer to use the more generalized term "food freedom" to describe one of the key benefits of the HCC, because a life *without* strict food rules is inherently freeing.

## The HCC and the Hunger–Fullness Scale

Traditional diets essentially teach us to ignore our body's hunger cues in favor of following whatever codex of random rules they prescribe. After years of overriding this innate wisdom, our body basically gives up talking to us and we stop getting the message. Are you "full" or has your body just succumbed to the abuse?

A framework like HCC helps give us ample opportunities to intuitively experience how hunger and fullness feel. And I mean literally *feel* them, not just understand the concept. Hunger and fullness have their own ebbs and flows that are greatly affected by what's on our plate. Think about how you feel after you eat a big bowl of plain salad greens vs. a big bowl of salad greens with some diced chicken, black beans, and walnuts on it. Or when you start your day with a bowl of plain oatmeal made with water vs. a bowl of oatmeal made with soy milk and topped with chia seeds, raspberries, and a dollop of peanut butter. These simple combos are critical when the goal is fueling our bodies with the nutrition we need to thrive while working *with* our hunger and satiety. Noticing these differences is a key aspect of being able to nourish your body with confidence.

If you're saying to yourself, *"But, Abbey, I'm so far removed from my body's hunger–fullness cues that I don't even know where to start!"* well, I have some good news. Putting aside certain medical conditions that require more mechanical feeding, most of us can train our brain to engage in this interoceptive feedback! Think of it like rewiring a house. The basic bones are all there (perhaps they've been buried in dust bunnies or been incorrectly wired by some shady home DIY guy). You just need to reconfigure a few things to get the whole place lighting up again.

One of the best tools to employ alongside our HCC is the Hunger–Fullness Scale, which helps you tap into and understand your body's natural hunger and satiety signals with the goal of mindful eating. The scale is typically from 1 to 10, where 1 is extreme hunger (you could eat a horse) and 10 is feeling uncomfortably full. Ideally, you aim to start eating when you are at a 3 or 4, before you get overly hungry or cranky. You then aim to stop eating at 6 or 7, where you are comfortably full but not stuffed.

Here's how to successfully use this scale to help you reconnect with some of your body's natural hunger and satiety cues:

- **Take a Pause.** Before eating, take a moment to assess where you fall on the Hunger–Fullness Scale. This can help you decide whether you're eating from true physical hunger or for other reasons, like boredom, sadness, or stress.
- **Reduce Distractions.** If you've ever sat down with a big bag of chips to binge-watch a whole season of *The Bachelor* in one go, you've probably only broken eye contact when you're fumbling with crumbs at the bottom of the bag. A lot of us are just not great at multitasking, so power down and make eating mindfully your mealtime priority.
- **Slow Down.** We're all busy people, so I get that sometimes luxuriating at an hour-long dinner is just not in the cards. Especially if you have kids who can barely sit down for five minutes at a time. That said, racing through a meal can not only wreak havoc on digestion, but it also doesn't give your brain enough time to register that you're full. So, slow down by chewing your food thoroughly, taking sips of water between bites, and breaking up your eating with dinnertime conversation.
- **Do a Midmeal Check-in.** Halfway through your meal, ask yourself where you now fall on the Hunger–Fullness Scale. Still have a solid appetite? Continue on until you reach that comfortably full, but not too stuffed, threshold.
- **Consider Journaling.** While I don't encourage you to obsessively track calories or macros (which can be a very slippery slope for a lot of people), tracking how you feel on the Hunger–Fullness Scale before and after meals can help you start to learn new eating patterns. How hungry were you before you started eating? What did you end up eating? Where did you rank in fullness at the end of your meal?

Now, no different than with intuitive eating, the Hunger–Fullness Scale should *not* be another hard-and-fast rule you need to break.

Sometimes, you're going to end up on the fringes of the scale and that is A-OK: You haven't failed; you're just living a normal vibrant life (where the ice cream was just too tasty to put down!). The Hunger–Fullness Scale is one of many tools in the toolboxes that we can use to collect data on how different hunger crushing combinations make you feel, to help you make future mealtime decisions. No guilt, no judgment, no moral weight. Just data to inform another delicious day.

### HCC and Diet Traps

If you recall from Chapter 2, we discussed all the common diet traps that so many of us have fallen into after years of yo-yo dieting and food rules. And the HCC can act as an antidote to every single one.

- **The Binge-Restrict Cycle.** One of the important benefits of using my Hunger Crushing Combo is to help you nip the binge-restrict-repent-repeat cycle in the bud. With an additive approach to nutrition, your favorite foods, like bread or crackers or chips or whatever, are not off-limits. You love white bread? The sky's the limit on how to enjoy white bread! Turn it into a satiating sandwich with turkey, arugula, and pesto. Make an open-faced avocado toast with a poached egg. Crisp it up into croutons for a big-ass salad. Or *gasp*, just eat it as is. When foods aren't inherently "bad" or "off-limits," they lose their power. They lose their irresistible allure. They become just another food.
- **Comfort or Emotional Eating.** Despite the fact that the conversation around comfort eating and comfort foods is almost always related to "junk," literally *any* food can be comforting. In Hungary, a hearty nutritious chicken paprikash is a commonly cited comfort food. In Portugal, a chorizo and kale stew called caldo verde is a top pick. In Jewish culture, it's a simple chicken soup! If Bubby made it, it's comfort food!

But as a culture we have communally decided that if we're down and out, we "deserve" to eat something "naughty" or "bad." Cue the midnight McDonalds run. When we remove the morality around food and put all foods on an equal playing field, we can make choices that *actually* feel good to us, not just physically, but emotionally too. We may find that our ultimate comfort food isn't French fries in gravy because we're so deprived of carbs, but rather, that it's our mother's gumbo that brings us true joy.

Am I suggesting that you're automatically never going to crave chocolate again or that you're going to start gnawing on carrots after a breakup? Let's not get crazy here! But when you allow yourself the freedom to eat foods judgment-free, you start to learn what actually fills your cup.

- **Satisfaction Hunt.** When foods aren't off-limits, and a scoop of raspberry ripple isn't such a carnal sin, you realize how little of these Naked Carbs or other treat foods you need to feel satisfied. So, rather than plowing through your whole pantry in an effort to "eat around your craving," you'll learn how to work your favorite foods into your diet in a balanced way.

- **Last Supper Syndrome.** Here's an easy one. The diet *doesn't* start tomorrow, because diets are a thing of your past. If you're not anticipating having to heavily restrict all of your favorite foods, there will never be a need to clear out all of the "junk" in an epic binge.

- **"Health Halo" Deception.** Part of the reason that we are often fooled by marketing tactics like Health Halos that call out specific "healthy"-sounding attributes in foods, is because we've lost touch with our bodies' true needs. We see the term "organic" and we think, "Oh, perfect, I can eat the whole box!" But after reading this book, and honing your interoceptive skills, you're not going to be fooled again. My Hunger

Crushing Combo will help you snatch the power away from stealthy food marketers and deliver it back to you and your body.

### Putting It All Together (on One Plate)

One of the most important things to remember is that foods are neither good nor bad, clean or toxic. They're just food. Food was never meant to fall into a category or be labeled a certain way or make us feel ashamed of our likes and dislikes. It was meant to do two things: nourish our bodies and bring us joy.

Furthermore, foods may not ever be nutritionally equal. I mean, we're never going to make a luscious slice of carrot cake have the same nutrient composition as a carrot (and even if we tried, that pretty much defeats the purpose). However, we can make all foods morally equal. How do we do that? By neutralizing the power they have over us.

My Hunger Crushing Combo puts all food on a level playing field. Nothing is off-limits, so there is no denial. And it does this by quite literally placing seemingly antagonistic foods on the same plate. A "fear food" or food that is traditionally bound by diet culture, and a "health food" can coexist in the same meal. No cheat days. No last supper binges. No miserable state of denial.

When previously restricted foods are no longer off-limits, they get knocked off their pedestal, robbed of their moral status, and become just another food. Our diet becomes the least interesting thing about us, and food no longer distracts us from all of the amazing things life has to offer. Finally, fueling your body "well" becomes as intuitive as brushing your teeth. That is food freedom, and my goodness, does it ever taste good.

**PART 2**

# THE HCC FOR YOUR LIFE AND YOUR GOALS

The beauty of the HCC is that it can be applied to any goal, any person, and in any stage of life. And it not only helps support your physical well-being, but also absolves you of the nagging guilt, fear, and shame we so often associate with food. So, regardless of your age, sex, body composition, or dietary preferences, you can experience unique improvements to your health by keeping three simple things in mind: Fiber. Protein. Healthy fats. One is great. Two is better. All three are amazing.

The general HCC framework theoretically celebrates all three of the Hunger Crushing Compound categories equally, encouraging you to focus on whichever feels best to you at that moment.

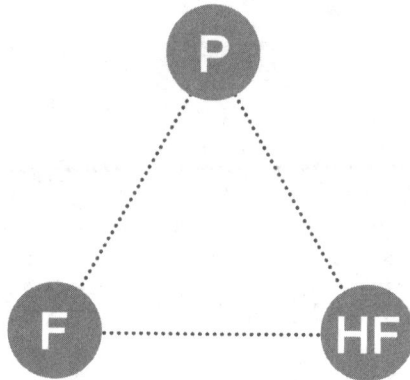

With that being said, I get a lot of questions about specific nutrition or health goals and how to best apply this framework using evidence-based practices. In the following chapters, I'm going to provide some suggestions on which Hunger Crushing Compounds we *specifically* want to focus *more* on to meet certain goals, while still not getting lost and trapped obsessing over the details. All of the HCCs are still in play, but based on the best practices in nutrition research, they may hold relatively different levels of importance in our meal planning. This is represented by different relative icon sizes in our Hunger Crushing Combo Triangle. This doesn't necessarily correlate to a percentage of calories from each category (for example, if protein is the largest icon, it doesn't mean over half your calories should be coming from protein). But rather, it gives you some direction on which of the three HCCs you should be most mindful about in your meals and snacks, so you aren't overwhelmed trying to juggle all three equally. Some goals may necessitate a greater attention to protein, whereas for others, focusing on fiber or fats may be advantageous. It's also important to me to flag that these chapters may contain specific scientific calculations and evidence-based optimal macro ranges that may seem like a departure from the gentle guidelines of the HCC approach. I share this only because I don't believe in censoring science, and I *always* come with receipts. This info is here if you are looking for the background science to better understand the guidelines and recommendations; none of this is a suggestion to do any of these calculations yourself or meticulously count out grams of protein to meet an arbitrary goal. So, even when there is more guidance and structure given, the main crux of the framework holds true: We add, we don't restrict. We aim to satisfy and satiate. And we approach all of our choices from a place of self-care.

Welcome to a new sustainable and enjoyable way to meet your goals.

# CHAPTER 6

· · · · · · · · · · · · · · · · · ·

# Not Another Diet:
# HCC for Weight-Loss Goals

have spent the past fifteen years taking down diet culture, and often that has meant being critical of our collective obsession with weight loss at any or all costs. Chances are, if you're here reading this book, you've likely been scammed and disillusioned by diet culture more than once.

But I haven't had to fight the diet industry alone. Over the past decade, we've seen a social movement toward greater acceptance of body diversity and various antidiet movements, which has been truly freeing for so many.

But where does that leave you, if you're trying to respect your body and want to reject the extreme fads and quick fixes that have failed you in the past, but you *still* want to lose weight? Are you just vain and shallow? Have you "failed" at being a good feminist? Have you "given in" to toxic social pressures? It can feel like you're crossing the picket line in front of everyone you love, admire, and trust.

That is not how we roll here. In the same way that guilt is not welcome at the dinner table, it also isn't helpful when it comes to your goals. So, while I will always denounce diet culture, I will unequivocally support those who want to lose weight. For any and every reason, as it is none of anyone's business to judge what is a valid motivator for change. At the end of the day, I want you to feel empowered in the choices you make about your body. And for some, that is going to mean losing weight. But before you do, I want you to ask yourself about **intention** and **approach**.

The **intention** should always be from a place of self-care, not self-punishment. Are you making changes to help improve your life in some way, or because you are "bad" and your coworker made a Miss Piggy joke at the work party? (*Honestly, F that guy!*) If you want to make changes that you can stick to for life, you must approach them from a place of body kindness and care. The **approach** must always be one that feels good. A weight-loss goal can quickly go from being health-centered to counting out your grapes. The mental health for physical health trade-in *never* nets out in the black. We want to approach weight-loss goals with a gentle additive approach that helps you build balanced meals that satiate and satisfy.

My Hunger Crushing Combo is your official toolbox, and the more specific guidelines in this chapter offer the best tools to accomplish the healthy weight-maintenance job.

## Risks of Intentional Weight Loss

I cannot let you dive into a chapter about weight-loss goals without a reminder that for many, the line between healthy weight-loss strategies and disordered eating is razor thin. Whereas one person might be able to just cut back on potato chips without a second moralizing thought, another person will find themselves living on a spin bike for two hours to "pay" for a single slice of pizza. If you have any suspicion that this could be a slippery slope for you, I suggest you skip this chapter or, at the very least, work one-on-one with a dietitian, to safely unpack those feelings first.

Even when you're going into a weight-loss diet with a neutral psychological relationship with food, there are physical risks associated with highly restrictive approaches.[1] Honestly, there are more dangerous (and often ridiculous) rapid weight-loss "hacks" popping up every day than there are episodes of *The Simpsons*, and most of them have ding-dong-diddily-squat benefits and risks grander than Marge's hair. Here are just a few of the potential threats of signing up for the extreme weight-loss diet du jour:

- Nutritional deficiencies
- Muscle loss
- Electrolyte imbalances
- Heart problems
- Gallstones
- Hormonal imbalances and amenorrhea[2]
- Loss of bone density[3]
- Disordered eating[4]

In addition to these very real and very harmful outcomes, restrictive dieting can also completely backfire by slowing your metabolism.

A prime case study of this is with the research that followed fourteen *Biggest Loser* reality show contestants for six years after the show.[5] It found that a third of contestants regained almost all of their lost weight, landing themselves within 1 percent of their starting weight. What was even more devastating was that their leptin levels (our fullness hormone) and basal metabolic rate were still depressed after six years at their next follow-up. Translation? These poor souls put themselves through hell and humiliation just to be hungrier, *and* now need to cut out an entire meal just to not gain *more* weight. To try to lose it again, they'd need to shave off around 500 calories (for a normal calorie deficit) *plus* another 600 to account for their metabolic decline!

Similarly, studies show that, within five years, people who have followed very low-calorie diets (1,200 calories or less) tend to regain between 26 and 121 percent of the weight lost (yes, that means some people end up heavier than where they started).[6] Even when we look at more moderate weight-management programs, we see an average regain rate of 30 to 35 percent.[7] Weight cycling, sometimes called yo-yo dieting, is not only hella frustrating, but with each kick at the can, it may increase the risk of insulin resistance, hypertension, and high cholesterol.[8]

## Benefits of Intentional Weight Loss

Despite all of the dangers of diet culture, it would be grossly negligent not to acknowledge the science in favor of maintaining a healthy weight. Research shows that for some folks with obesity, even a modest weight loss of 5 to 15 percent of their body weight can improve many obesity-related complications.[9] And speaking of obesity, a quick reminder that despite the shortcomings of such words as "overweight" and "obese" (see "Why BMI Is Kinda BS," page 137), I will be using these terms frequently in this chapter to explain the research to date. I also want to clarify that the potential benefits of intentional weight loss are *not* universal and almost exclusively apply only to folks who have excess body fat. If you're already lean or at your healthiest weight, additional weight loss is more likely to do more harm than good. While everyone's unique outcomes will vary, here are some potential perks to taking steps to achieve and maintain your healthiest happiest weight. Weight loss may

- Reduce risk of type 2 diabetes[10]
- Reduce risk of heart disease[11]

- Reduce risk of certain cancers (endometrial, esophageal, renal, and pancreatic adenocarcinomas; hepatocellular carcinoma; gastric cardia cancer; meningioma; multiple myeloma; and colorectal, postmenopausal breast, ovarian, gallbladder, and thyroid cancers)[12]
- Enhance mobility and joint health[13]
- Improve respiratory function[14]
- Improve digestive health[15]
- Support a healthy immune system[16]
- Improve energy levels and sleep[17]
- Improve mental health[18]
- Support a long, happy, healthy life[19]

## Why BMI Is Kinda BS

Body mass index (BMI) has been widely used as a screening tool in research to help group individuals into weight categories that may put them at risk for chronic disease. BMI is a simple metric calculation of body weight (kg) divided by height ($m^2$). And despite the fact that we've been using it to classify obesity and as a catch-all proxy for body fat, nutritional status, and disease risk since the nineteenth century, it's honestly . . . kinda crap. It was designed by a statistician for a life insurance company, based on data from white "healthy" men, and while it is *somewhat* useful for the average white population, it's just not accurate on an individual basis. For one, it doesn't differentiate between weight from fat and weight from muscle. So, a bodybuilder who has a BMI of 30 and superlow 10 percent body fat could technically be classified as "obese." It also doesn't account for how fat is distributed, and as we now know, it's largely visceral fat that is associated with health concerns. Remember the "fat but fit paradox" (page 74)? It's very possible for someone with a "healthy" BMI and lower body weight to have high amounts of inflammatory visceral fat. It also doesn't account for differences in body composition across ages, sexes, and ethnic groups, and has been shown to be grossly inaccurate for assessing the risk of people of color.

Combining BMI with waist circumference can be helpful, because it can better evaluate abdominal obesity (visceral fat) and related cardiometabolic risks vs. going by BMI alone. Adding other measurements, like body fat percentage, muscle mass, and biomarkers like blood pressure, blood fats, and blood sugar control provides even more data points to more comprehensively evaluate someone's health status and chronic disease risk. All this to say, simply having one measurement (like BMI) isn't enough to get an accurate picture of your health.

## Fat Loss vs. Weight Loss

Before we go further, I want to clarify something that is super-duper important when it comes to the benefits of weight loss. They're not actually benefits of *weight* loss; the true benefit lies predominantly in a combination of *fat* loss and lean muscle mass preservation (or growth).

As we've discussed throughout Part 1, most of the dangers of carrying excess weight relate to the abdominal fat that surrounds our organs (a.k.a. visceral fat).

So, reducing excess body fat, especially inflammatory visceral fat, is undoubtedly advantageous, as it's one of the main drivers of metabolic disease. And while aerobic exercise has been shown to help reduce visceral fat, there is no diet to help "spot-reduce" fat.[20] Otherwise, we'd all have Barbie doll figures with tiny waists, big breasts, and round bubble butts. For most of us, those aren't the cards we were dealt. To lose visceral fat, we just need to lose fat in general. Sorry, boobs; you're probably going to go, too.

While you might have to put up with an A cup when you want a C, you don't want to lose fat at the expense of muscle mass. Muscle is the cornerstone of vitality, and once it's gone, it's a hell of a journey to get it back.

Research suggests that we can gain about ½ to 2 pounds of muscle mass per month with a well-planned nutrition and exercise regimen in the first one to two years of resistance training.[21] Although building more muscle will always be advantageous, even just maintaining what we've got is an important goal. Adults start to fight against natural muscle loss beginning as early as our thirties, where we can expect a decline of 3 to 8 percent per decade.[22] At around age seventy-five, our muscle strength continues to be lost at a rate of 3 to 4 percent per year in men and 2.5 to 3 percent per year in women.[23] This means that, between the ages of thirty and eighty-five, a 150-pound adult who does not regularly engage in strength training to counteract these losses may end up losing up to 33 pounds of muscle! *Yikes on bikes!* When it comes to maintaining a healthy body composition, nature is already working against us; the last thing we want is for our diet to deal another big blow. If managing your weight as you age is the goal, minimizing muscle loss throughout your journey should be top of mind. Here's why:

Lean muscle tissue is metabolically active, and "costs" more calories than fat to maintain. Each kilogram (2¼ pounds) of muscle increases your basal metabolic rate by 13 to 22 calories. And this is just the effect on calorie burn if you just sat on your tush all day. In reality, more muscle means more "calorically expensive" mass to lug around, both when doing daily activities and when engaging in actual exercise. So, your boost in calorie burn is actually more like an extra 20 to 40 calories per day for every kilogram of muscle that you add, depending on how active you are.[24] In contrast, the more muscle you lose (either from aging, dieting, inactivity, or other factors), the slower your metabolism, and the more difficult it becomes to lose or maintain your weight.

Muscle tissue is also closely involved in glucose metabolism.[25] The more muscle tissue, the more cavernous the "sink" for glucose to drain from the blood, reducing the risk of insulin resistance and type 2 diabetes. If you recall from Chapter 3, this also feeds into the risk of obesity because insulin resistance can increase visceral fat, fueling this vicious cycle of metabolic dysfunction. It's all bad news bears.

Now, it's superimportant to note that all bodies are good bodies, and metabolically "healthy" bodies come in all sorts of different shapes, sizes, and compositions. Some people will naturally carry more fat, whereas others carry more muscle, even if they do the exact same fitness routines! But when we look at longitudinal population research, there is a strong correlation between higher body fat and the risk of health problems, particularly chronic illnesses like heart disease.[26] In contrast, more muscle seems to be protective against these issues, particularly for women! The bottom line is, regardless of the number on the scale, the more muscle you have, the greater the defense against the diseases we are trying to avoid.

### Fat Burning vs. Body Fat Loss

From weight-loss pills and potions to fasted workouts to keto diet plans, you've probably been drawn in by the promise of a specific hack's "fat-burning" potential. But here's an unfortunate truth if you've ever heard one: *Fat burning is a bust.* Let me explain:

There *are* legitimate ways to put your body into "fat-burning mode," or to boost the relative proportion of fat being "burned" instead of carbohydrates, for example. This is the entire premise of the keto diet, and we also see it with intermittent fasting, exercising before eating, and popular weight-loss supplements like conjugated linoleic acid (CLA) and green tea extract.[27] All of these approaches can legitimately enhance fat burning!

Here comes the big fat BUT: Increasing the relative burning of fat *does not* mean you're losing weight or even burning body fat **if total calorie intake stays the same.** In fact, when you dive into the studies on all of these popular "fat-burning" hacks, you'll see that this doesn't actually result in *any* difference in weight loss or body fat percentage.

The bottom line is this: Weight and fat loss will always come down to a calorie deficit, not any one well-marketed hack. And we don't *just* want to see the number on the scale go down at any or all costs. We want to reduce visceral fat and increase muscle, to improve our metabolic health and longevity. And while any weight-loss diet can increase the risk of muscle loss, you're at an especially high risk if

- You are already in the normal or underweight BMI category and have less fat to lose. Lower-weight folks will often lose up to 35 percent fat-free mass when trying to lose weight![28] *Oof!*
- You're losing weight at a faster than recommended rate (more than 1% of your body weight per week).
- You're intermittent fasting, especially doing full-day fasting or an extreme "OMAD" (one meal a day) diet.
- You're not including resistance exercise (strength training) in your routine.
- You're not getting enough protein.
- You're already over the age of sixty-five.

Aside from your age, the rest of these risk factors of muscle loss are within your control, so the approach you take to your weight-loss journey matters. This is the difference between losing weight with a juice cleanse vs. a balanced nutrient-dense way of eating, as what's encouraged by the Hunger Crushing Combo. Doing the delicate dance to lose fat and preserve muscle requires a much more careful approach than a haphazard calorie deficit. It takes a gentle tactic and self-caring intention.

## Achieving a (Healthy) Calorie Deficit

Weight loss is rarely easy, but it is (at least theoretically) quite simple: It will always come down to energy balance.

$$\text{Calorie Input} - \text{Calorie Output} = \text{Calorie Balance}$$

On the left side of the equation, 100 percent of our **calorie input** comes from the foods or drinks you're putting into your body to provide energy, sustenance, and nutrition.

**Calorie output** depends on many more variables. Your basal metabolic rate (BMR) is the calories you need for basic functions (things like breathing, your heart beating, or thinking). It makes up 60 to 75 percent of the total number of calories you burn each day.[29] Your daily activities of life (nonexercise activity thermogenesis, a.k.a. NEAT), such as washing dishes, walking to the mailbox, getting dressed, or cleaning the house, make up another 10 to 50 percent.[30] Then, 8 to 10 percent of daily calories are burned through what's called the thermic effect of food (TEF), meaning the energy required to eat and digest. And that leaves us with 5 to 15 percent from exercise.

How many calories you need to consume in a day just to maintain your current body weight will depend on your age, sex, body composition, genetics, hormone levels, physical activity, and more. There are dozens of online calculators based on various equations that aim to help determine how many calories you should consume in a day (see the box "Equations to Estimate Your Calorie Needs").

# Equations to Estimate Your Calorie Needs

In nutrition practice, a lot of experts will get a rough pulse on calorie needs by plunking some data into a total daily energy expenditure (TDEE) equation. Keyword: rough. There are pros and cons to each of the different energy equation calculators, but a lot of my colleagues and I prefer the Cunningham calculation, because it takes into account lean body mass vs. fat mass, which can greatly improve its accuracy.

**To calculate energy needs for women:**

LBM (lean body mass) = total body weight (kg) × (1 – body fat percentage)

RMR (resting metabolic rate) = 500 + [22 × LBM (lean body mass in kg)]

TDEE (total daily energy expenditure) = RMR × activity factor

**Activity factors:**

Sedentary (little to no exercise): RMR × 1.2

Lightly active (light exercise/sports 1 to 3 days/week): RMR × 1.375

Moderately active (moderate exercise/sports 3 to 5 days/ week): RMR × 1.55

Very active (hard exercise/sports 6 to 7 days a week): RMR × 1.725

Superactive (very hard exercise/physical job): RMR × 1.9

Now, let's do some math with an example. Let's say we've got a thirty-year-old female named Jen, who weighs 158 pounds (70 kg), has an average body fat percentage of 25 percent, and is moderately active playing tennis 4 times a week.

LBM = 70 × (1 − 0.25) = 52.5 kg
RMR = 500 + (22 × 52.5) = 1,655 calories/day
TDEE = 1,655 × 1.55 = 2,565.25 calories/day

Using the Cunningham equation, Jen expends about 2,565 calories a day, and would need to consume approximately the same amount of calories to maintain her current body weight.

I share this equation and example solely as background knowledge to better understand the complexity of calorie needs, not as a suggestion to revert back to your calorie-counting ways. You're here for a reason, and it's certainly not to do more mental math.

Here's the thing: The numbers spit out by an online calculator are a very crude estimate of your *true unique* needs. Depending on which calculation you use and how you plug in activity factors, you can expect to see variations between 300 and 500 calories a day! If you were following that religiously with no internal input from your body, that inaccuracy could potentially even result in weight gain! This is why I do *not* like relying on any of these external directives for determining how much and when to eat.

We also can't perfectly predict how many calories you need to "cut" to see consistent weight loss. If you recall from Chapter 2, the whole *"cut 3,500 calories and you'll lose a pound of fat"* that we've drilled into our brain is an oversimplification. So, even though most diets recommend a daily calorie deficit of around 500 calories (since 500 × 7 = 3,500), how many calories *you* can safely cut is highly individualized. In the field of dietetics, most of my colleagues may use a theoretical calorie equation only as a starting point to hypothesize the amount of calories needed for a calorie deficit. The rest will come down to trial and error, and feedback from the body to craft and adjust the plan. We start with making small changes to evaluate the outcome on weight (and often, even just writing down your daily intake for your dietitian to review will result in weight loss). And then we can gently tweak the dials to land in a safe weight-loss sweet spot.

What do I mean by *safe*? Our clinical obesity guidelines generally recommend a steady weight-loss rate of 0.5 to 1 percent of our total body weight, or 1 to 2 pounds per week max.[31] Anything greater than this, we're at higher risk of breaking down our muscles as fuel. Remember, we don't want to lose *just any* weight! We certainly don't want to lose muscle that will help us maintain our weight loss over time. And the slower the weight-loss pace, the lower the risk of cutting into our gains.

Okay now, if you're having involuntary eye twitches every time I mention numbers or say "calorie deficit," I got you. The word "deficit" always gives me the ick. It denotes denial, deprivation, and generally having less of what we want. But it absolutely doesn't have to feel like any of those things.

The beauty of the Hunger Crushing Combo is that it can help you naturally create a calorie deficit. It's a sneaky calorie deficit. No calculations, no counting, no spiraling into weighing out your peas.

And that comes down to satiety and satisfaction.

## The HCC Formula for Healthy, Sustainable Weight Loss

While there is no one-size-fits-all diet when it comes to weight loss, several key insights have emerged from nutrition research that can give us some solid guidance on best practices. Namely, that we should be leaning heavily on our Hunger Crushing Compounds to naturally edge out less satiating Naked Carbs. Protein is a nonnegotiable to maintain muscle in calorie deficit; high-volume, high-fiber carbs help make said calorie deficit easier; and healthy fats can be carefully curated to bring satisfaction to calorie-reduced meals.

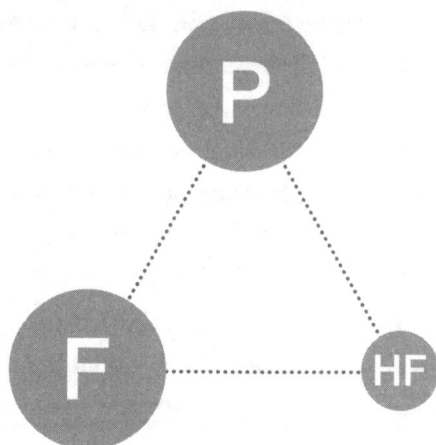

**Protein**

If you recall, protein is king of the satiety hierarchy, which is why it needs to be one of our top priorities when losing weight. Unlike fat and carb intake, variations in protein intake are what greatly affect fat-loss rates. Protein slows down our digestion and stimulates the release of satiety hormones like peptide YY and GLP-1, helping curb appetite, while offering just 4 calories per gram. We also need more protein to stimulate muscle synthesis when we're in a caloric deficit, so a higher protein intake helps spare muscle mass from being broken down as fuel.[32] If we're looking to lose fat, not metabolic muscle, we need to do a delicate dance of feeding our body fewer calories than it needs to maintain its current weight, while still making sure those muscles get preferentially fed.

Our basic dietary guidelines suggest aiming to get 10 to 35 percent of your daily calories from protein, to support general health, but 10 to 35 percent is a huge range, reflective of the inherent variability in how different bodies respond to food![33] For someone consuming 2,000 calories, that could be 50 to 175 grams a day! When fat loss is the goal, aiming for the upper end of that range is the ideal play. Research suggests going from a diet that's 10 to 15 percent protein to one that is 20 to 30 percent protein can result in a threefold bump in fat loss.[34] Another study found that when people doubled their protein from 15 to 30 percent of their total calories, they spontaneously ate approximately 400 fewer calories overall.[35] In dietetic practice, another way of communicating these approximate protein goals is to use our total body weight, with research suggesting aiming for at least 1.8 grams/kg of body weight (adjusted for a BMI of 30 if considered in the "obese" category).[36] So, for a 158-pound woman, this could mean around 125 grams of protein a day. Yes, you could do a quick calculation based on your body weight, to give you a very rough idea of what your approximate needs might be. But for most people, a good place to start for weight loss is to aim for a "meal dose" of protein at all meals (20 to 35 grams), and at least a "snack dose" (8 to 20 grams) for most, if not all snacks. This also aligns nicely with optimizing the use of protein for repair, maintenance, and growth of tissue like muscle.

I don't want you to have to obsessively count or measure anything, so you'll find charts in Chapter 11 that will help you eyeball "meal dose" portions on a plate.

### Carbohydrates & Fiber

We can't just live off protein, which is where its weight-loss bosom buddy, fiber, comes into play. Research suggests that, when held against a variety of variables, including race, age, and other macronutrients, fiber intake was the most strongly predictive of weight loss and diet adherence.[37]

The RDA for total fiber intake for adult men and women is 38 grams and 25 grams per day, respectively.[38] But nearly 95 percent of adults aren't even meeting this minimum, and for a lot of people, the optimal fiber intake for weight loss is even higher.[39] One small study (with predominantly female participants) found that when participants upped their fiber intake from 16.6 to 28 grams per day, they felt less hungry and more satisfied, and their calories were naturally slashed by 300 per day.[40] So, if weight loss is your goal, you should be aiming for a "meal dose" of *at least* 6 to 12 grams of fiber at all meals and *at least* half of that at snacks (3 to 6 grams as a "snack dose"). You'll find a chart of visual cues with specifics in Chapter 11.

But what about Naked Carbs? As we now well know, Naked Carbs are easier to overeat because they lack Hunger Crushing Compounds, which can get in the way of maintaining our calorie deficit. So, while I don't want you to cut out Naked Carbs, you will want to load them up with Hunger Crushing Compounds (especially fiber and protein), so you can feel satisfied from a more moderate portion. For example, if you used to have three big handfuls of potato chips as a snack, now you might choose to mindfully include just one handful as you bulk up your plate with HCC-rich foods like sliced veggies with tzatziki. I want you to find a way to incorporate the Naked Carbs that bring you the most pleasure bang for your caloric buck.

### Healthy Fats

We've already reclaimed fat from the 1990s' smear campaign (for a refresh, revisit Chapter 4), but you may be wondering how fat fits in with weight loss. Fat is higher in calories (9 kcal/g) than carbs and protein (4 kcal/g, respectively), but it is also very satiating *and* emotionally satisfying. So, to get the most value from those extra calories, you'll want to focus on choosing dual-citizenship fats (e.g., full-fat yogurt, avocado, salmon, or nuts and nut butter) more often over solo artists (e.g., cooking oil). I'm not suggesting you shouldn't cook with oil (*boiled chicken breasts and steamed Brussels sprouts give me state-owned retirement home vibes*). But this is where we want to employ our SMART use of added oils, usually around a thumbtip size, to help with cooking and flavor without adding hundreds of extra calories to each meal. Chapter 11 has visual cues and specifics.

## What If the Scale Doesn't Budge?

If you recall from Chapter 2, your body gets a little pissy when it's put on a strict diet. Even a gentle approach like using an adapted HCC framework can be met with resistance, pushback, and frustration. And if that scale is not moving at that sought-after 1 to 2 pounds-a-week pace, you may be tempted to pull out one of your old tricks and live off green juice and broth-based soup. Instead, I want you to ask yourself the following question with compassion and kindness: *Have I been prioritizing protein and fiber at every meal?*

If you feel you've been hitting those meal and snack doses we discussed and the scale has still stalled, the next consideration is the sources and portions of Naked Carbs in your diet. A lot of people will ask me, *"Abbey, how much is too much or too often when it comes to sweets, treats, and other less nutritious Naked Carbs?"* And the answer in the context of a weight-loss goal is, *It depends.* If you've been losing weight while having white bread at breakfast and a bowl of ice cream at night, then amazing! Keep at it! But if you've plateaued or are gaining, it might be time to tweak the Naked Carb portions or frequency. For one person's journey, this might mean edging out three cookies by serving one alongside a bowl of strawberries or glass of milk. For another person, it might mean mostly enjoying higher-fiber carbs like fruit as an after-dinner sweet, with a more decadent dessert a couple of times a week.

To take the personalization even further, what may be necessary to elicit the weight-loss results someone desires might just not be enjoyable, sustainable, or healthy. So, adjusting expectations and reorienting values become critical. And if you feel the eating pattern that you need to take on to trigger weight loss is starting to feel restrictive or distressing, it may be helpful to shift the focus away from the diet, at least momentarily. Instead, consider working with a registered dietitian to focus on other important weight-management tools like exercise, sleep, stress management, and supplements. We will chat about this in more detail in the pages to come.

## The HCC for GLP-Is and Weight-Loss Drugs

As briefly introduced in Chapter 2, GLP-1 agonists like semaglutide (brand names Ozempic, Wegovy, and Rybelsus), tirzepatide (brand names Mounjaro and Zepbound), and liraglutide (brand name Saxenda) are some of the most powerful weight-loss medications we've ever seen.

A lot of folks who turn to GLP-1 agonists do so after years of struggling with their weight and blood sugar management. And while these medications are clearly quite effective with these goals by reducing appetite, slowing gastric emptying, and stabilizing blood sugar regulation hormones, one of the less expected and monumental outcomes is in reducing "food noise." Food noise isn't just thinking about what you're going to have for dinner while you're still at work. It's an all-consuming, inescapable, and debilitating racket in the brain that can only be quieted (at least temporarily) with food. One of the ways GLP-1 agonists are thought to help people curb appetite and get overeating under control is by acting directly on brain receptors involved in pleasure and affecting the perception of food as a reward.[41] So, not only can this obviously make weight loss easier, but it also helps free up your mental energy for other activities, goals, and things that bring you joy. You can imagine how life-changing this can be!

While the Hunger Crushing Combo Triangle still ultimately applies to folks who are using adjunct medications like GLP-1 agonists, some important considerations should play into your choices.

First of all, GLP-1s' appetite suppression effects often come as a package deal with a number of digestive maladies. Namely, severe nausea, vomiting, constipation, and diarrhea. For some, this can present a whole new quandary around not being able to eat *enough* to meet basic nutrition needs. I know that, if you've struggled with overeating your whole life, it's hard to imagine a scenario where you're physically malnourished, but this paradoxical outcome does occur![42] So, with limited bandwidth to even want to eat and an obvious desire to still meet your body's needs for optimal functioning, **every food choice counts**. Opt for smaller, more frequent, nutrient-dense meals to quell nausea and meet your needs.

**Protein** becomes a nonnegotiable for every meal and snack. Since GLP-1 agonists often induce weight loss beyond the 1 percent weekly recommended pace, loss of lean muscle mass (and strength) is a significant risk.[43] One study found that up to 39 percent of weight loss was from lean mass, not because of the medication itself, but simply due to the rate at which weight is lost.[44] Rapid loss of lean tissue may also explain why some patients report excess hair loss and skin laxity (what the media has offensively pet-named "Ozempic face") while taking these medications.

Another nutrition-mediated side effect of GLP-1s is constipation and bloating, thanks to their role in slowing down digestion in the gut. And this is where **fiber** comes into play. All fiber is good fiber when it comes to supporting digestion, but focus on lower FODMAP foods rich in insoluble fiber (e.g., quinoa, carrots, seeds, green beans, and kiwi) to add bulk to stool without bloating and gas.

In the other corner of the calorie-density ring is **fat**. Fats can provide a lot of nutrition in a small package, but if we were to spend our days drinking coffee loaded with heavy cream, we might completely override the medication's effectiveness in promoting weight loss. So, this is another one of those delicate dances, and one that can be addressed by focusing on nutrient-dense, dual-citizen HCCs. For example, full-fat yogurt and cottage cheese, fatty fish, nuts and seeds, and avocado all offer great nutrition bang for your appetite buck. Remember, when weight loss medication is in play, every food choice matters.

I know that it might at first sound asinine to tell you not to undereat when you're on a drug to try to help you essentially undereat to create a calorie deficit, but sustainable weight loss is a marathon, not a sprint, even when you have pharmaceutical support! So, ensuring adequate nutrients, calories, and protein is crucial to your health and success.

## Favorite Foods for Weight Loss

One of the most challenging things for many people pursuing weight loss is envisioning what their new meal or snack plate looks like and how to make that a reality. Using the HCC may make logical sense, but having some examples of foods that help support weight loss can help you kick off your journey with confidence. Keep in mind that any food can be a weight loss–friendly food when it's worked into a diet with a modest calorie deficit. Here are just a few examples that offer great nutrition for your caloric buck to help you support your goals:

- **Eggs.** Two eggs provide 13 grams of protein and 11 grams of fat for 150 calories. From a simple morning scramble, to baked in casseroles, to poached on toast, there's no shortage of delicious ways to enjoy eggs.
- **Cottage Cheese.** Cottage cheese offers phenomenal satiety, with a ½-cup portion offering a whopping 12 grams of protein in a 90-calorie package. Serve it sweet with berries and honey, or savory with a swirl of pesto and chopped veggies.
- **Greek Yogurt.** With 12 grams of protein per ½ cup, research shows that yogurt may help reduce appetite by increasing circulating hormones GLP-1 and peptide YY.[45] Use Greek yogurt as a base in smoothie bowls, fruit parfaits, and dips.

- **Leafy Greens.** Leafy greens are low in calories and high in water, fiber, vitamins, minerals, and antioxidants. Try them raw and chopped for salads, added to soups and wraps, sautéed with a little garlic and olive oil, or tossed into your protein shake.

- **Raspberries.** Research suggests that berries may offer unique benefits for weight management by helping support a healthy gut microbiome, appetite management, and thermogenesis.[46] Raspberries are particularly powerful in this department, thanks to their remarkable 8 grams of fiber per cup! Enjoy raspberries as a quick midmorning snack, or add to oatmeal, salads, smoothies, yogurt, or baked goods.

- **Apples.** Apples are a staple in any weight-management regimen, because they're naturally sweet, high in fiber (providing 4 to 5 grams each) and, like berries, they contain thermogenesis-activating polyphenols (especially in the peel!). Toss an apple into your lunch box for work, throw it into salads, or add it to protein oats for breakfast!

- **Legumes.** Legumes like peas, beans (including soybeans), and lentils are fabulous sources of plant-based protein and fiber. Because of their dual citizenship, they digest slowly, keep you fuller longer, and help balance blood sugar levels. Meatless Monday is a great start, but try slowly increasing your meatless meals by swapping lentils or beans for ground beef in chilis, tacos, and stir-fries.

- **Fish.** Fish and seafood are a fantastic source of satiating protein, with 23 to 25 grams per 3½-ounce serving! Aim for two or three servings per week for optimal benefits, serving it baked, poached, grilled, or from a can, for easy sandwiches and wraps.

- **Chia seeds.** As a built-in HCC, research suggests that, when combined with a calorie deficit, chia seeds can offer some major weight-loss perks.[47] One ounce gets you 5 grams of protein, 9 grams of healthy fats (including omega-3s), and 10 grams of fiber! Wowsers! Sprinkle onto salads, add to muffin and pancake batters, and toss into smoothies, yogurt, and oatmeal. If you don't eat eggs, you can use chia seeds to make vegan eggs that work as a great binding agent in baked goods (mix 1 tablespoon of chia seeds with 2 tablespoons of water to make one "egg").

## An Example HCC Day

The simplest way to get started is to keep the HCC Weight-Loss Triangle in mind when you build your meal. What foods should you be focusing on and what can take a back seat? Using this as a judgment-free starting point, you can then collect data on how this diet pattern makes you feel. Are you a bit constipated? Maybe you need to pull back on the protein and add more veg! Are you battling muscle soreness days after a workout? This might be the time to add an extra high-protein snack! Are you just generally exhausted and hungry? You might actually need *more* carbs and calories! And most important, does this way of eating feel like something that you can enjoy for life? What and how much you eat on a diet are important for weight loss, but your ability to eat that way for life is the *most* critical determinant of long-term success.

Remember, the total amount of food you eat in a day is surprisingly stable, so what may be "a lot" to one person, would be "too little" for another. So, whatever your calorie needs, here's what a sample day of eating the HCC way *might* look like for someone looking to lose weight:

Breakfast: Eggs scrambled with a scoop of cottage cheese and handful of spinach served with a bowl of raspberries

Snack: Cottage cheese with blueberries

Lunch: Bountiful green salad with roasted chickpeas, quinoa, avocado, and balsamic vinaigrette

Snack: Apple slices, graham cracker cookie with cinnamon Greek yogurt dip

Dinner: Chicken breast tacos with guacamole and high-fiber tortillas, served with cabbage slaw

Snack: Air-popped popcorn with a glass of fortified soy milk

Remember, *this is not your meal plan!* This is merely an example, to show you how to build balanced meals using the Weight-Loss HCC Triangle without obsessively counting every damn thing. To determine your unique calorie and macronutrient needs, I will always recommend working with a registered dietitian. They will be able to provide a comprehensive evaluation of your history, goals, and preferences, and help you design a personalized low-risk plan for success.

## To Supplement or Not?

Now that you have a good idea of how different areas of your everyday lifestyle are contributing to your weight-loss journey, you might be curious about all the supplements that are marketed to you. I've definitely seen far more questionable products on the market than science-backed ones. Not to mention, we ideally want to try to get the bulk of our nutrition from whole foods, where we can. But life happens, and there are a lot of reasons why it's not always easy! In this case, working a few evidence-based supplements into your routine can help you take the anxiety and guesswork out of eating well to meet your goals. Always speak to your health-care provider and/or registered dietitian to determine any contraindications with any medications you may be taking and/or for personalized guidance about the right supplements for you. Here are a few I frequently recommend.

- **Soluble Fiber.** Soluble fiber supplements like partially hydrolyzed guar gum (PHGG), psyllium husk, glucomannan, pectin, and inulin can be effective tools in supporting weight-loss goals by keeping you fuller longer. Just be aware that fiber supplements are notorious for causing digestive distress, so it's imperative that you start with a small amount and slowly work your way up over a week or two. For example, if the supplement's recommended dosage is 10 grams, I would start with 2 grams and slowly increase as tolerated.
- **Protein Powder.** Protein foods arguably require the most time, energy, and skill to prepare. You can't just gnaw on a chicken breast straight from the fridge; you've got to do some work first! So, for those of us who don't have the bandwidth to bust out our Jamie Oliver cookbooks three times a day, protein powder comes in clutch. But like any other supplement, not all protein powders are created equal. Whey protein is the gold standard for many people, but in addition to not being an option for those who don't consume animal products, whey tends to cause digestive distress and acne in some people. This is actually the reason I created my own plant-based protein powder, Neue Theory. Most plant-based protein powders are low in the key muscle-building amino acid leucine. So, if choosing plant-based, look for one that adds additional leucine, as we do with Neue Theory.
- **Vitamin D.** Vitamin D doesn't cause weight loss, but adequate vitamin D stores do seem to play a role in a variety of metabolic processes that help enable it. Studies suggest that vitamin D may influence the expression of genes involved in fat metabolism and insulin sensitivity, both of which may increase fat storage over time.[48] Speak to your doctor about taking a supplement with at least 1,000 IU as a simple step to maintain optimal levels for supporting weight loss.

- **Probiotics.** There are hundreds (if not thousands) of probiotic strains, each with its own specialty superpower. But *Lactobacillus* strains tend to be the genera that are most studied for weight and fat loss. One study found that twelve weeks of *Lactobacillus gasseri* supplementation reduced belly fat by 8.5 percent, along with other significant reductions in waist and hip circumferences, and BMI.[49] There is still so much we don't know about the role of probiotic supplementation on weight loss, but they are generally a very low-risk supplement to experiment with. When buying a probiotic supplement, make sure to look for one that has two to ten billion CFUs (colony-forming units) per dose, and store them according to their instructions (which for some strains may require refrigeration).

### An Important Note on Supplements

The supplement industry is a bit of the Wild West, in that supplements aren't regulated by the US Food and Drug Administration (FDA) in the same way as pharmaceuticals. This means supplements are basically produced "on scout's honor" by the manufacturer, placed on shelves, and sold to consumers until enough reports of adverse effects come in to warrant closer regulatory inspection. For that reason, I always recommend looking for supplements that bear a third-party icon or seal indicating they have been tested by an independent lab to make sure they contain what they claim and in safe amounts. Since third-party testing is not mandatory and it costs brands a lot of money to do it properly, if you don't see a clear statement on the brand's packaging or website, it's best to choose another product.

## Lifestyle Strategies

Balanced eating is arguably one of the most important controllable factors for maintaining a healthy weight, but it can't be the only maneuver in our playbook. Especially if (or when) weight loss stalls. Here are some of the most important complementary lifestyle strategies to put in play today:

- **Aerobic Exercise.** Get this: Intentional exercise actually makes up only 5 to 15 percent of your *total* energy expenditure. In other words, if all the calories your body burns in a day total around 2,000, only 100 to 300 of them are from that time you spent sweating it out in that $30 class (+ *the $15 smoothie afterward*). This is why it's so important we stop thinking of exercise as the grueling punishment for our dietary sins. When we integrate daily movement we love into a gentle calorie-reduced diet that we can sustain, we *do* see synergistic benefits for weight management and body composition.[50]

  Exercise seems to be particularly important for helping people maintain their weight loss, and it is consistently one of the top reported behaviors among those who have successfully lost large amounts of weight and kept it off long term.[51] Most research suggests that burning between 200 and 350 calories per day from exercise helps minimize weight regain.[52] In light of this, experts recommend adults aim for a minimum of 150 to 300 minutes (2½ to 5 hours) per week of moderate-intensity exercise, 75 to 150 minutes (1¼ to 2½ hours) per week of vigorous-intensity aerobic physical activity, or an equivalent combination to support overall health and disease prevention.[53] For weight loss, this gets bumped up to 225 to 420 minutes (3¾ to 7 hours) of moderate-intensity exercise per week, or 40 to 60 minutes per day.[54]

If these numbers feel overwhelming or you're new to regular exercise, remember, *all movement is good movement.* So, choose an activity that brings you joy! Maybe that's jogging with your stroller, dropping into a group fitness class, taking up martial arts, or going skiing with your friends. Let your daily movement complement your diet, not sabotage it.

- **Resistance Training.** Cardio may burn calories in the moment, but resistance training builds the muscle that keeps burning calories long after you hop off that Peloton. One study found that after twenty-four weeks of weight training, men and women saw a 9 percent and 4 percent boost in resting metabolism, respectively.[55] We also burn a few extra calories in the hours immediately after a weight-training session; the more intense the workout, the greater the "after-burn" effect.[56] While everyone's going to have their preferences with exercise, it's important that we don't swing far too right or left on the #TeamCardio vs. #TeamStrength debate. Research clearly shows that folks who do both cardio *and* weight training (rather than just one over the other) see the greatest weight loss effects.[57] Variety is also important to keep yourself out of the workout slump: In addition to more aerobic-style workouts, experts recommend spending at least two days per week focusing on strengthening all of your major muscle groups (chest, arms, back, shoulders, legs, and core). So, pick up some heavy stuff and put it back down (and, like, repeat that a dozen times or so). This could mean working with dumbbells, resistance bands, bodyweight movements, weight-bearing machines, or getting creative pushing tires or boxes guerrilla-workout style. It doesn't have to be fancy or expensive to work!

- **Sleep Hygiene.** Sleep is our body's designated time to rest, repair, and rejuvenate. Skimping on shut-eye is like showing up to Wonka's chocolate factory for day one of your weight-loss diet; it can be done, but man, it's gonna be a slog. Research shows that sleep deprivation, even just one night of the tossy-turnies, can increase the hunger hormone ghrelin and lower the satiety hormone leptin.[58] Studies also show that undersleeping can stimulate the reward center of the brain to respond more aggressively to high-sugar, high-fat foods (*cue the midnight M&M's pantry raid*).[59] Not surprisingly, prospective research has found that people who sleep less than five hours a night are 35 percent more likely to gain more than 11 pounds over six years, and it's mostly that unwanted visceral fat.[60]

So is that an invitation to hit the snooze button on repeat? Not so fast, fellow sleepy sheepies. As with everything in wellness, there's also too much of a good thing. Although undersleeping is arguably more problematic, sleeping more than nine hours a night is also associated with weight gain, with about 25 percent increased risk of gaining 11 pounds over six years. This is why experts recommend aiming for seven to eight hours of quality sleep per night, a goalpost that can be best achieved with a few key sleep hygiene hacks:

- *Follow a consistent sleep-wake schedule.* This means going to sleep and waking up at the same time every day . . . yes, even on the weekends. (*Trust me, you're going to love joining the six p.m. dinner reservation gang!*)
- *Avoid stimulation at night.* Some of the most common activities that can make it harder to fall asleep when done too close to bedtime include eating a heavy, high-fat meal; engaging in vigorous sweaty exercise; drinking caffeine or alcohol; and heavy use of electronic screens. Save your Vanderpump reunion for the treadmill and bust out the

old-school paperbacks at night in bed. Research consistently shows that the blue light emitted from most of our
electronics (smartphones, tablets, HD TVs) all disrupt
the production of our body's natural sleep hormone, melatonin, making it more difficult to wind down.[61]

- *Create a sleep-promoting environment.* Consider adding blackout blinds, calm darker room colors (e.g., blues,
grays, and purples), cozy bedding or pillows, a white noise
machine, and a cool crisp temperature (between 60° and
67°F is optimal for boosting natural melatonin).[62]

- **Stress Management.** Telling someone to "stop being
stressed" feels borderline offensive these days. It seems like
there are countless reasons to feel worried and anxious and
very few opportunities to relax. That means it's up to us to
consciously build in time to engage in stress management as
a long-term investment in our health. You may be stressed
right now because of lack of time (and therefore, carving out
an hour for therapy feels counterintuitive), but giving yourself that push to prioritize yourself is key to preventing burn-
out, especially if you want to lose weight. Making changes to
your diet without addressing the stress you already have (or
the stress those changes are causing you) is like trying to ride
a bike with no wheels. It's going to be a very turbulent ride.

Now, to be clear: Some stress is actually good for us.
Acute forms of stress are vital inborn survival mechanisms,
and theoretically, this kind of stress would likely increase
weight loss, since adrenaline downregulates appetite. We
also see a transient boost in metabolism in those moments of
heart-racing panic. If I had a bear tailing me, you can *bet* I'm
going to be running faster than I have in any Barry's Boot-
camp class.

But most of us aren't experiencing the "gotcha" scaries on the regular. Instead, we're largely experiencing chronic stress of compounding pressures coming from all angles: work, money, relationships, kids, family, health, and more. And it's that slow-building omnipresent stress that radiates through your body, pulsating in the background at all times. That's the kind of stress that makes losing weight harder by releasing a whole slew of hormones, including the oh-so-demonized cortisol. Cortisol has this tricky little quirk where it selectively prevents the breakdown of belly fat (a.k.a. that dangerous visceral fat) while promoting insulin resistance and revving up our hunger hormones like ghrelin.[63] And we're not just hungry for anything, we're going straight for the Naked Carbs. Research actually shows that high-sugar, high-fat foods can provide a temporary reprieve from a cortisol spike.[64] This explains why we often find ourselves at the bottom of a tube of Pringles before we're even halfway through the first episode of our favorite true crime show.

Here's the annoying irony: Dieting is an actual stressor on the body.[65] Research suggests that the greater the calorie deficit, the higher the stress-induced cortisol.[66] And it's not just a physical stressor from deprivation, undernutrition, and raging hanger. Dieting can be stressful emotionally (food cravings), socially (skipping events and dinners), financially ($200 cleanse), and more. This is one of the reasons that I recommend a gentle additive approach like my Hunger Crushing Combo. We have more than enough to stress over; let's not let our diet tip the scales. And for all those demands, here are some key stress management tools to keep in your toolbox.

- Practicing mindfulness meditation
- Listening to calming or uplifting music

- ◆ Going for a nature walk
- ◆ Learning to say no and set personal boundaries
- ◆ Minimizing exposure to global news and social media (if this is a trigger for you)
- ◆ Trying guided relaxation techniques, like progressive muscle relaxation, imagery, or tai chi
- ◆ Practicing yoga or taking a stretching class
- ◆ Connecting with others regularly (especially people in your life who encourage and support you)

- **Hydration.** It shouldn't come as a surprise to you that water is your BFF when you're trying to lose weight.[67] Your hydration needs will be unique and variable, based on activity, metabolism, age, and more, but as a rough guideline, women and men should aim, respectively, for 2 and 3 liters (about 2¼ and 3¼ quarts) daily.
- **Low to Moderate Alcohol.** If we just think about satiety bang for your caloric buck, alcohol is a bit of a bust. Whereas carbs and protein provide 4 calories per gram, alcohol has 7 (almost as much as fat, which comes in at 9 calories per gram). However, unlike fat, carbs, and protein, alcohol's calories come without any satiety or nutrition perks at all.

  When you consume alcohol, your body prioritizes metabolizing and eliminating the toxic ethanol as quickly as it can. That means dietary fats, carbohydrates, and proteins get put on the metabolizing back burner and get stored as body fat while they wait their turn.[68]

  Alcohol also increases our appetite by increasing our hunger hormone ghrelin while decreasing the satiety hormone leptin.[69] Plus, it affects our brain's reward and pleasure neurotransmitters like dopamine, increasing the desire specifically for high-calorie, highly palatable foods.[70] So, we're more likely to stop for greasy "street meat" after the bar than go home and crunch on midnight carrots.

How much is too much? Moderate alcohol intake is defined by the American Heart Association as up to two drinks per day for men and up to one drink per day for women.[71] Keep in mind that your standard drink will add around 150 calories (and no fullness factor), so treat alcohol as similar to Naked Carbs. The Canadian guidelines (Canada's Guidance on Alcohol and Health) recently cracked down even harder after reviewing the expected health effects of weekly alcohol intake.[72] They've concluded that adults should be drinking no more than two standard alcoholic drinks per week, to reduce the risk of cancer, heart disease, and other severe alcohol-related consequences.

Overall, less is more with alcohol, but I'm never going to tell anyone to not have a celebratory glass of wine or summer spritzer on the patio. So, work those little pleasures into your week in moderation, monitor progress, and adjust as needed.

If you think you have a problem with alcohol consumption, I encourage you to seek outside support (consider the 24/7 SAMHSA National Helpline: 1-800-662-HELP [4357]). And if you don't drink alcohol, there's no reason to start (*not even for those antioxidants in wine!*).

## Wrapping Up the HCC for Weight Management

The weight-loss world is overwhelming AF. Every new diet contradicts the last you tried, each with its own set of persuasive before-and-afters, anecdotes, and carefully curated "evidence." The truth is, any diet or protocol that puts you in a calorie deficit can result in weight loss. The question you have to ask yourself is, *At what cost? Can I do this for the rest of my life? Do I feel healthy and happy, or depleted and depressed?* The best diet is the one that feels the most intuitive to you, and that's why my Hunger Crushing Combo has helped so many people on their journeys to a healthier happier life. Approach this next leg of your adventure with empathy, kindness, and curiosity. Collect data on how different Hunger Crushing Compounds make you feel, how different combos affect your results, and how this way of eating may feel different emotionally, psychologically, and socially as compared to every "diet" that came before it. Because this isn't just another diet. It's *your* diet uniquely designed to enhance your life and help you reach your goals. Make it work for you.

# CHAPTER 7

· · · · · · · · · · · · · · · · ·

# Flattening the Curve:
# HCC for Insulin Resistance,
# Diabetes & PCOS Management Goals

If you've been told your blood sugars are elevated or have been diagnosed with insulin resistance, prediabetes, diabetes, or polycystic ovary syndrome (PCOS), and you want to know how to manage those through nutrition, this is the chapter for you.

There are a number of factors at play when it comes to your risk of insulin resistance including genetics, inactivity, age, and stress, just to name a few. But excess body fat, particularly around the midsection, can play a pretty significant role. For that reason, the Hunger Crushing Combo Triangle and recommendations from the previous chapter on weight loss are all relevant for this population too. That said, there are unique nutrition considerations for insulin resistance that go far beyond the frustrating and often useless advice to *just lose some weight.* So, consider thumbing through Chapter 6, and using Chapter 7 as your extension pack!

## The HCC Formula for Insulin Resistance

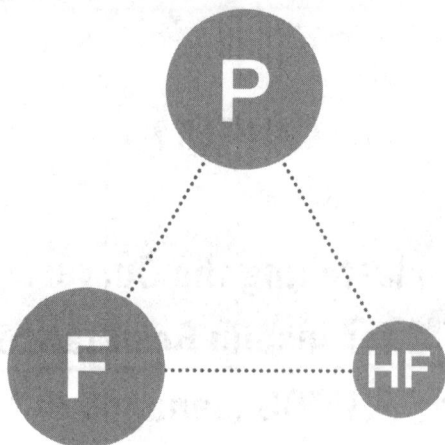

I know what you're expecting this section will lead with. *No. Carbs. Ever.*

Yeah . . . no, we're past that.

Since carbohydrates are the main contributor to blood sugar and insulin spikes, I appreciate that cutting them out completely seems like the most effective solution for folks with or at risk of type 2 diabetes. But managing insulin resistance isn't *just* about lowering blood sugars after any one given meal. It's about reducing the risk of type 2 diabetes, heart disease, obesity, neuropathy, and countless other chronic diseases that can severely interfere with quality of life.

Carbs don't *cause* diabetes, and when we're talking specifically about higher-fiber carbs, they can actually be protective. For example, a high-fiber, carbohydrate-rich diet has been shown to significantly improve postmeal blood sugars, insulin response, and cardiovascular risk factors. And while starting your day consistently with Cocoa Pebbles might not be advised, research suggests that low- or no-carb diets aren't necessarily the best choice for diabetes or blood sugar management either.[1] Now, of course, if you're content to live the rest of your life deconstructing sandwiches and scraping the toppings from your pizza crust, I love that journey for you. But there are a lot of blood sugar–stabilizing benefits to fiber-rich carbs, especially when combined with their HCC bosom buddy, protein (and some healthy fats)!

### Carbohydrates & Fiber

If you recall from Chapter 3, fiber (along with its sidekick, protein) is a major headliner when it comes to blood sugar management. It helps slow down the digestion of sugar and coats the intestinal lining, promoting a more leisurely release of glucose into the bloodstream. It feeds all our good gut bacteria their favorite prebiotic snacks, releasing short-chain fatty acids (SCFAs) and reducing inflammation. And it keeps us fuller longer, getting us through that three p.m. energy slump without three trips to the communal staff room doughnut box. *Honestly, I could write a Taylor Swift–style anthology of ode-to-fiber love songs, and still have content for the vault.*

As with our weight-loss recommendations, you'll want to aim for at least 6 to 12 grams of fiber at all meals and at least 3 to 6 grams at snacks. (See page 254 for visual portion cues.)

The timing of our fiber consumption in the meal may also offer a slight blood sugar–stabilizing edge. That is, if it makes sense, having a fiber-rich food *before* you consume Naked Carbs may help lower peak blood sugar by up to almost 50 percent (see the science of meal order, on page 82).[2] If you recall, however, the research isn't definitive on how much more advantageous it might be to consume veggies twenty minutes before rice, compared to simply enjoying Hunger Crushing Compounds *and* Naked Carbs in a normal mixed meal. So, this is *not* a recommendation to obsessively dissect your chicken Caesar wrap at the staff luncheon. But if you're given the option to start a meal with a fresh salad before diving into the pasta main, you may get an extra leg up on blood sugar control.

All fiber is helpful in some capacity for insulin resistance, but soluble fiber offers a unique edge by forming a gel in the gut to slow down gut transit, and thereby, sugar absorption.[3] And guess where soluble fiber is found? Plants, baby! In fact, any conversation about blood sugar management needs to start with plants, because fiber is only found in plant-based foods: fruits, veggies, nuts, seeds, whole grains, and legumes. Each of these food categories has its own unique super-powers when it comes to reducing or managing insulin resistance.

- **Fruit & Vegetables.** There are very few things that we can claim as "fact" in the world of nutrition, but the value of fruits and veggies is pretty much undisputed: for general good health, and specifically, for reducing the risk of type 2 diabetes.[4] Not only are they both great sources of fiber, but that fiber is bound in a food matrix with vitamins, minerals, and antioxidants that have incredible benefits for boosting insulin sensitivity, lowering inflammation, and fighting disease-causing oxidative damage. Notice I'm talking about veggies *and* fruit here. I get that a lot of us grew up in the Atkins era, with our moms leaving half a banana to collect fruit flies because it would be "too much sugar" to eat the whole thing. But according to a massive seven-year study on half a million adults, fresh fruit consumption is associated with significantly lower risk of diabetes, and among those with diabetes, lower risk of death and major vascular complications.[5] The more fruit, the lower the risk! Choose higher-fiber options (e.g., berries and pears) more often, and alternate colors (green, white, red, orange, yellow, blue, and purple) for the greatest range of health perks.
- **Whole Grains.** Whole grains are carb-rich foods like whole wheat, rye, oats, hulled barley, millet, and quinoa, which have all three parts of the natural grain intact: the bran, germ, and endosperm. When food manufacturers make "white" grains (e.g., white bread, white rice, white pasta, etc.), they're stripping the grain of its beneficial bran and germ. Tasty

(when we're talking classic PB&J on Wonder Bread), but it will never have the blood sugar–stabilizing benefits of the OG whole package. Choosing grains with the words "100% whole grain" as the first item in the ingredient list will yield the best blood sugar–lowering response.

Now, I'm not forgetting about other nutrient-dense plant foods. Nuts, seeds, and legumes are also fantastic sources of fiber, while offering dual citizenship with healthy fats and/or protein (and we will talk more about them in a hot minute).

**Protein**
Protein and fiber are quite the power couple when it comes to blood sugar management. Like fiber, protein slows the digestion and release of sugars into the blood, but also stimulates insulin to shunt those sugars into our hungry cells. It is the building block of muscle (a key consumer of blood glucose), and keeps us fuller longer (even when in a calorie deficit). Since the vast majority of folks with insulin resistance and/or type 2 diabetes may benefit from fat loss (particularly visceral fat loss), the general protein "dose" recommendations outlined on page 147 apply here, too: 20 to 35 grams per meal and 8 to 20 grams per snack, spread out throughout the day, for stable blood sugars and energy management. And remember, this isn't a militant fitness model prep diet. No one needs to be weighing out their egg whites to hit their protein goals. A "meal dose" is about the size of your palm for most lean animal protein and protein-dense plants like tofu, and the size of a fist for most other plant-based proteins like legumes and high-protein dairy. Most folks can delete their My Fitness Pal, and simply keep the visual cues on page 254 top of mind when building their plate.

Speaking of different sources of protein, research does consistently show that there are benefits, particularly for insulin resistance, to replacing animal proteins with plant-forward meals more often.[6]

According to one large meta-analysis, plant proteins (plus fermented dairy like yogurt) offer protection against type 2 diabetes; red and processed meats increase the risk; and lean options like poultry and fish have no effect.[7]

There are several reasons that plant-based proteins outperform meat for insulin resistance.[8] First, they're lower in saturated fat. Excess intake of saturated fat causes chronic inflammation, interferes with insulin signaling pathways, and increases fat accumulation in the liver and muscles, all of which contribute to insulin resistance.[9] One hundred grams of rib-eye steak has 10 grams of saturated fat, whereas the same portion of firm tofu has 1 gram. Mind the gap, my friends (*'cause she's quite a big gap*).

Second, plant-based proteins double as sources of fiber, a dual-citizen twofer deal you just can't get in poultry or beef. Remember that fiber and protein are coconspirators in blood sugar management: You get satiety and blood sugar–stabilizing benefits from both constituents, the muscle-building gains of protein, *and* the gut health perks of fiber.

Plant proteins also tend to be packaged with various phytochemicals and antioxidants that fight chronic inflammation, whereas animal proteins (particularly red and processed meats) contribute pro-inflammatory compounds like nitrosamines, advanced glycation end-products (AGEs), and heme iron (when consumed in excess).[10]

Based on this evidence, it's pretty clear that opting for more plant-based proteins is best for improving insulin sensitivity and lowering your risk of diabetes and complications. When choosing protein foods to build your HCC plate, choose plant proteins like these:

- Legumes, like lentils, chickpeas, black beans, green peas, and split peas
- Soy foods, like tofu, tempeh, and edamame
- Seitan, which is a meat alternative made from vital wheat gluten

Now, I want to make it clear that I am not suggesting you need to go fully vegan; it does not take a drastic diet change to see dramatic improvements in blood sugars. So, start with just one meat to meatless meal swap per week. That could be as intuitive as bean tacos instead of beef, or tofu curry instead of pork. Once you've gained a bit of confidence in your vegetarian cooking, try to swap out one more meal. Eventually, aim for less than two servings of red meat per week (and opt for lean cuts with minimal visible fat), and enjoy processed meats less frequently, on special occasions. In other words, say yes to a celebratory July 4 hot dog (with extra banana peppers, please!), but pass on the weekday BLT drive-through ritual.

### Healthy Fats for Insulin Resistance

If you did a side-by-side analysis of our HCC Triangle for weight loss vs. insulin resistance, you'll see that they're almost completely identical. But if we wanted to follow the playbook, you'd see that the focus on healthy fats is a little more pronounced on this side of the tracks. Here's why:

When healthy weight loss is our goal (and there aren't other major metabolic factors at play like diabetes), our top priority is to create a calorie deficit (and do it as effortlessly and enjoyably as possible). To do that, fat (being the most calorie-dense macro) and Naked Carbs (being the least satiating macro) are typically where we can dig.

The value of healthy fats, however, is amplified when blood sugar mismanagement is in play. Since chronic inflammation is one of the predominant catalysts to insulin resistance, focusing on anti-inflammatory healthy fats can directly improve your insulin sensitivity. If you recall from Chapter 1, we're talking predominantly about MUFAs (monounsaturated fats) and PUFAs (polyunsaturated fats), most notably our beloved omega-3s.

Omega-3s help reduce chronic inflammation in the body, which explains why research has found a strong correlation between higher omega-3 intakes and lower risk of type 2 diabetes.[11] Diets rich in mono-unsaturated fats also seem to be metabolically protective, and despite being calorie dense, are not associated with increased risk of weight gain![12] So, think like our friends in the Mediterranean Blue Zones by focusing on marine- and plant-based whole-food sources like fatty fish, nuts, seeds, avocados, and olives.

## What About the Saturated Fat in Dairy?

The relationship between dairy intake, insulin resistance, and diabetes is as complicated as Ross and Rachel's love story. Some studies suggest that consuming full-fat dairy products is associated with a lower risk of insulin resistance and type 2 diabetes; others, that only low-fat dairy products are beneficial; and the rest, that there's no significant impact either way. Overall, more research is needed, but here's what you need to know for your HCCs.

There are a myriad of different fatty acids in animal foods, but unlike red meat, for example, dairy is rich in short-chain fatty acids that make it less likely to contribute to chronic disease.[13] There's also a dense array of nutrients (e.g., protein, calcium, and other minerals) in dairy that contribute to the "whole food matrix" that affects how these fats are metabolized.[14] This is why our dairy dual citizens (e.g., yogurt, milk, and cheese) have more favorable impacts on health compared to more concentrated forms of dairy fat (e.g., butter and heavy cream).[15]

My take is not to fear dairy fat, but to focus on dual-citizen dairy fats like full-fat yogurt, cottage cheese, and cheese, that pack in blood sugar–stabilizing protein.

## HCC for PCOS

Polycystic ovary syndrome (PCOS) is a hormonal disorder affecting 4 to 20 percent of folks with ovaries.[16] Please note that for simplicity (and often to reflect the binary nature of scientific research), I will be using noninclusive language (i.e., women or females) when discussing PCOS, but I fully acknowledge that this section applies to many trans men and nonbinary people as well.

PCOS is characterized by irregular menstrual periods, excess androgen levels (a.k.a. male hormones, e.g., testosterone), and multiple cysts on the ovaries that can ultimately impair fertility. In fact, PCOS is the leading cause of female infertility.[17] As an infertility warrior myself, I know firsthand the frustration and devastation of struggling to conceive.

While not part of the official diagnostic criteria, insulin resistance is often a hallmark feature of PCOS, with more than half of folks with PCOS developing type 2 diabetes by age forty.[18] Elevated insulin levels also contribute to the symptoms of PCOS by stimulating the ovaries to produce more androgens, impairing fertility, and leading to other not-so-glamorous signature features like unwanted facial hair and weight gain. In fact, unwanted weight gain, or difficulty losing weight, is one of the biggest challenges I hear from folks with PCOS.

The Hunger Crushing Combo Triangle for PCOS is ultimately the same as what we would recommend for insulin resistance and/or weight loss, to help reduce the risk of type 2 diabetes, improve appetite regulation, reduce inflammation, and reach or maintain a healthy weight.

### Protein for PCOS

Protein is a cyster's BFF, with the ability to significantly reduce fasting insulin and insulin resistance, and support fat-loss goals.[19]

## Fiber for PCOS

In addition to improving insulin sensitivity and weight-loss outcomes, the role of fiber in supporting a healthy gut microbiome is paramount. Research suggests that the combination of high androgens and insulin resistance in PCOS can significantly increase the risk of gut dysbiosis.[20] Since an impaired gut microbiome may increase the risk of obesity, we want to focus on fueling the gut with high-fiber plants.

## Healthy Fats for PCOS

The evidence in support of a diet rich in omega-3 fats also appears to be helpful in managing PCOS symptoms, for all of the same reasons we discussed earlier concerning general insulin resistance and type 2 diabetes.[21] Omega-3s help combat the chronic inflammation that is characteristic of PCOS, improve insulin sensitivity, and reduce the risk of heart disease (which is at double the risk for folks with PCOS).[22] Some researchers even say the evidence of omega-3 benefits for women with PCOS is so strong that it should be considered a "novel drug" for PCOS patients.[23] The greatest dietary sources of omega-3 fats come from fatty fish, fish oils, flaxseeds, chia seeds, and walnuts.

### Should You Cut Out Dairy for PCOS?

The blogosphere is flush with recommendations for folks with PCOS to swear off dairy for life, pointing to its potentially inflammatory effects. But as with everything in nutrition, the research is conflicting and best practices are highly individualized. Generally speaking, full fat may have a real edge.

Dairy is a mixture of protein, carbohydrates (lactose), and fat. When we take away the fat (as we see with 0 percent or skim options), we're removing one of the two key blood sugar–buffering agents that help temper inflammation and insulin spikes. Skim

dairy also contains relatively greater concentrations of androgens and insulin-like growth factor (IGF-1), which increases oil
production and impairs ovarian function. This explains why some
research suggests that consuming fermented full-fat dairy options
over skim or low fat may actually have a protective effect against
infertility and hormone-related acne.[24] These effects may be small,
and your unique reactions to dairy may vary, so experiment to see
how your symptoms improve with different types and amounts
of dairy. And if the fat content doesn't seem to play a major role
(or you're lactose intolerant), no sweat! There are plenty of great
nondairy alternatives to explore. But the bottom line is, don't let
the dairy *fat* hold you back.

## Our Favorite HCC Foods for Insulin Resistance, Type 2 Diabetes, and PCOS

Research suggests certain HCC foods may offer a unique nutritional
edge, without denial or deprivation. So, in addition to all of those in
our weight-loss chapter, here are some additional faves:

- **Fatty Fish & Fish Oil.** Studies show that a diet rich in
  omega-3-rich fatty fish, like salmon, tuna, mackerel, halibut,
  and sardines, may help reduce inflammation, triglycerides,
  and insulin resistance.[25] To optimize your omega-3s from
  whole foods, the American Heart Association recommends
  eating two servings of fatty fish per week.[26]
- **Oats.** Oatmeal has taken a bit of a beating in the media
  over the past few years, with some anticarb and carnivore
  circles calling it the "worst breakfast you can eat." I respectfully disagree (*that title is firmly reserved for my dog's kib-
  ble*). The unique fiber in oats (beta-glucan) has been shown

to slow digestion, stabilize blood sugar, and offer powerful anti-inflammatory perks.[27] Compared to instant oats, steel-cut oats will always have an edge, because the minimal processing results in a slower, more tempered blood sugar rise.

- **Pears.** Pears have spent their life in the shadows of their more popular cousin, apples, but when it comes to insulin resistance, they are truly *elite*. Onc medium-size pear contains an impressive 5.5 grams of blood sugar–stabilizing fiber, which along with its unique cocktail of polyphenols, can help slow down carb digestion and absorption. Throw pears onto salad, into oats or yogurt, or simply eat them as part of a balanced snack.

- **Cruciferous Veggies and Leafy Greens.** Countless studies confirm that the more vegetables folks with diabetes consume, the better their blood sugar control.[28] Cruciferous and green vegetables, including spinach, kale, Brussels sprouts, broccoli, cauliflower, and Swiss chard, are exceptionally beneficial, thanks to their fusion of antioxidants, fiber, and phytochemicals. Taken together, these powerful plant components have been shown to help improve insulin sensitivity, appetite regulation, and inflammation management.[29] Try switching up the veggies you buy each week to boost antioxidant and fiber diversity and further optimize the anti-inflammatory effects.

- **Avocado.** The viral avocado toast trend might feel passé in the TikTok years, but when it comes to insulin resistance, these fruits are never going out of style. Avocados are a powerful dual citizen packing a whopping 10 grams of fiber and 19 grams of healthy fats (plus a bonus 3 grams of protein) per fruit.

- **Walnuts.** Nuts are a built-in Hunger Crushing Combo all on their own, with walnuts clocking in with the most significant dose of anti-inflammatory omega-3s. Tree nut consumption (including walnuts, almonds, hazelnuts, and pistachios) has been linked to improved blood sugar levels and lower risk of heart disease and death.[30] The most significant risk reduction seems to be when consuming at least 2 ounces of tree nuts per day (e.g., 12 to 15 walnut halves), so add them to salads, yogurt, and oats, or keep a little container in your purse for a crunchy midday snack![31]

- **Vinegar.** Start whipping up some tangy vinaigrettes, because adding vinegar to your daily routine may help temper those blood sugar spikes! We have some surprisingly strong evidence that the acetic acid in balsamic, malt, and cider vinegar, a.k.a. ACV (among other vinegars), can slow digestion, inhibit sugar digestion enzymes, improve satiety, and reduce the blood sugar response of a carb-containing meal.[32] Whip up a simple cider vinaigrette by combining equal parts ACV to extra-virgin olive oil, a squirt of grainy mustard, and salt and freshly ground black pepper to taste.

## HCC Example Day for Insulin Resistance, Diabetes & PCOS

Remember, folks with insulin resistance are not a homogenous group. Your calorie needs will be unique, and the amount of carbohydrates you can consume (or what you need to pair it with) to avoid a spike and crash will require some experimenting. So, for the love of avocado toast, don't turn this into a month-long meal plan. This is a mere example of what a day of balanced eating with insulin resistance might look like, keeping our HCC Triangle in mind.

Breakfast: Veggie omelet with whole-grain sourdough toast
Snack: Small bowl of overnight oats with protein powder and berries

Lunch: Bountiful kale salad with roasted salmon, walnuts, wild rice, and cider vinaigrette

Snack: Cheese stick and sliced pear

Dinner: High-fiber legume pasta noodles with chicken breast and two heaping handfuls of sautéed vegetables or greens

Snack: Small bowl chocolate chia pudding made with Greek yogurt with berries

## Supplements to Consider for Insulin Resistance, Diabetes & PCOS

Food plays an integral role in meal-to-meal blood sugar management and long-term insulin sensitivity. But I'm all about ways to alleviate the mental burden of eating "perfectly" for health, which is where sometimes medication (read on) and/or supplements can come into play. Here's a list of some popular blood sugar–balancing options (and my thoughts on whether they're worth the hype):

- **Berberine.** Berberine is often described as "nature's Ozempic" (*a bit of false advertising, if you ask me, but that's a rant for another day*). It's a bioactive compound found naturally in a number of plants that "works" by naturally increasing production and release of GLP-1. Yep, the same hormone that GLP-1 agonists like Ozempic utilize to turn their blood sugar and weight management tricks. One systematic review and meta-analysis concluded that berberine supplementation (0.9 to 2.4 grams per day) reduced fasting glucose by 0.82 mmol/l and HbA1c by 0.63 percent.[33] For reference, Ozempic lowers fasting glucose by around 2.0 mmol/l and A1c by around 1 percent, so though berberine certainly is not a replacement or equivalent, the results are still promising.[34] That said, most of the data we do have on berberine is of low methodological value, so we are a long way from confidently recommending patients swap their medication for supplements. As always, speak to your doctor about your unique needs.

- **Myo-inositol.** Similar to B vitamins, this naturally occurring compound acts as a secondary messenger in insulin-signaling pathways. Research on folks with insulin resistance, diabetes, PCOS, and other metabolic disorders suggests that adding 2 grams twice per day may help improve insulin sensitivity and promote regular ovulation in women with PCOS.[35] It may also help manage some of the other pesky side effects of PCOS like acne and excess hair growth. When choosing a myo-inositol supplement, look for one that is combined with a small amount of d-chiro-inositol in a ratio of 40:1.[36]

- **Resveratrol.** Recent research on this powerful antioxidant (found in red wine and berries) has found that resveratrol supplements significantly reduced testosterone, luteinizing hormone, and dehydroepiandrosterone sulfate (DHEAS) in women with PCOS, three markers associated with excess body hair, acne, and infertility.[37] While the studies used between 800 and 1,500 mg per day, we don't have insight on best practice for dosage, so always work with a dietitian to determine whether it's right for you.

- **Omega-3s.** You've seen me rhapsodize on the benefits of fatty fish more than once in the previous chapters, but if you're vegetarian, vegan, or just *can't* deal with the potent perfume of a salmon steak, an omega-3 supplement is worth considering. Omega-3 supplements have been shown to be promising for insulin resistance and diabetes, with a small effect on fasting glucose and a moderate effect on insulin resistance.[38] And we see similar benefits for the PCOS population as well.[39]

We ideally want to aim for 0.5 to 1 gram of combined EPA and DHA omega-3s daily, which could be met with either two or three servings of fatty fish per week, a third party–tested supplement, or a combination of both.[40] Some individuals may benefit from higher doses of supplements, so speak to your doctor about your unique benefit and risk considerations.

- **Supplemental Fiber.** We all should try to get our roughage from foods first (let's eat those plants!), but if you're struggling to get your fill, adding a scoop of soluble fiber before a meal has been shown to help flatten the blood sugar curve.[41] Popular fiber types include psyllium, inulin, partially hydrolyzed guar gum, flaxseeds, cellulose, and wheat dextrin (just to name a few). The daily dosage of fiber supplements can vary greatly by brand and fiber variety, so check the label, start with one-quarter of the suggested scoop size, and work your way up.

- **Mulberry Extract.** Rich in anti-inflammatory antioxidants, mulberry extract has been shown to help reduce blood glucose and insulin.[42] While most studies use a dose around 250 mg per day, we still haven't determined an optimal protocol for blood sugar management, so always work with a dietitian if considering adding it to your stack.

## Other Blood Sugar Management Tools & Considerations

Managing insulin resistance, reducing the risk of diabetes, and quieting the unpleasant side effects of PCOS is far more nuanced than just popping a pill or eating more fish, and it's certainly more complicated than the blanket recommendation to just go lose some weight. Let's review some other key tools to help you improve your overall metabolic health.

- **Exercise.** If you recall from Chapter 7, exercise offers one of the greatest ROIs for blood sugar management. Research suggests that walking for just thirty minutes after a high-sugar meal can reduce peak blood sugar by 13 percent and total glucose response by 10 percent![43] Even a three-minute quickie exercise "snack" can help! Ideally, we want to hit a minimum of 150 to 300 minutes per week of moderate-intensity activity, 75 to 150 minutes per week of vigorous-intensity aerobic physical activity, or an equivalent combination. We also need at least two days per week of resistance training to build more muscle mass to sop up the excess sugar in our blood.

- **Eating Like a King at Breakfast.** If you're in a calorie deficit, it doesn't matter what time of the day you consume your food. That said, eating like a king at breakfast and a pauper at dinner (and the hours that follow) may have some metabolic advantages. Thanks to our natural circadian rhythm, insulin sensitivity is higher during daylight than it is after the sun goes down. In other words, our cells are just more effectively able to absorb and utilize carbs earlier in the day. This makes total sense when you consider that our body would likely benefit more from those energizing carbs when we're active during daytime vs. when we're ass-in-recliner marathoning out *Desperate Housewives* at night. This means that you'll likely see a lower blood sugar spike if you eat your toast at nine a.m. than you would by eating that same piece of bread at nine p.m. Get the most out of your day with a hearty, well-balanced breakfast that includes protein *and* high-fiber carbs.

- **Second Meal Effect.** Research has found that when you consume carbs at two consecutive meals, the blood sugar spike after the second meal is less pronounced, even when the carb load is exactly the same![44] Basically, the first meal "wakes up" the pancreas to get to work faster so it's more prepared to pump out insulin for meal two. When planning how to spread out carbs in the day, it may be advantageous to focus them in our breakfast meal (when our insulin sensitivity is greatest), and our lunch (when our body is better "primed" to respond), tapering off for dinner and evening snacks.

- **Sleep Hygiene.** In Chapter 6, we covered the association between poor sleep and weight gain that indirectly impacts metabolic health, but skimping on shut-eye can affect blood sugar *directly*, as well.[45] Because deep REM sleep helps boost insulin sensitivity the next morning, studies have linked inadequate sleep duration, poor sleep quality, and sleep disorders like insomnia and sleep apnea to type 2 diabetes and PCOS.[46] Folks, sleep is sexy, don't let hustle culture tell you otherwise, so aim for seven to eight hours of restful sleep per night (and check out pages 159–161 for sleep hygiene tips).[47]

- **Stress Management.** There is a clear and undisputed link between stress and the risk of diabetes thanks to the role of cortisol in glucose mismanagement and unhealthy coping strategies (e.g., smoking, drinking, or eating less-nutritious foods).[48] While just "not being stressed" isn't helpful, and sometimes the thought of adding a stress-relieving practice to your already full to-do list is also well . . . *stressful*, the long-term capital gains may be worth your while. One review of the literature found that mindfulness stress-reducing activities and yoga reduced fasting blood glucose by about 17 percent in those with diabetes.[49] Find an activity that helps you better manage your stress, whether that be meditation, journaling, deep breathing, talking to a friend, or working with a mental health professional. If it feels like self-care, it will absolutely help.

- **Limit Sweetened Drinks.** High-sugar beverages, like soda, sweet tea, sweetened coffee drinks, and fruit juice, are consistently associated with an increased risk of type 2 diabetes.[50] When plain water gets boring, you can try infusing it with some fresh lemon or cucumber slices, or opt for herbal teas and unsweetened seltzers.

## What About Artificial Sweeteners?

Artificial or nonnutritive sweeteners (a.k.a. the blue, yellow, and pink packets at the coffee shop, and the base of most diet and "zero-calorie" drinks) provide the sweetness so many people crave without the added sugar or calories. There's been a lot of back and forth on artificial sweeteners, with "clean eating" enthusiasts pointing to research linking heavy artificial sweetener consumption with insulin resistance and obesity.[51] But it's important to point out that this could partially be due to what we call "reverse causality": the reality that many folks who consume these sweeteners do so *because* they already have or are at risk of metabolic disease and are taking steps to reduce their sugar consumption by choosing something like Coke Zero over full-sugar Coke.

There may still be some validity to these concerns as some evidence suggests that the sweetness of artificial sweeteners may trigger a small release of insulin and may also negatively affect the gut microbiome.[52] But I wouldn't freak out if you use a little of the artificially sweet stuff in your coffee or enjoy the occasional diet soda. Every food and nutrition choice requires a risk-benefit analysis. And while the research we have on humans and the dangers of sweeteners is largely exploratory, contradictory, and far from conclusive, there is *good* evidence that swapping out sugar in favor of artificial sweeteners can be an effective weight-loss

and blood sugar–management strategy.[53] Now, that's not a prescription on my part to drink or consume *more* of them. I suggest
treating all (naturally or artificially) sweet beverages similarly by
limiting consumption and, more often, choosing naturally sweet
whole foods like fruit, which come bound up with Hunger Crushing Compounds.

- **Avoid or Limit Alcohol and Cigarette Smoking.** Whereas
  alcohol can cause a transient drop in blood sugar, smoking
  and heavy alcohol use can further inflammation, and ultimately promote insulin resistance.[54] When it comes to alcohol specifically, unless you're a dirty martini fan (*I personally
  just can't get into olive-flavored booze*), alcohol tends to come
  neatly packaged with juice, syrups, sodas, or the carbohydrates inherent in the liqueurs, wine, or beer. Work with your
  doctor on quitting smoking, and if you do choose to imbibe
  an occasional drink, be mindful of mixers and lean more
  heavily on sparkling water, citrus, herbs, and bitters for flavor.
- **Don't Go Crazy on Caffeine.** I have a general rule in nutrition counseling, and that is I never tell people to change how
  they like their coffee. For a lot of people (*myself included*),
  the morning coffee (or tea) ritual is sacred. It shall not be
  F'ed with (*unless, of course, you want to interact with a pissy
  Abbey all day*). And coffee isn't necessarily a no-no for diabetes. Actually, the research is rather confusing. In short, while
  caffeine does appear to *transiently* increase blood sugar levels and impair insulin sensitivity, there is also a lot of good
  research suggesting that regular coffee consumption may
  reduce the risk of diabetes and prediabetes long-term.[55] Keep
  in mind, we're talking about black coffee (without sugar), not
  a java chip Frappuccino with extra whipped cream. I'm also

not suggesting you use this little fun factoid as a reason to jitter yourself through your own personal pot of coffee every day. Pushing yourself past your own personal optimal "Gold-ilocks dose" can increase symptoms of anxiety, impair sleep, and potentially even increase heart disease risk.[56] But if you love your coffee ritual, and it's not negatively affecting you in other ways, rest assured it's absolutely dietitian (and mompre-neur) approved.

- **Blood Sugar–Management Medication.** The details of diabetes medication are outside the scope of this book, but I think it's important to note that leaning on medication to help manage your blood sugars is *not* a moral failure. It isn't taking the "easy way out." The most common antidiabetic medications include metformin, GLP-1 agonists (see page 150 for nutrition tips if using these medications), and insulin therapy. Speak to your doctor about whether medication is appropriate for you.

## Wrapping Up the HCC for Diabetes and Insulin Resistance

We want our bodies to run a pretty tight ship when it comes to insu-lin and blood sugar management. And while our genetics will make this easier or more challenging, the Hunger Crushing Combo is one of the most impactful tools we have for supporting whatever hand we got dealt. It's always ideal to work one-on-one with a registered dietitian to help manage your insulin resistance, but until you can, my HCC is a safe, evidence-based place to start.

# CHAPTER 8

. . . . . . . . . . . . . . . .

# Strength and Endurance: HCC for Sports & Fitness Nutrition

Whether you're training for your fourth Spartan race, embarking on a couch-to-5K program, or consider yourself more of a Weekend Warrior, the HCC can be applied to your specific athletic needs.

Exercise can *very* crudely be divided into two main camps: (1) strength and power activities, and (2) endurance and cardio-based activities. Each offers a distinct form of challenge to your body that targets different areas of your health and fitness. The main objective of strength or power training (e.g., lifting weights, exercise machines, doing bodyweight exercises, or using resistance bands) is to increase muscle mass, strength, and power, whereas endurance exercise (e.g., jogging, playing tennis, or joining your gym pals to kick some butt at morning boot camp) is more geared toward boosting your cardiovascular stamina.

All activity needs adequate fuel, but proper nutrition is particularly critical when we're working toward specific fitness or sports-related goals. When our activity levels go up, so too do our calorie and specific nutrient needs. But before you pull out your phone to re-download that calorie-counting app you deleted after reading Part 1, I want you to consider a gentler way. As with previous chapters, I will be sharing the evidence-based calculations for the different macronutrients as "background" knowledge. And while nutrition often does need to be a bit more intentional in more active folks, you don't need to count every bite. The beauty of this framework is that once you've collected enough data on your own body's response to food and activity, it can all eventually operate in the background, shifting you toward a pattern of eating that fuels you and your activity best.

## The HCC Formula for Muscle Gain, Strength & Power Activities

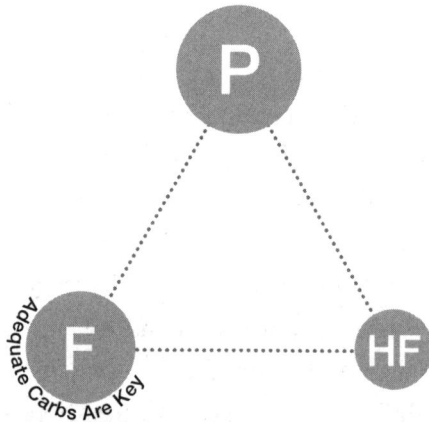

Different activities can require wildly variable nutrient inputs. If you're training for a specific event or sport, it's always advised to work with a dietitian trained in sports nutrition to determine your unique needs. But when we look at best practices for muscle growth, the stereotype does ring true: Protein is kinda a big deal. What might surprise you, however, is that carbs are not that far behind it, followed by fat and then fiber. Yep, when we're looking to bulk, we actually don't necessarily *want* to crush our hunger. At least not until our muscles have gotten their fill.

### Protein for Muscle Gain

Resistance or strength training exercise may account for about 87 percent of muscle maintenance and growth, but adequate protein is imperative to getting the most out of your time in the gym.[1] Resistance training triggers our muscle cells to take up more amino acids (the building blocks of protein) to help grow and strengthen the muscle fibers.[2] This requires consistent training to, or close to, the point of muscle failure, along with recovery and rest time (which is actually when muscles grow), stress management, and, of course, adequate calories and protein.

Naturally, pop culture references of greased-up muscle men grunting in the gym might lead you to believe that to get results, you need to pound back a full boiled chicken and a carton of raw eggs every day. *I don't want to yuck someone's yum, but let's not get crazy here.* In reality, protein goals for muscle gains aren't actually that different than for weight loss: 1.6 to 2.2 grams per kilogram (2¼ pounds) of body weight per day (adjusted for a BMI of 30 if considered in the "obese" category), or 20 to 30 percent of calories from protein.[3] Keep in mind that the higher end of this range (2.2 g) is not necessarily *better* or more *optimal* than the lower (1.6 g), and where you land will depend greatly on your unique needs. But if you read Chapter 6, you'll recall the research on weight loss suggests around 30 percent of calories from protein, which does seem to be even *more* than the 20 percent minimum for muscle growth. *Whaaaat?* The difference comes down to the fact that when weight loss is the primary goal, your daily calorie intake will be lower to create a calorie deficit than it would be when you're maintaining your weight or gaining muscle. To demonstrate the potential difference between these seemingly similar (but actually very different) goals, if your baseline needs were 2,300 calories, a weight-loss diet may recommend 1,800 calories and 135 grams of protein, whereas a muscle gain diet may recommend 2,700 calories and 135 grams of protein. See: similar total protein requirements, but very different distributions.

And speaking of distributions, let's talk about **protein timing**. Gym bros have long stressed the importance of the "anabolic window": the suggestion that there is a short period (typically thirty minutes to an hour) after exercise, during which the body is allegedly more "accepting" of protein for muscle recovery and growth. But recent research suggests that the window is more like four hours *around* your workout, and that muscle protein synthesis can extend even twenty-four to forty-eight hours postexercise.[4] That means you can get yourself home, have a shower, and *then* eat your eggs.

As for **protein spacing**, most research suggests that we can most efficiently utilize a certain amount of protein at once for building muscle, 0.3 to 0.4 g of protein per kilogram (2¼ pounds) of body weight per meal.[5,6] This is why most nutrition experts recommend spreading your protein among four or five meals and snacks to yield 20 to 35 grams of protein per meal (what I described as a "meal dose" on page 171).[7] But a recent study revealed that even when participants were given a whopping 100-gram portion of protein in one meal, it didn't just get converted to fat when their body hit the 25-gram mark; the muscle protein synthesis was just prolonged over more time.[8]

What this tells us is that achieving our total daily protein needs is *the most important* consideration for muscle growth. Spacing and timing can also contribute but are predominantly advantageous for satiety, blood sugar management, and energy-stabilizing perks.

## Are High-Protein Diets Bad for You?

While I have been over here singing the praises of protein, there have long been concerns that a high-protein diet may be "dangerous" for your kidneys. So, is your double–egg white omelet going to be your demise? Naw, you're good. Although a high-protein diet can increase the workload of the kidneys (as they are in charge of clearing out any protein by-products), as long as your kidneys are healthy, they're more than able to do their job.[9] Of course, if you do have decreased kidney function, you should speak to your doctor or dietitian about the amount of protein you can safely consume.

As for sources of protein, there are some important distinctions and guidelines to consider if muscle growth is your goal. Animal-based proteins (e.g., eggs, chicken, beef, fish) are all high-quality complete proteins (see Chapter 1 for a refresher course on complete proteins), whereas most major plant-based proteins (with the exception of soy, quinoa, amaranth, buckwheat, hemp, chia, nutritional yeast, and mycoprotein such as that found in Quorn) are incomplete. Good news for my plant-based friends: Your body is really freaking smart. Not only is there a variety of plant-based proteins that are rich in key muscle-building amino acids (e.g., soy, pea, lentils, chickpeas, and hemp seeds), but your body keeps a little reservoir of amino acids at the ready to employ for building muscle and other tissues. And research comparing high-protein vegan and omnivore diets confirms that muscle gains are comparable when macros and training protocols are held equal.[10] If you want to eat a vegan or vegetarian diet, the key is to consume a variety of plant-based proteins to cover all your amino acid bases.

## Carbohydrates & Fiber for Muscle Gain

Protein may be essential for muscle growth, but carbs are still our body's preferred source of energy for exercise, whether it's a sweaty HIIT class, long bike ride, or an iron-pumping session in the gym. It's therefore important that we consume carbs to replenish our muscle glycogen stores (a.k.a. our storage carbohydrates) that get depleted after a heavy lifting sesh. If we blow through the carbs in our preworkout meal *and* deplete our glycogen reserve tank, we're just not likely going to have the chutzpah to push ourselves to the point where muscle fibers can tear and repair. Carbs are also protein sparing. When enough carbs (and total calories) are available, our body is less likely to break down muscle protein to be used as energy, leaving that protein to do what it does best: get dem gains! Our clinical best practice guidelines for bodybuilding and muscle growth still do suggest consuming 1.2 grams of carbohydrates per kilogram (2¼ pounds) of body weight every hour (for around 4 hours) after training, to support training intensity and optimize muscle glycogen recovery.[11] For a 135-pound adult, that would be about 72 grams of carbs or 1½ cups of cooked white rice. And, yes, I said white rice. A Naked Carb *gasp*. And it has to do with fiber.

Okay, okay, I know this seems wacky. I've spent all these pages waxing poetic about my romantic tryst with fiber. And no matter what your body composition goal, fiber is incredibly important. But when that mountain of raw kale inevitably edges out our chicken or fish (and bloats us up like Wonka's blueberry girl), we're going to have a hard time meeting our protein and calorie needs. We also know that fiber can blunt the insulin response. This is great if you're trying to manage your blood sugars, but not ideal if you want to drive protein and carbohydrates from your postworkout meal into your tired muscles super-duper stat.

Bottom line: Carbs (both Naked and high-fiber varieties) can be a useful tool for helping fuel more rigorous training sessions, support recovery, and spare muscle from being broken down as fuel. Research generally suggests at least 3 grams of carbohydrates per kilogram (2¼ pounds) of body weight per day for gaining muscle and strength, plus the typical 25 to 38 grams of fiber per day.[12] That would equate to *at least* 180 grams of carbs per day for a 135-pound individual or between 45 and 65 percent of their calories from carbs.[13]

The key is choosing higher-*carb* fiber sources and fiber-protein dual citizens, whenever possible. When you are thinking about carbs for building muscle, think about choosing such foods as oats, quinoa, sweet potatoes, apples, berries, chickpeas, and lentils more often.

### Healthy Fats for Muscle Gain

There is no question that getting adequate fat in the diet is important for brain health, cellular function, and hormone production, including muscle-supporting hormones like testosterone. And this does spill over into its role in bulking as well by increasing growth factors that support muscle growth.[14]

That said, there's only so much we should need to fuss over in life, and how many grams of fat you're getting is just not it. If you're consuming adequate calories to meet your muscle growth needs (and you're not intentionally choosing only fat-free foods), fat can be an afterthought. When it comes to healthy fats, aim to include some higher-fat protein sources like salmon, tuna, eggs, hemp hearts, and full-fat Greek yogurt (a.k.a. some of our favorite dual citizens!) into your daily menu.

## HCC Example Day for Muscle Gain, Strength & Power Activities

Bodybuilding culture can admittedly seem at odds with our food freedom philosophy. It often appears militant, repetitive, and bland AF. And while there's no denying that professional athletes may need to be more mindful about specific macros, it doesn't have to run your life. Rather than obsessively counting every gram of protein that you might get in a thin smear of hummus, keep the visual cues from page 254 top of mind. Here's an example of how our hypothetical adult might space out their daily protein for optimal gains:

> Breakfast: Protein oats made with oatmeal, whipped egg whites, hemp hearts, and banana
>
> Snack: Protein shake with peanut butter and jam on whole-grain toast
>
> Lunch: Taco power bowl with ground chicken taco meat, black beans, rice, tomatoes, guacamole, and shredded cabbage
>
> Snack: Bowl of popcorn and a handful of shelled edamame
>
> Dinner: Beef and broccoli stir-fry with teriyaki noodles and cashews
>
> Snack: Bowl of cottage cheese with sour cherries and honey

## The HCC Formula for Endurance Activities

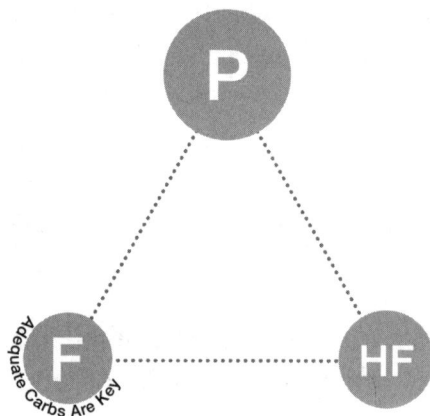

P

F        HF

Adequate Carbs Are Key

Endurance sports require cardiovascular stamina, aerobic capacity, and a sustained physical effort over an extended period of time. We're talking long-distance running, cycling, and swimming, as well as team sports that require long practices or such activities as hockey, lacrosse, soccer, and cheerleading. And while the protein requirements are exceptionally high here, the most important nutritional consideration for endurance activity is *not* a Hunger Crushing Compound. Yep, it's time for a much-needed ode to carbs.

### Carbohydrates & Fiber for Endurance

Carbs are the body's preferred fuel source during exercise. After using up the carbs consumed immediately pretraining, we ramp up our use of stored glucose (glycogen) to fuel our training. After 90 to 120 minutes of continuous exercise, those stores run dry, which is when athletes run the risk of "bonking" or "hitting the wall" as the body scrambles to come up with an alternative, less-efficient energy source (that is, protein or fat). The goal is to spare precious glycogen in the liver and keep a steady influx of carbs available to our muscles, so we can perform harder, longer sessions. And to do that, we often like to reach for lower-fiber, easily digestible carbs (yep, Naked Carbs) before, during, and immediately after exercise.

- **Carb Types & Timing.** How many carbs you need to support your training or activity depends on intensity, duration, and individual metabolic responses. That said, best practice suggests that your average one- to three-hour endurance activity would require a daily intake of 3 to 10 grams of carbs per kilogram (2¼ pounds) of body weight, making up 45 to 55 percent for men, and 55 to 65 percent of most women's total calories.[15] For our hypothetical 135-pound female, that's 180 to 600 grams of carbs per day. But it's how those carbs are distributed (and in what form) that really matters.

  In the HCC model, we use the terms "Naked Carbs" and "HCC Fiber-Rich Carbs" to describe carb types, but the sports world usually classifies them as "simple" or "complex." Simple carbs are more quickly digested because they're low in fiber and made up of one or two sugar molecules bound together, such as higher-sugar, lower-fiber fruit like bananas, grapes, mangoes, raisins, or foods with added sugars. Complex carbs are made of three or more sugar molecules and generally are rich in fiber, starch, or both, so they usually take longer to digest. Examples would include whole grains like oats, hulled barley, or quinoa; legumes like beans or lentils; and starchy vegetables like sweet potatoes, corn, or peas. You really don't need to overthink it too much; with sports nutrition specifically, the "best" foods for you depend mostly on your unique needs and response.

Let's start with your **pretraining fuel.** If there's time for a full meal one to four hours before activity, you'll want to build a balanced plate made predominantly of "complex" carbohydrates with a bit of fiber and lean protein, and a smaller amount of fat. The closer you are to game time, the less fiber, fat, and protein you actually want. Some people may prefer to train fasted (with no carbs on board), which is fine if it works for you, but if your activity lasts any longer than ninety minutes, it's likely to hurt your performance.

- **Immediately before** an endurance activity, a lot of folks like to lean on simple or Naked Carbs for fast-acting energy, but working in some "complex" carbs can also be useful, particularly when there's also a weight-management goal in place. That said, this is *not* the time for a bowl of farty high-fiber, low-carbohydrate cauliflower or a greasy cheeseburger, because gas, abdominal pain, and the overwhelming urge to poop are not going to help you beat your best time. So, it's always a good idea to trial different carb sources to determine what is best tolerated and most likely to help you perform your best. Now is also the time to get in your hydration with either water or a sports drink (see our Supplements section on page 203).

- **During exercise,** top-ups of fluid and simple Naked Carbs may be necessary to prevent glycogen depletion and a big bad bonk, especially if you're training for over ninety minutes and want to maintain good performance throughout your session. Best practices suggest getting in around 30 to 60 grams of high glycemic index simple Naked Carbs per hour from sources like a ripe banana, sports drinks, gels, or chews.[16] If it's an option, spreading your carbs into smaller consistent ten- to fifteen-minute snack intervals that keep your blood sugar levels relatively consistent throughout the activity are better than one or two bigger loads that could result in digestion distress.[17] Now, let's say you made it past the finish line (congrats!), but it's not quite time for that much-needed nap.

- **Fueling your body *after*** endurance exercise is a crucial act of self-care and recovery. Consuming carbs immediately postexercise can significantly improve recovery and performance in subsequent sessions.[18] So, think of your postactivity carb meal as the actual final leg of your marathon or race (*except this one can be completed on your couch!*). Endurance athletes should aim for about 1.2 grams of carbs per kilogram (2¼ pounds) of body weight within thirty minutes of the big push (so for a 135-pound woman, about two bananas or 1⅓ cups of rice), and to repeat with another carb "dose" every hour for four to five hours, to replenish those glycogen stores.

Okay, *now* you can nap.

### Protein for Endurance

At this point, it seems clear that the star of the show for endurance sports is unequivocally carbs. That doesn't mean we throw our HCC framework out the window. The protein needs of an endurance athlete are also very high, ideally aiming for around 1.8 grams of protein per kilogram (2¼ pounds) of body weight or 15 percent of total calories, whichever is the greater amount.

Timing matters with protein too. The most important consideration is to spread out protein evenly throughout the day, to help maximize muscle protein synthesis and optimize recovery and adaptations to your training.[19] At least three to four hours before a training session, include a "meal dose" (see page 147) of protein, or 20 to 35 grams. If you have a source of protein within one to two hours of training, make it a "half" to "full dose" of quickly digesting protein like whey protein powder, egg whites, chicken, or Greek yogurt, so it's not sitting in your stomach, jostling around, while you're on the move. Again, experiment ahead of time to see what foods, portions, and timing work best for you. During exercise, you can likely stick to carbs unless you're doing a long bout of activity over three hours long. Finally, following your activity, you'll want another "full dose" to help replace any protein you used as fuel during exercise, repair all those micro muscle tears, and promote the building of new proteins like mitochondria.

**Healthy Fats for Endurance**
Healthy fats definitely take a back seat when training for endurance. In fact, we want to avoid fat in close proximity to or during training, to reduce the risk of bloating or gastrointestinal distress midactivity, and to ensure that the mobilization of those much-needed carbs isn't handicapped or slowed down. That said, dietary fat can play a protective role in supporting healthy hormonal balance for women, and anti-inflammatory omega-3 fats specifically may help support recovery. We therefore have to just be a little more strategic and intentional about choosing anti-inflammatory healthy fats (e.g., salmon, nuts, seeds, and avocado) most often, and working them in *around* our heavy training or activity days, to meet our needs.

## HCC Example Day for Endurance

The best foods for engaging in an endurance sport or activity are going to be highly individualized, and figuring out the best foods to fuel your activity will take experimentation and practice. So, use this as inspiration, ideally while working with a dietitian to craft the best game day plan for you:

Breakfast: Bowl of oatmeal, raisins, and almonds with hard-boiled eggs

Pretraining Snack: Whole-grain toast with almond butter and banana

Midtraining Fuel (if needed): Ripe banana or raisins as needed, plus sips of water and electrolyte drinks

Posttraining Snack: Protein shake and banana

Lunch: Sandwich with chicken, avocado, and vegetables, with sweet potato fries

Dinner: Spaghetti lentil bolognese with side salad

Snack: Whole-grain crackers with garlic, herb, and cottage cheese dip

## Favorite Foods for Sports Nutrition

There are no "magic" #fitspo foods that are going to put you at the top of your game, but these beloved staples in the fitness community may be worth working into rotation:

- **Bananas.** Superripe bananas are often regarded as a perfect portable package of nutrition for fueling pre-, during, and posttraining. They are a rich source of quick-digesting simple carbs and a great source of critical electrolytes like magnesium and potassium. Whereas greener bananas are high in prebiotic fiber and resistant starch, and better for blood sugar management throughout the day away from training, ripe bananas offer quicker, more efficient energy and are less likely to cause gastrointestinal distress.

- **Raisins.** Portable, affordable, and a concentrated source of simple carbohydrates, raisins are another fantastic pre-, during, or postworkout snack. And like the equally accessible banana, they're absolutely evidence based.[20] One study comparing raisins and a sports gel supplement before an hour-long cycling session found that the unassuming raisin offered the same outcomes for performance, blood sugar, and fat-burning levels as the supplement![21] Raisins are a great base for a shelf-stable energy mix, and are fantastic toppers for oats, Greek yogurt, or cottage cheese.

- **Dairy.** Dairy provides all essential amino acids necessary for muscle repair and growth, with its two main forms, casein and whey, offering distinct benefits.[22] Whey protein is quickly digested and absorbed, making it ideal for preworkout meals and postworkout recovery. Casein protein, on the other hand, digests more slowly so as to provide a steady release of amino acids over several hours. Dairy is also loaded with other exercise supporting nutrients like electrolytes (e.g., potassium, calcium, and magnesium), phosphorus, and B vitamins. And different dairy-based foods offer different perks. One study found that combining Greek yogurt with resistance training significantly improved strength, muscle thickness, and fat-free mass, while reducing body fat better than a carbohydrate-based placebo.[23] Alternatively, cottage cheese is a classic bodybuilding bedtime snack because the main protein, casein, helps reduce muscle breakdown and enhance protein synthesis while fasting overnight.[24] Add milk, cottage cheese, or Greek yogurt to smoothies, pancakes or muffin recipes; or use as a base for nutrient-rich breakfast bowls.

- **Eggs.** Muscle-man archetype Arnold Schwarzenegger famously claimed that, in his glory days, he was eating *fifteen eggs a day*. And as excessive and tedious as that sounds, his ritual was at least *somewhat* grounded in truth. With 7 grams of protein per egg, and key muscle-supporting nutrients (e.g., cholesterol, vitamin D, and B vitamins), eggs are like a muscle-building supplement in a perfect little package. For a double-protein experience, try scrambling a scoop of cottage cheese into your eggs!

- **White Rice.** White rice is a high-GI, fast-absorbing carb that the body can use for immediate fuel, to store as glycogen for the next big push, or to spare muscle from being used as fuel. And because it isn't high in fiber, it's unlikely to cause gas, bloating, or urgency during a heavy training session. Because nobody wants *the runs* when they're actually trying to, um . . . run.

## Supplements to Consider for Fitness & Sports Goals

If there was ever a population who should consider supplementing, it's this one. Nutrient needs are high, the right macro split is more critical to hit, and most folks have to choose between spending time in the kitchen to pan-fry *another* chicken breast, or spending time training or in the gym. Supplements can help make fueling your body for the activities you love easier and more intuitive, and assist you in achieving greater balance in life outside your fitness goals! Here are some of the most commonly used additions to consider in your stack.

- **Protein Powder.** The protein needs of anyone training to increase endurance, strength, or muscle mass are relatively high, so protein powder is and always will be a fitness staple. Whey protein (from dairy) is considered the gold standard because it contains all of the essential amino acids, is rich in the most important muscle-building amino acid, leucine, and is most similar to human skeletal muscle. It is also rapidly digested and metabolized into individual amino acids, to be able to feed those freshly worked hangry muscles stat.

Unfortunately, a lot of folks find that whey protein can cause digestive distress and other unpleasant side effects like acne. It's also not appropriate for those who choose to avoid animal products. This is where high-quality plant-based protein supplements can come into play, particularly those that utilize a combination of protein sources and/or added amino acids, like leucine. Plant protein is naturally much lower in leucine than whey, so it's advantageous to look for a protein brand that has at least 2 grams of leucine to fill the gap. (This is exactly why we added leucine to my Neue Theory protein powder, and others should really be following suit.)[25]

## What About BCAAs?

We know that leucine, isoleucine, and valine, the three branched-chain amino acids (BCAAs), are important for muscle protein synthesis, but assuming we're getting enough of these in the protein we eat or through a high-quality protein powder, is there any benefit to supplementing with *more*? For most folks, probably not. While the benefits of supplementing with BCAAs for performance and body composition are negligible at best, they may, however, help reduce muscle soreness in resistance athletes (less so for endurance sports).[26] If you find you get some enhanced muscle recovery postworkout by adding BCAAs into your stack, amazing! But otherwise, focusing on high-quality, BCAA-rich protein sources (e.g., chicken, beef, fish, eggs, dairy, and protein powder) will likely do the trick.

- **Creatine.** Creatine is a chain of three amino acids that our body produces and that can also be consumed from meat and seafood. On average, men's bodies produce 1 gram of creatine per day, whereas women biosynthesize a bit less, about 0.8 grams per day. If we consume meat and/or seafood, we get about 1 to 2 grams per day from our diet, so most omnivores' creatine stores sit at around 60 to 80 percent full. Women tend to fall on the lower end of this range because, on average, their diets are lower in creatine than men's. Ditto for vegetarians and vegans, whose stores generally only reach 55 to 65 percent saturation.

The goal of creatine supplementation is to get these stores as close to 100 percent as possible, to improve strength and exercise performance. It's most often used in bodybuilding, powerlifting, sprinting, cycling, rowing, and other sports that require intermittent or explosive movements. And it really does work! Creatine has been shown to lead to improvements in strength, exercise performance, and sprinting time in men and women, with no reports of detrimental outcomes.[27] The general guideline for use is a "loading" phase of 0.3 grams per kilogram (2¼ pounds) of body weight for five to seven days (around 20 grams per day), followed by a maintenance dose of 0.03 grams per kilogram (around 5 grams daily).[28]

- **Carb Gels & Drinks.** Whether you're looking to quickly replenish glycogen stores posttraining, or need a rapid source of energy before or during a long cardio sesh, a carb-based sports gel or drink can help get the job done. Athletes can often benefit from a concentrated source of Naked Carbs without any protein, fat, or fiber to slow down their action, as well as from the extra hydration. Gels usually contain 20 to 30 grams of simple carbs per packet, whereas sports drinks usually contain 14 to 20 grams per 8-ounce serving. Different brands may also include electrolytes, caffeine, and amino acids, so speak to your dietitian or coach about your unique needs.

- **Omega-3s.** Omega-3s help enhance oxygen delivery (to get oxygen more quickly to the muscles), support cell membrane fluidity (which boosts energy production in the muscle cells), and are inherently anti-inflammatory (allowing for better recovery).[29] Although some studies show no clear benefit of omega-3 supplementation, many others demonstrate improvements in explosive power, $VO_2$ max, submaximal heart rate (HR), fatigue and muscle soreness, with longer-term treatments (e.g., eight weeks) sometimes contributing cardiovascular and endurance perks.[30] Different individuals require different optimal dosages, and there is no standard recommendation for adults. However, many health organizations support an intake of 0.5 to 1 gram per day of combined EPA and DHA, and research shows there are no adverse effects from taking up to 1 gram of DHA per day, or up to 1.8 grams of EPA for most people.[31]

- **Beet Products.** Beets contain dietary nitrates ($NO_3$), which get converted into nitric oxide (NO) in the body, to help dilate blood vessels and improve oxygen delivery to working muscles. In other words, it makes physical activity feel easier, so that you can perform at a higher intensity for a longer period of time. Research has found that beet juice or powder may enhance muscle power output, and reduce muscle fatigue during training.[32] Most studies see benefits from dosages of 1½ to 2 cups of beet juice, 55 ml (2 ounces) of beet concentrate, one large beet, 20 to 40 grams of beet powder, or another source of 300 to 800 mg of plant-based nitrates. Experiment with adding it to your smoothies, oats, or yogurt.[33]

- **Caffeine.** A lot of us depend on caffeine just to get ourselves to walk a mere ten steps to our car in the morning, never mind to help us muster up the motivation for a 10K run. But the mechanism of benefit here is basically the same. Research has shown that consuming around 3 mg of caffeine per kilogram (2¼ pounds) of body weight does enhance performance across endurance, power-based, team, and skill-based sports.[34] The International Society of Sports Nutrition (ISSN) suggests a dosage of 3 to 6 mg of caffeine per kilogram of body mass, usually sixty minutes before activity, with the risk of side effects at or above 9 mg/kg outweighing the perks.[35]

- **Beta-alanine.** Beta-alanine is a nonessential amino acid often used for fueling high-intensity exercise or activities that depend on muscle endurance by helping delay muscle fatigue and pain. According to the ISSN, daily supplementation of 4 to 6 grams for two to four weeks can improve exercise performance, particularly for trials lasting one to four minutes.[36]

- **Electrolytes.** More than just $H_2O$, hydration requires a delicate balance of electrolytes (e.g., sodium, potassium, calcium, magnesium, and chloride) to regulate fluid balance. Sodium and potassium are particularly important for muscle contraction and preventing severe muscle cramping or spasms. If you've ever watched a competitive bodybuilder literally lock up on stage midpose, looking like a greased-up wax figure, it's because they've dehydrated themselves to make their muscles look as defined as possible. Cue the gaggle of *more* greased-up muscle-men to carry their buddy offstage.

    Fluid and electrolyte needs can be particularly high for athletes who are performing at high intensities, at elevated altitudes, or in the extreme heat. Research suggests that electrolyte supplements that combine fluid, carbohydrates, and sodium (along with other electrolytes in less critical amounts) can help improve performance and enhance recovery.[37] A general rule of thumb is to consume about 2 cups of fluid one to two hours before an event, and continue to hydrate with water to replace sweat losses during exercise. If you're engaging in high-intensity workouts, endurance exercise lasting over an hour, or any activities in hot, humid, or high-altitude conditions, consider an electrolyte replacement that offers 30 to 60 grams of carbohydrates, 0.5 to 1 liter of water, and 250 to 700 mg of sodium per hour.[38]

## Lifestyle Strategies for Sports Nutrition

It goes without saying that no one ever won a triathlon simply by watching other athletes practice on TV. To get stronger, faster, bigger, or better, you have to put in the work. Obviously, nutrition plays an integral part in how well your body responds to said work, but a number of other key factors are influencing your results, as well.

- **Sleep Hygiene.** Despite the well-documented importance of restorative sleep for athletic performance, cognition, immunity, general health, and reducing the risk of injuries, athletes consistently get worse shut-eye than the general population.[39] If you're struggling with nighttime sleep, consider shifting your training to earlier in the day, avoid stimulant supplements in the afternoon, and sneak in twenty- to ninety-minute power naps, which have been shown to help improve performance after a subpar night of ZZZs.[40]
- **Rest & Recovery Days.** Depending on the intensity and training cycle, it's generally recommended to work in one to two rest days per week, to prevent overtraining. And remember, nutrition needs to be prioritized even on rest days! This doesn't mean significantly reducing your calorie intake on days you're not working out. Rest days may burn fewer overall calories than training days, but you still require a balance of

protein, fats, and fiber-rich carbs (vs. the Naked Carbs that come in clutch on performance days). Staying hydrated is also key.

## Wrapping Up: The HCC for Fueling Sports Performance and Recovery

Exercise and nutrition go hand in hand when it comes to any health-related goal, including those aimed at bolstering our athletic training and performance, improving strength or endurance, and supporting postexercise and rest day recovery. The Hunger Crushing Combo is a true MVP for helping you achieve your goals on and off the court, gym, or track without running your life.

# CHAPTER 9

·················

# Healthy Aging:
# HCC for Perimenopause,
# Menopause, and Beyond

If you're a woman in your midforties to early fifties, you may be reaching this last definingly female era, characterized largely by the end of a woman's menstrual cycles and fertility. And if you're thinking, *"Woo hoo! We're saving on birth control and hundreds of dollars from monthly tampons!"* hold your horses, Mama, because it's not exactly a free ride. Here's what actually goes down.

First up, perimenopause, which is finally receiving its due both in research and in popular media. "Perimenopause" refers to the transitional phase before menopause, marking the time during which a woman's body naturally shifts toward the end of her reproductive years. And like its literal translation ("around menopause"), it's annoyingly ambiguous and indistinct, meaning there is no clear test that you're "in it." Some signs like sleep disturbances, weight gain, or mood swings can easily be explained away by life circumstances and stage (e.g., the fact that a lot of us will still have young kids and stressful careers when the transition starts!). There also isn't a precise age for entering perimenopause. It is often sometime in our forties, but could also start a whole decade before!

During this four- to ten-plus-year journey from perimenopause to menopause, our ovaries start to produce less estrogen, progesterone, and testosterone. Unfortunately, this comes with increased risk of obesity, metabolic syndrome, heart disease, and osteoporosis, along with such not-so-fabulous symptoms as hot flashes, night sweats, vaginal dryness, mood swings, insomnia, brain fog, and changes in libido. Not exactly a good setup for the life I envisioned when my kids are finally sleeping in their own beds.

While perimenopause and menopause are of course normal natural parts of life, for many women, they can negatively affect *quality* of said life. In some cases, hormone therapy or other medications may be recommended, but supporting this season with my Hunger Crushing Combo can absolutely help. And ideally, we put these motions into play well before we have our final cycle. If you're past your postpartum days, or in your mid- to late thirties or older (whichever comes first), this chapter is for you.

## Dietary Patterns During Perimenopause & Menopause

With half of the population slated to eventually experience the hormonal roller coaster that is perimenopause and menopause, there's a good reason to want to better understand how our diet may help or cause harm during this pilgrimage.

Not surprisingly, foods that are low in Hunger Crushing Compounds don't set us up for happy, healthy, hot flash–free aging. Research shows that a diet rich in highly processed foods may intensify such menopause symptoms as hot flashes, brain fog, and vaginal dryness, whereas eating more whole fruits and vegetables calms these common complaints.[1]

Other research on the beloved Mediterranean diet (a whole-food diet rich in plant protein, fish, olive oil, fruits, and vegetables, and low in processed and red meats) confirms the power of nutrition in softening the P-to-M transition, helping reduce everything from hot flashes to osteoporosis to breast cancer to cognitive decline.[2]

Food can be incredibly powerful in fighting the not-so-comfy heat wave! Let's bring it back to our Hunger Crushing Combo Triangle to help you better understand what matters most.

## The HCC Formula for Perimenopause and Menopause

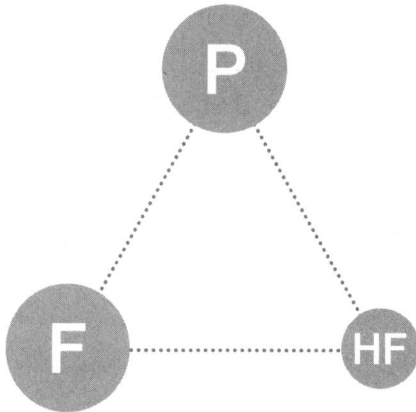

When it comes to a balanced diet for getting through the years of the Great Pause, the Hunger Crushing Combo framework does it all (*other than maybe making your teenage or adult kids want to hang out on a Friday night to teach you what terms like "simp" or "slap" mean*). But prioritizing balanced meals rich in protein, fiber, and healthy fats helps reduce the risk of muscle and bone loss, visceral fat gain, and blood sugar and blood lipid (cholesterol) dysregulation, while offering bonus perks for mood regulation, hot flashes, and night sweats. Let's dive in.

### Protein for Perimenopause and Menopause

It's inevitable that our body will naturally change as we age, and we should be celebrating and honoring it through those many beautiful seasons. But, alas, some quirks inherent in these changes leave something to be desired. Protein can't fix all of our middle-age problems, but in the context of perimenopause and menopause, it definitely can help with a few that matter most: loss of muscle mass, bone mineral density, and weight gain (most concerningly, that visceral fat around our waists).

I know thirty-year-olds like to complain that their metabolism has gone to sh*t, because they used to be able to eat Big Macs in their twenties without gaining a pound. But research actually shows that our metabolism stays remarkably stable between the ages of twenty to sixty, and *then* it starts to decline by less than 1 percent per year after that.[3]

If we want to slow that decline, prevent excess weight gain, and maintain muscle mass as we age, we need to prioritize protein, ideally 1.2 to 1.6 grams of protein per kilogram (2¼ pounds) of body weight.[4] For our 135-pound female friend, that would be between 72 and 96 grams per day (ideally on the upper end, depending on total calories). So, you want to make sure you're including a "meal dose" of protein (that is, 20 to 35 grams) at all three meals, plus half of that in snacks (see page 254 for your visual cues).

Protein (and the muscle mass it helps build) isn't just important for supporting a healthy metabolism and body composition as we age. It also makes up approximately 30 percent of our bone tissue, which is put at risk during perimenopause and menopause as our estrogen levels decline, increasing the risk of osteoporosis, fractures, and falls.

Thankfully, again, protein's up for the job. One large cohort study following a massive group of women for thirty-two years found that intake of dairy protein and plant protein specifically (but not total or animal protein) significantly reduced the risk of hip fractures.[5] Dairy protein like that found in Greek yogurt and cottage cheese is bound up with other bone-building nutrients like calcium, magnesium, phosphorus, and vitamin D.

As for plant-based proteins, the most readily available, versatile, and bioavailable form is soy, as found in tofu, tempeh, edamame, soy milk, and countless "faux meat" foods. Soy protein is rich in unique phytoestrogen compounds, called isoflavones, which mimic the effect of endogenous estrogen in the body. Since declining estrogen levels play a role in muscle loss and belly fat retention during perimenopause and menopause, "replacing" endogenous estrogen with the phytoestrogens in soy protein may help minimize these effects.[6]

The effects of the isoflavones in soy don't only help thwart some of the unwanted body composition changes associated with the estrogen falloff, but they may also help temper a wide range of menopause gripes, including hot flashes and vaginal dryness.[7]

So, when choosing protein during the perimenopause transition and postmenopause, aim for plant-based most often, with ideally at least one serving of whole-food soy per day. After plant-based protein, fill the rest of your meals with dairy, eggs, and poultry, and limit red and processed meat to less than two 3- to 4-ounce cooked servings per week.

### Fiber and Carbs for Perimenopause and Menopause

One of the inherent superpowers of plant-based proteins is that they are all dual citizens with fiber, which can help counteract the effect of our declining estrogen during this season of life. Estrogen is inherently cardioprotective and helps regulate our blood sugars. So, less estrogen means increased "bad" LDL cholesterol and insulin resistance. Estrogen also plays a critical role in fat distribution, and when it takes a nosedive, we see a shift in fat storage from the hips and thighs toward the belly area. The problem with this isn't so much that you can no longer find a comfortable pair of pants to wear, but that this visceral fat increases the risk of heart disease and insulin resistance. And guess what? The insulin resistance then further exacerbates the gain in belly fat! It's all a very messy cycle (that would be a hell of a lot messier if I gave you *all* the complicated science-y details). But all you need to know is that fiber understands the assignment. Fiber slows the absorption of carbs to provide more stable blood sugars and insulin responses, keeps you fuller longer to support a healthy weight, and helps reduce total cholesterol and "bad" LDL cholesterol.[8] Research has also found that hot flashes occur most often when blood sugar levels drop, so maintaining more stable levels with fiber-rich carbs may help reduce the unpleasant sweats.[9] It's a win-win-win situation.

In addition to our dual-citizen plant-based proteins, we ideally want to focus on a variety of antioxidant and anti-inflammatory–rich colorful fruits and vegetables that not only help reduce the risk of chronic disease, but have also been shown to quell specific menopause symptoms like poor concentration, insomnia, headaches, depression, and irregularity.[10] While, of course, there is room for Naked Carbs in every stage of life, as we move through perimenopause and beyond, we may notice they don't always play so nice. A big slice of birthday cake with extra frosting just hits different by age fifty-five (*and not the good different*). Indigestion, postsugar fatigue, mood swings, constipation, sleep disruption, and sensitive teeth may just naturally coax us into making more fiber-rich carbohydrate choices to help mitigate the unpleasantries. Don't punish yourself for making choices that used to feel good to you in your younger years. You're still settling into a new phase of life, and that takes time to re-collect data on what foods help you live your best postmenopausal life.

Healthy Fats for Perimenopause & Menopause

Some emerging research points to the benefits of a low-fat diet for menopause, largely to counter the effects of estrogen declines on fat storage and weight gain. But remember that healthy eating is about a lot more than just macros and calories, and that not all fats are created equal. And this holds particularly true when the goal is to counteract pesky "pause" symptoms. For example, one study on the Mediterranean diet and menopause found that extra-virgin olive oil was associated with reduced depressive mood, irritability, anxiety, and tiredness.[11] Likewise, another study found that, unlike animal-based saturated fats, monounsaturated fats lowered the risk of cognitive decline in postmenopausal women.[12]

Unsaturated healthy fats also help counter the elevated risk of heart disease and inflammation that are part and parcel with this phase of life.

Ultimately, what all of this tells us is that we will just want to be more intentional about our fat choices during perimenopause through to full menopause. That means choosing whole-food dual-citizen healthy fats that offer mad menopause-managing bang for their caloric buck, and limiting high-fat fried foods, fatty cuts of meat, and ultra-processed meats like bacon or sausage.

## Our Favorite HCC Foods for Managing Perimenopause and Menopause Symptoms

There is no magical "hormone diet" that will rewind time to your grade 12 prom (*thank G-d*) and restore your body to a fertile myrtle of the past. So, while we can't stop the perimenopause train reaching its final destination, we can make intentional food choices that address some of the unpleasant side-effect hurdles along the way. Here are some of my favorite Hunger Crushing Combo foods that are particularly powerful in this season of life.

## Does Soy Cause Breast Cancer?

You've probably caught wind of one of the most pervasive myths about soy out there: that it causes breast cancer. And at first blush, the concern seems legit! Since estrogen can promote the growth of estrogen receptor–positive breast cancer, and soy contains phytoestrogens that mimic endogenous estrogen, it makes sense that the more of these estrogen look-alikes, the greater the risk of cancer! Not so fast. The effects of phytoestrogens are more nuanced than that. The best-quality research we have now shows that they can potentially *lower* the risk of breast cancer.[13] If you are at risk of breast cancer, of course, speak to your health-care team about an appropriate amount of soy for you, but otherwise, rest assured, the totality of the research is on soy's side.

- **Edamame, Tofu, and Other Soy-Based Foods.** As discussed on page 215, soy-based foods like tofu, tempeh, edamame, and soy milk contain unique compounds called isoflavones, a type of phytoestrogen that mimics the body's estrogen in beneficial ways. As our natural estrogen levels decline, upping our intake of soy may reduce the risk of bone and muscle loss, plus specific symptoms like hot flashes, anxiety, and depression.[14] And because many soy foods are also low in saturated fat and cholesterol, while rich in fiber, protein, healthy fats, antioxidants, and phytosterols, they may also help lower LDL cholesterol and risk of heart disease, stabilize blood sugars, and help you maintain a healthy weight. Although there are no official recommendations for soy intake during perimenopause or menopause, research suggests a daily intake of 40 mg total isoflavones derived from whole soybeans, which translates to around ¼ cup of whole soybeans or 3.5 (extra-firm) to 7 (silken) ounces of tofu for tackling menopause symptoms.[15] Incorporate more meatless meals into your week by adding tofu to stir-fries, edamame to salads, and soy milk to smoothies and oats.

- **Cruciferous Vegetables.** Kale, broccoli, cauliflower, Brussels sprouts, cabbage, and their ilk contain unique estrogen-modulating compounds, which research suggests may help reduce perimenopause and menopause symptoms.[16] They're also rich in fiber and bone-supporting nutrients like calcium and vitamin K, to help counter the increased risk of osteoporosis.

- **Almonds.** While a delicious nut mix is a convenient way to sneak in nutrient variety, of all the nuts in the jar, almonds are a menopause management star. Like soy, they're a natural source of phytoestrogens (for hot flashes), calcium (for bones), and vitamin E (for immune function), with research showing countless benefits for inflammation, heart health, blood pressure, and weight management.[17] And even though nuts are calorie dense, studies suggest that including nuts as part of a healthy diet pattern doesn't lead to weight gain.[18] In fact, when consumed in conscious serving sizes (a "standard" serving is around an ounce, or twenty almonds), they may actually support weight loss and help reduce waist circumference.[19] Add nuts to salads, oatmeal, yogurt, and baked goods, and keep a small container in your car or work desk for a satiating snack.

- **Flaxseeds.** Flaxseeds are uniquely rich in phytoestrogen compounds called lignans that research suggests may help reduce the frequency and severity of hot flashes and vaginal dryness.[20] Try adding ground flaxseeds and flax meal to baked goods, oats, smoothies, and pancakes!

- **Fortified Dairy.** Dairy is one of the best dietary sources of such bone-supporting nutrients as protein, calcium, phosphorus, potassium, magnesium, and, when fortified, vitamin D, and is uniquely beneficial for supporting a healthy body composition as we age.[21] Choose higher-protein dual-citizen dairy sources like Greek yogurt, kefir, and cottage cheese most often.

- **Citrus Fruit.** Packed with antioxidants for heart health, fiber for satiety and blood sugar management, plus bone-supporting calcium and magnesium, citrus fruit is a favorite for this season of life. And thanks to its anti-inflammatory immune-supporting nutrients, some research suggests it may reduce the risk of menopausal symptoms by up to 77 percent.[22] Some women do find that acidic foods may exacerbate bladder control symptoms, so keep a symptom journal, and stay hydrated to mitigate the risk.

## HCC Example Day for Perimenopause and Menopause

You've made it past the thankless days of young parenthood and "grindset" work culture; now it's time that you make nutrition choices that are devotedly and unapologetically for *you*! The sky's the limit, queen! But here's a very simple guideline to get you started:

> Breakfast: Soy milk smoothie with Greek yogurt, ground flax-seed, and berries
> Snack: Mandarin orange, roasted edamame, and almonds
> Lunch: Quinoa salmon salad with diced vegetables, avocado, and crumbled cheese

Snack: Strawberries with dip made of silken tofu, melted dark chocolate, and almond butter

Dinner: Tempeh cauliflower–sweet potato lettuce wraps with peanut sauce

Snack: Hummus with whole-grain crackers with a cup of ultra-filtered milk (which offers 5 grams more protein per cup compared with regular)

## Foods That May Trigger Menopause Symptoms

Menopause symptom triggers are highly individualized and sometimes totally random, but when we look at population research, we see some patterns emerge.

**Coffee, tea, and other forms of caffeine** may increase urinary incontinence (by acting as a bladder irritant and diuretic), hot flashes, and core body temperature.[23] Experiment with cutting back or switching to decaf to see whether you get symptom relief.

**Alcohol** can also exacerbate hot flashes and night sweats, while interfering with your already compromised sleep quality.[24]

**Spicy foods** can act as a vasodilator to mimic or aggravate hot flashes.

**High-sugar foods** can result in a blood sugar spike and subsequent crash, which research shows is what can often trigger hot flashes.[25] If you're enjoying dessert postdinner, dressing it up in layers of HCCs is your best bet for dry sheets.

## Supplements to Consider During Perimenopause and Menopause

Food always comes first, but when health concerns rise and calorie needs decline as they do with maturity and age, a simple supplement regimen may be a supporting feature of self-care.

- **Omega-3s.** If you've read through most of these chapters, you know that a lot of folks don't meet their omega-3 needs from food alone. Although the research on specific menopause symptoms and omega-3s is mixed, they do seem most promising for helping to reduce night sweats and depressive symptoms.[26] While there is no official omega-3 dosage for menopause, most research suggests somewhere in the neighborhood of 500 to 1,000 mg daily if you're not consuming at least two to three weekly servings of fatty fish.[27]

- **Creatine.** Creatine is one of the safest and most well-studied supplements, and it has unique benefits for women as we venture through perimenopause and beyond.[28] When combined with resistance training, creatine supplementation during menopause has been shown to counteract our estrogen-related declines in muscle, bone, and strength.[29] The general guideline for dosing is a "loading" phase of 0.3 g/kg for five to seven days, or around 20 grams per day, then a maintenance dose of 0.03 g/kg, or 5 grams daily. If you experience bloating or side effects, you can skip the loading phase; it might just take longer to see the desirable effects while training.

- **Vitamin D.** A critical component of healthy bones, vitamin D also plays a role in supporting immunity, mood, mental health, muscle function, heart health, blood sugars, and more. And for folks in the early stages of perimenopause, there is even some emerging research linking greater intakes of vitamin D to lower risk of early menopause.[30] Since most of our vitamin D$_3$ comes from sunlight, not food, a lot of women can benefit from a supplement, ideally one that also includes vitamin K$_2$, which works synergistically to optimize calcium metabolism. There is a very wide range in appropriate dosages depending if there is a deficiency to correct, so it's ideal to have your levels tested before deciding the right dosage for you.

## What About Calcium Supplements?

When we think about bone health, we likely all go straight to calcium. It's recommended that healthy perimenopausal and menopausal women aim for at least 1,200 mg of calcium daily, which can be easily obtained through such dietary sources as leafy greens, dairy products, fortified plant milks, fish, and calcium-set tofu. Won't taking a supplement do the same thing? In this case, we're not sure. Research suggests that calcium supplements do not seem to lower the risk of fractures in older adults.[31] Not to mention, some research has found that calcium supplementation of 1,000 mg per day or more may increase the risk of cardiovascular disease in postmenopausal women by 15 percent.[32] Speak to your doctor to weigh the risks and benefits for you. And if you do supplement, space it apart from meals that are already high in calcium, since your body can absorb only so much at once.[33]

### Lifestyle Considerations During Perimenopause and Menopause

In addition to nutrition, other everyday lifestyle habits can play a role in minimizing symptoms and mitigating abrupt body changes that leave you feeling more *ugh* than *ahhhh*.

- **Hydration.** The big Pause slows down a number of key bodily processes (e.g., regularity and digestion, detoxification, cellular metabolism, skin healing, body temperature regulation, and more), making proper hydration more important than ever! While the amount of fluids you need in a day is highly individualized, a good baseline is around 33 ml/kg/day, or just over 2 liters (about 70 ounces) for a 70 kg (158-pound) woman.[34] Start every morning with a 16-ounce glass to get a head start, then set reminders every hour to take a few sips. You might also want to experiment with tapering your consumption a few hours before bed, to prevent frequent toilet trips that can further disrupt sleep.

- **Sleep Hygiene.** Here's a not-so-fun little factoid: Your hot flashes are actually causing more hot flashes! Yep, there's a vicious cycle whereby hot flashes can interfere with quality sleep, but not sleeping can actually make your symptoms worse! Poor sleep can also magnify mood swings, brain fog, cognitive decline, and weight gain, while impairing healthy bone turnover and repair.[35] Craft a healthy bedtime routine by avoiding screen time, caffeine, and alcohol before bed; maintaining a comfortable dark, cool, and quiet sleeping environment; sticking to a consistent bed and wake-up schedule; incorporating a relaxation ritual like a meditation or deep breathing; and limiting high-sugar or high-fat foods and excess fluids a few hours before bed.

- **Daily Movement.** In addition to its role in weight management, exercise may help reduce the severity of hot flashes, mood swings, depression, and sleep disturbances.[36] Weight-bearing exercises, like climbing stairs, jumping rope, doing aerobics, or strength training, can also be particularly important for preventing muscle and bone loss, and reducing your risk of osteoporosis. Find a handful of activities that you enjoy that can be incorporated into your routine daily to reach a weekly total of 150 minutes of moderate-intensity aerobics and at least two weekly sessions of strength-training exercises.

- **Avoid Smoking.** You don't need a millennial dietitian nagging you about the dangers of smoking. You've probably got a GP, partner, siblings, and maybe even a few adult kids lecturing you about your increased risk of cancer, lung disease, and heart disease (which are already heightened during menopause). But here's another one: Smoking may be making your menopause symptoms worse, leading to more severe hot flashes, mood swings, and vaginal dryness.[37] If you smoke and are having trouble quitting, contact your health-care provider or call a national smoking quitline like 1-800-QUIT-NOW for help.

- **Aromatherapy.** The world of aromatherapy can (and often does) teeter into grifty snake-oil MLM territory if left unchecked, but when it comes to menopause, there is actually some science to back it up. In one study, researchers found that inhaling 0.1 to 0.5 percent neroli (a.k.a. *Citrus aurantium*, or bitter orange) oil for 5 minutes twice daily led to improvements in sexual desire, blood pressure, cortisol, and estrogen concentrations, compared to the control, all of which the authors credited to the relaxing ritual.[38] Another study found that after four weeks of twice-daily use, sleep quality scores more than doubled![39] While we don't know if this is a placebo effect or how long these results would last, if it adds to your Zen, essential oils may be a low-risk wellness ritual to try.

## Wrapping Up: Managing Perimenopause and Menopause Your Way

Mainstream science has really done women dirty by *not* investing more money, time, and influence into understanding how to help us through this tumultuous female era. As a result, menopause can be a particularly vulnerable time for women to be sucked into predatory pseudoscience territory, looking for solutions that work. And while a lot of alternative remedies are likely benign, they can become dangerous when they distract us from evidence-based strategies and gentle recommendations that we can incorporate into our lives long term. Use this chapter as a starting point to have meaningful conversations with your health-care team about which solutions may be right for you.

# CHAPTER 10

. . . . . . . . . . . . . . . . . . .

# Raising Healthy Happy Eaters:
# HCC for Kids

If you're at an age where you're now trying to raise your own family in a world deeply steeped in diet culture, you probably remember your time in the "clean plate club" well. Whether we were bullied into eating past the point of fullness because *"all those other kids in Africa are starving"* or we watched our mom grimace with every glimpse in the mirror, a lot of us are just coming to and unearthing the damage that these early life lessons may have done. Loads of studies suggest that children of moms who diet are more likely to experience a negative body image, poor self-esteem, and disordered eating, and to become chronic dieters themselves.[1,2] In fact, moms' concerns about their body and weight is the third-leading cause of body image problems among young children. And this is not a dig at your mom. I'm sure that she (like you) was doing what she believed (and was taught by her mom) was best. Generational diet culture runs damn deep. But when we know better, we can do better. And if there's one recurring goal I hear from women who are fighting their own battles against diet culture, it is to end the generational diet cycle with them.

Easier said than done. In the age of social media, the diet culture battles our parents had to fight are now compounded by an endless stream of "experts" telling us that our kids' Cheerios are jacked up on pesticides (they're not) and their baby carrots are steeped in pure bleach (also false). Sugar is bad, dairy is bad, gluten is bad, oils are bad, even conventionally grown apples are a danger to childhood! So, even if we've been able to free *ourselves* of the shackles of *our own* food guilt, now we're pinned down with crushing self-reproach over our inability to get our kids to drink bone broth.

I promise you, the kids will be all right. My goal for you in this chapter is to give you the confidence and clarity to raise a competent eater with a healthy relationship with food, without its becoming your full-time job.

## The Division of Responsibility

When we're in the early days of shaping our little ones' relationship with food, the *what* to eat is far less important than the *how*. And that comes down to what is widely known as Satter's Division of Responsibility in Feeding (sDOR).[3]

The sDOR was developed by dietitian and family therapist Ellyn Satter, who noticed that a lot of dinnertime power struggles between parents and children seemed to arise when parents were being either too controlling (*"You can't leave the table until your plate is clean"*) or too lax (*"Sure, have another bag of chips right before dinner"*). In essence, Satter sought to create a balanced approach to feeding that respected both parents' role in providing structure, and a child's autonomy in deciding what feels right for their body.

Studies show that children supported with sDOR develop more diverse food preferences, are more likely to maintain calorie balance to meet (but not exceed) their needs, and tend to follow more appropriate growth trajectories.[4]

The sDOR emphasizes very clear roles for parents and children when it comes to mealtime. Parents' responsibilities would include **what**, **when**, and **where** the child eats, and a child's responsibility would be to determine **how much** to eat, or whether to eat at all.

Now, I know what you're thinking, *"I'm just supposed to let little Billy starve if he doesn't like the chicken I made?"* and I get it, I'm a Jewish mother. The thought of my kids' just choosing to go on a hunger strike for funsies is triggering AF. But the goal of the sDOR is to ensure mealtimes are a safe space for our kids to explore new foods, find joy in eating, and feed their bodies on their terms.

**Your Feeding Responsibilities**

I know, you're thinking, *"Ugh, more responsibilities? I'm drowning in to-dos as is."* But I promise, I'm about to take a huge burden off your plate. That is, what and how much your kids decide to eat are no longer in your jurisdiction. Want to offload that job onto your children with confidence? Here's what you need to do first:

- **What: Be Considerate Without Catering.** Ever feel like a short-order cook? Thankfully, the sDOR is designed not just to help support our littles, but to make *our* lives easier and less stressful too. When meal planning, start by asking yourself, *What would bring me joy to make and eat?* Mama, you deserve a break from chicken nuggets and fries too. So, under the directives of sDOR, one of the most important things to consider when meal planning is to *be considerate without catering.* This means offering a variety of foods from different food groups (ideally three to five meal components), all served family-style, so that kids can make choices at their own pace without pressure.

    It's also important that the options on the table balance familiar well-liked "safe" foods, with foods that may be new or that they're still "learning to like." Often, "safe" foods are carbohydrate-based options like rice, pasta, potatoes, or bread. It's ideal that there is enough of these foods to go around with extra to spare, in the event your kiddo isn't feeling up to trying the chicken skewers or mushrooms on the table. Kids' bodies are remarkably resilient (and as we will soon find out, they need a lot of carbs!). But when I'm feeling a little anxious at the sight of my kid's beige plate, I remind myself of this:

*I would rather my kids be open to eating broccoli all through their decades of adulthood, than turning them off veggies for life just because I was desperate to sneak in some vitamin C when they were four. What matters now is that I have given them the tools in a safe, low-pressure, supportive environment that gives them the autonomy to trust and respect their own body wisdom.*

- **When: Meals and Snack Times.** Kids thrive on routine, and knowing that they will reliably be fed at specific times in the day provides them with the sense of security they need to move through the day without obsessing over food. Ideally, there is enough time between meals and snacks for them to come to the table with an appetite, but not so much time that they're melting down (or can't meet their total calorie needs). Find a schedule that works for you, but in my house, it looks a bit like this:

  - 7:00 a.m.: Breakfast
  - 9:30 a.m.: Snack
  - Noon: Lunch
  - 3:00 p.m.: Snack
  - 5:30 p.m.: Dinner
  - 7:30 p.m.: Snack

- **Where: Family Matters.** Of course, there will be nights when you're raw-dawging cold pizza over the steering wheel as you cart the kids from school to hockey to ballet, but part of the superpower of using sDOR is the sit-down family meal.

    An ideal eating environment should be calm, predictable, and comfortable, and free of distracting tablets, TV, phones, or toys. If we don't want mealtimes to be a fight, we need to turn the battlefield into a sanctuary where our kids can show up with a smile, nourish their bodies, and build critical life-long skills.

In response to your supportive and considerate approach to the **what**, **when**, and **where** for mealtimes, your kids can

- Reap the social, emotional, and physical rewards of family meals
- Learn to enjoy a wide variety of foods at their own comfortable pace
- Maintain their inherent intuitive eating skills
- Eat in amounts that complement their hunger and fullness cues necessary to support growth
- Grow predictably into their natural body size.

### Is sDOR Appropriate for All Children?

For some children, particularly neurodivergent kids with low interoceptive skills, who may struggle to recognize internal hunger and fullness cues, additional support may be needed to help them cultivate healthy eating habits and achieve nutritional adequacy beyond using sDOR. In such cases, gentle reminders around eating schedules, maintaining consistent, structured meal- and snack times, and visual cues can help them better understand their bodies' needs. Parents and caregivers may also provide extra guidance in identifying hunger and fullness, fostering a supportive environment for developing healthy, mindful eating habits tailored to their child's needs.

## What If My Kid Is "Overweight"?

It can be incredibly unsettling and triggering to be told that your child is "overweight" and needs to be put on a weight-loss diet. And while it's not my place to override the recommendations of your child's pediatrician, I urge you to think about the long game, as the food and body messages we send to our kids today can have lifelong repercussions. Children put on diets are more likely to be classified as overweight or obese as adults, *and* are more likely to suffer lower self-esteem, body dissatisfaction, and depression.[5] And even the most multidisciplinary, long-term, specialty clinic weight interventions may be only marginally "effective" for kids.[6]

Childhood is a time of rapid growth and development, and dieting during these critical growth years can increase the risk of nutritional deficiencies, which in turn can impair physical growth and cognitive development.

When children are offered a variety of nutritious foods (as outlined by the HCC), and allowed to make choices without pressure or heavy manipulation (as recommended by sDOR), they are better able to grow into the body shape and size that's genetically best for them. If you are concerned about your child's health, I encourage you to review your **what, when,** and **where** responsibilities and best practices, and see whether any adjustments can be made to the eating experience to help your child get back in touch with their body's true needs.

## The HCC Formula for Healthy
## Kids and Adolescents

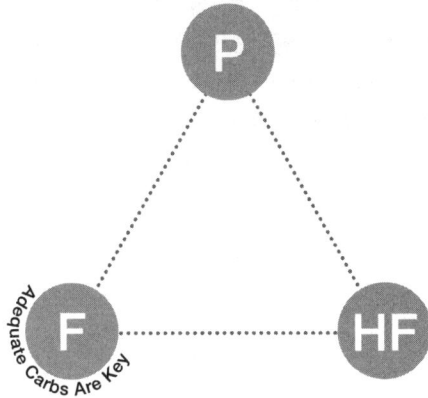

Ask one hundred parents what the most common phrase they hear from their kids, and if it's not *NO!* it surely has something to do with food.

*"I'm hungry!" "I need a snack!" "What's for dinner?"*

Honestly, I've got two boys; these words make up the background music of my life. But, yeah, kids need to pack a lot of calories into a small body. Compared to adults, children need more micronutrients and a *lot* more calories relative to their body size. The challenge is, there's only so much room to pack those calories into that little tum, so kids' meals typically need to be at least a third more calorie dense than those of their adult caregivers.

And when kids hit puberty, well, you better take out a second mortgage, because your grocery bill is about to get wild. Calorie and macronutrient needs differ significantly between childhood and puberty due to rapid growth, hormonal changes, and increased physical development that occurs during this transitional season. For instance, on average, adolescent girls' and boys' needs can increase, respectively, to 2,500 and 3,000 calories per day.[7]

What this means for you is that kids' meals don't have to always look perfectly balanced or nutritious; they can afford (and need) the extra calories in that moat of ketchup they built around their hamburger. And it's okay if it seems as if, some days, they eat more sugary dip than the dipper. Calories are king when it comes to feeding kids, and one of the easiest and most reliable sources of calories is carbs.

### (Naked) Carbs and Kids

Cookies. Candy. Cupcakes. Kids like sweet stuff. And while, of course, there's a social or learned component to this (see "Naked Carbs for Fun," pages 235–236), this preference is largely believed to have important evolutionary and biological purposes. For example, if newborns were not born attracted to sweet flavors, they might not be innately drawn to the breast or bottle for a taste of Mom's carbohydrate-rich milk or formula. Likewise, as kids undergo rapid development, their inherent drive for sweet foods helps provide their brain's preferred source of fuel! So, the next time your child begs for a second cookie, consider preordering the next size up in pants, because a growth spurt might be under way!

Even without a supersprout season in the works, kids just need a lot of carbs. For most kids, 50 to 65 percent of their total calories will come from carbohydrates, which for your average-size preschooler is between 140 and 175 grams per day.

And, of course, the ideal scenario is that we fulfill our kids' physiological need for carbs (and their innate preference for sweetness) with Hunger Crushing Compound–rich whole foods. Trust me; that is all part of the long game of teaching our kids to maintain their innate body wisdom and become healthy, competent eaters. And if you're on day five of chicken fingers and frozen fries this week, we will get there, I promise.

But one of the most humbling lessons I've had to learn as a parent who is also a nutrition professional, is that there's "ideal," and then . . .

*there's kids.* You can't change them, you can't predict their next moves, and you can't force them to follow any sort of parenting playbook. So, while you and I both know that a dense seedy whole-grain sourdough loaf may be more nutritious than Wonder Bread, the latter is A-OK.

In fact, Naked Carbs can be an important tool for helping kids meet their relatively high calorie and carbohydrate needs. And although we've kept this category relatively generic throughout the book, for kids specifically, I like to further divide Naked Carbs into two distinct and important categories: Naked Carbs for Energy, and Naked Carbs for Fun.

- **Naked Carbs for Energy.** Common "safe" foods for kids are also (typically) simple carb-based foods. White rice, white pasta, white bread. All of these options may be *more* "naked" than their whole-grain counterparts, but they don't typically contain *added* sugar, and they still provide important nutrition for kids! For example, 1 cup of white pasta contains 2.5 grams of fiber and 8 grams of protein, plus 40 grams of energizing carbs and important micronutrients like B vitamins and iron! In some cases, the whole-grain alternative isn't even *that* superior anyway. For example, brown rice has just 0.5 gram more protein and 1.3 grams more fiber per half-cup compared to white! Do not let 1 gram of fiber be the difference between your kiddo's eating their dinner, and their pushing it around their plate.
- **Naked Carbs for Fun.** These are foods that are rich in (or mostly) added sugar like cupcakes, cookies, and ice cream. Here's a hot take that you probably won't see in many mom groups online: These are important too. Maybe not *essential* from a physiological perspective, as we know that excess added sugar displaces key nutrients for growing bodies. But we're in this for the long game, and as we've discussed ad

nauseam in Part 1 of this book, restriction only breeds desire, obsession, and, eventually, an unhealthy relationship with food.

Research has found that children who are restricted of "fun foods" like desserts and Naked Carb snacks end up eating *more* of these foods when they get the chance, compared to the kids who are allowed regular access.[8] And as you probably know (if you're reading this book), these early "nutrition" lessons can endure through adulthood.

So, for the same reason that we want to offer multiple and continuous exposures to new nutritious foods we'd eventually like our littles to enjoy, we also want to offer exposure to fun foods. The goal is to rob these foods of their power and give kids ample "practice" in collecting data on how these foods make their bodies feel. Here are some tips to do just that:

- *Serve dessert with the meal.* When we tell kids they need to eat X number of bites before they can get dessert, it teaches them that they must fill up on dinner, and then eat *past* the point of natural fullness by eating dessert. It also reinforces that desserts are fundamentally *different* and *better* than rice or chicken, and therefore, warrant obsession and preoccupation. To teach kids that all foods are morally equal, Satter recommends putting everything on the same plate. No bribes, no rewards, no bite-for-bite deals. Serve a single portion of dessert at each person's place when you set the table, and then allow everyone (yourself included) to eat their meal in whatever order they want.
- *Occasionally serve unlimited sweets at snack time.* Every once in a while, put out a plate of cookies, serve it with a glass of milk, cheese, or berries, and allow your kid to

eat their fill. This helps reduce the "forbidden fruit" effect by reducing scarcity mentality, teaches self-regulation and body autonomy, and allows kids to see food through a morally neutral lens.

• *Pro tip:* All of these work for adults who are struggling with their relationship with sugar, too, so make it a family affair!

## Fiber and Kids

Kids' fiber recommendations are actually pretty high: around 19 grams of fiber per day for one to three years old, and 25 grams per day for four to 8 years old. As we discussed earlier in the book, most adults aren't even meeting these numbers, so how the heck will my kid, whose body has been basically built by Goldfish?

The good news is, plenty of kid-approved foods are rich in fiber, and they're probably already (happily) eating them. Here are some examples:

Green peas (1 cup)—9 grams fiber
Raspberries (1 cup)—8 grams fiber
Smoothie (with berries)—6 to 8 grams fiber
Pear (medium)—5.5 grams fiber
Avocado (½ fruit)—5 grams fiber
Chickpea/legume pasta (2 ounces dry)—5 grams fiber
Granola bar—3 to 5 grams fiber
Apple (medium)—4.5 grams fiber
Fig bars (2 bars)—4 grams fiber
Trail mix (¼ cup)—4 grams fiber
Sweet potato (medium)—4 grams fiber
Russet potato (medium)—4 grams fiber
Oatmeal (1 cup cooked)—4 grams fiber

> Popcorn (3 cups popped)—3.6 grams fiber
> Carrots (1 cup)—3.6 grams fiber
> Banana (medium)—3 grams fiber
> Strawberries (1 cup)—3 grams fiber

Remember, unlike with adult weight-loss goals where *voluminous* high-fiber foods can come in clutch, we don't want to prematurely fill up our children on water, or they may have a hard time meeting their high-energy needs. So, it can be helpful to lean into *higher-calorie* fiber sources (e.g., whole grains, potatoes, and sweet potatoes), or dual-citizen fiber sources (e.g., avocado, nut butter, legumes, and seeds). And when lower-calorie, fiber-rich foods like vegetables are on the table (and I strongly recommend that they are), don't be shy about adding in extra fats (e.g., dips, olive oil, butter, or cheese).

**Protein for Kids**

Kids' protein needs are relatively modest. Based on the current evidence, children between the ages of four and thirteen years and fourteen to eighteen years, respectively, require 0.41 and 0.39 grams of protein per pound of body weight per day. For a 50-pound child, that's only 22 grams! Now, of course, if your teen is a rising track star or budding ballerina, check with their pediatrician to make sure their nutrients are on track, but on average, protein for kids is kinda no big whoop. Even if your picky eater refuses to try the "official" protein sources on the table (a.k.a. chicken, fish, tofu, beans, etc.), if they're eating enough calories, they're more than likely meeting their basic protein needs.

Here are some examples of the protein content of your kids' go-to foods, to put your mind at ease:

> Greek yogurt (½ cup) = 12 grams protein
> Pepperoni pizza (1 slice) = 9 to 12 grams protein

Chicken nuggets (4 or 5 pieces) = 8 to 11 grams protein

Milk (1 cup) = 8 grams protein

String cheese = 8 grams protein

White pasta (1 cup cooked) = 8 grams protein

Peanut butter (2 tablespoons) = 7 to 8 grams protein

Corn (1 cup) = 5 grams protein

Potatoes (1 medium) = 4 grams protein

Hummus (2 tablespoons) = 2.5 grams protein

White bread (1 slice) = 2 to 3 grams protein

Protein-rich foods come supercharged with some key nutrients for optimal growth as part of their food matrix. Namely, zinc, calcium, vitamin D, and perhaps most important, iron. Iron deficiency affects 7 to 16 percent of kids and teens, so making an intentional effort to offer protein sources that are higher in iron can help kids meet their needs (see page 114 for great options).

**Healthy Fats for Kids**

If parenthood has taught me anything that's helped enhance my own food freedom journey, it has been to *embrace full fat*. As we've already established, we need to pack a lot of calories into those little busy bodies, and since fats are the most *calorie dense* of the macronutrients, they're an economical and efficient choice.

Fat also makes food taste good. When kids make the brave leap from a food exposure sitting dormant on the table, to an actual mouth-chew-swallow milestone event, we want to make sure it tastes as damn good as possible, so they're up to try it again. Want your kids to try (and actually *like*) broccoli? Skip the low-fat unsalted steamed florets and throw a handful of cheese on those greens! Want them to eat their morning oatmeal? Add a spoonful of melted butter or a drizzle of cream (and maybe a few sprinkles for the *fun factor*). Introducing salad? Give them as much dressing or dip as they please! Don't hand your picky kid an astringent 0 percent fat plain Greek yogurt when you're far more likely to have a repeat customer after they taste a full-fat variety.

There are also unique benefits of certain fats for this stage of life, particularly for the rapidly developing brain (which is nearly 60 percent fat!). DHA omega-3 fats seem to be the most critical for supporting brain development, visual acuity, and mental performance, so try to work salmon, trout, or DHA-enriched eggs into the family menu more often.[9]

## Building Healthy Meals with sDOR and HCC

Listen, I get that this might be a radically different feeding approach to what you grew up with or have been currently utilizing at home. But if you take a step back, I hope you can see how a low-pressure strategy like sDOR can actually help alleviate some dinnertime anxiety.

Here are some important takeaway tips to help you integrate the feeding method of sDOR with the nutrition framework of HCC:

- **Exposure, Exposure, Exposure.** On average, it can take kids eight to ten exposures of a food before they accept it.[10] Be patient, this does take time.
- **Don't Be Afraid to Add "Unhealthy" Things to Make "Healthy" Foods Taste Good.** The quotation marks are absolutely critical here, because you'll find that even foods that have been demonized as "unhealthy" may be essential to getting your kid the nutrition they need. Do not be afraid to *add* fun foods to your child's meals! Try dips, oils, butter, and cheese for veggies; sweet, sticky glazes on fish and poultry; and sauces on *everything*! Oh, and don't forget about the sprinkles or chocolate chips in oats and yogurt! Make food fun!

- **Offer Choices from All Hunger Crushing Compound Categories.** I always recommend serving meals family style when kids are still learning to like a variety of foods (and inevitably going through picky phases). When possible, it's ideal to offer three to five different meal components for them to explore. Here are some examples:

  - *Protein:* Chicken, yogurt, milk, tofu, edamame, hamburger, salmon
  - *Fat:* Added fats and oils (salad dressing, cooking oil, melted butter), avocado, nut or seed butter, fatty fish
  - *Fiber:* Fruit, vegetables, whole grains, legumes
  - *Safe food (Naked Carbs):* Bun, bread, rice, taco shells, wraps, noodles, pasta, baked French fries

- **Upgrade Simple Carb "Safe Foods" with Hunger Crushing Cooking Hacks.** There are a lot of easy ways to add a little extra nutrition to your kid's favorite foods. Here are just a few of my favorites:

  - *White rice:* Cook your grains with bone broth instead of water to add 8 grams of protein per cup.
  - *Orange juice:* Puree ⅓ cup of silken tofu or Greek yogurt with fruit juice for a Creamsicle-like smoothie with an extra 3 to 7 grams of protein.
  - *Plain tomato pasta:* Puree lentils into your tomato sauce for 4 to 5 grams each of fiber and protein.
  - *Pancakes:* Use pureed cottage cheese in place of some of the liquid to add an extra 5 grams of protein to your chocolate chip pancakes.

- *Boxed mac and cheese:* Add pureed cottage cheese to the contents of the cheese seasoning pack to add extra creaminess and 7 grams of protein.
- *Tomato soup:* Puree white beans into tomato soup for an extra 3 to 4 grams each of fiber and protein.

## Simple Family Meal Examples

When you're dealing with fussy kids *and* limited mental energy to scour Pinterest for a new viral recipe to try, having some simple meal ideas you can fall back on is key. These are just some examples to illustrate how to use the HCC, sDOR, and the tips I've shared in this chapter. I stuck to some meal themes here to spark my own inspiration, but don't worry if the meal components on your table don't "make sense." Some nights it's going to be a real hodge-podge, and that's totally okay.

| | |
|---|---|
| Meatless Monday | Potato (Safe food/Fiber) |
| | Butter (Fat) |
| | Cheese (Protein/Healthy Fat) |
| | Sour cream (Fat) |
| | Bean chili cooked in olive oil (Protein/Fiber/Healthy Fat) |
| | Corn (Safe food/Fiber) |
| Taco Tuesday | Ground beef cooked in olive oil (Protein/Healthy Fat) |
| | Sautéed bell peppers (Fiber) |
| | Lettuce (Fiber) |
| | Corn (Safe food/Fiber) |
| | Guacamole (Fiber/Healthy Fat) |
| | Sour cream (Fat) |
| | Corn tortilla shells (Safe food/Naked Carbs) |
| Salmon Bowl | Salmon (Protein/Healthy Fat) |
| | Teriyaki sauce (Safe food/Naked Carbs) |
| | Rice (Safe food/Naked Carbs) |
| | Buttered broccoli (Fiber/Fat) |
| | Edamame (Protein/Fiber/Healthy Fat) |

| | |
|---|---|
| Pasta Night | Spaghetti (Safe food/Naked Carbs)<br>Zucchini "noodles" cooked in olive oil (Fiber/Healthy Fat)<br>Turkey meatballs (Protein)<br>Olive oil tomato sauce (Healthy Fat)<br>Cheese (Healthy Fat/Protein) |
| Pizza Night | Cheesy pita pizza (Safe food/Naked Carb/Protein/Healthy Fat)<br>Salad with cheese and dressing (Fiber/Protein/Healthy Fat) |
| Breakfast for Dinner | Scrambled eggs cooked in olive oil (Protein/Healthy Fat)<br>Toast (Safe food/Naked Carbs)<br>Peanut butter (Healthy Fat/Protein)<br>Berries (Safe food/Fiber)<br>Turkey bacon cooked in olive oil (Protein/Healthy Fat) |
| Pub Food Night | Chicken tenders (Protein)<br>Sweet dipping sauce (Safe food/Naked Carbs)<br>Baked fries in olive oil (Safe food/Naked Carb/Healthy Fat)<br>Carrot and celery sticks (Fiber)<br>Ranch dip (Fat) |

## Favorite Foods for Kids

Here's a good mom joke for you. What's the best food for kids? *Whatever food they will actually eat.* HA! All kids will have days where they only eat bagels, or bananas, or yogurt tubes, and we just kinda have to roll with those quirky hyperfixations and phases. But here are some of my favorite foods for growing bodies to throw into rotation:

- **Avocado.** Avocados are a popular first food in baby-feeding circles for a reason, and they can be an incredible tool to utilize as kids grow. They're calorie-dense, easy to eat, and are dual citizens with a solid dose of both fiber and healthy monounsaturated fats. Smash avocado into guacamole for a superdip that's likely more nutrient-dense than the dipper, or puree with citrus for a creamy salad dressing. My son's favorite snack is something he calls "candy avocado," which is simply a halved avocado filled with balsamic glaze that he can (*literally*) dig into with a spoon!

- **Super "Sprinkles" (Hemp, Chia, Flax).** If you're struggling with picky eating or a limited appetite, choosing foods that offer big nutrition in an itty-bitty package is quite the hack. Hemp hearts, chia seeds, and flaxseeds are triple-threat HCCs, offering varying amounts of protein, fiber, and healthy fats, including those brain-building omega-3s. They're also all pretty neutral in taste, smell, and texture, so like that old lady with her hot sauce, you can put that sh*t on everything. And don't be afraid of the whole *hemp* thing. The hulled seeds naturally do not contain cannabinoids, so these are not going to get your toddler high (*they're likely feral enough just the way they are*). So, try throwing flax into muffins, chia into smoothies, and hemp hearts into oats, to give every baby bite a big nutrition boost.

- **Nuts & Nut Butter.** A lot of us '80s and '90s kids can probably credit most of our growth solely to PB&J sandwiches. They're delicious, reliable, inexpensive, and nutrient-dense—the OG Hunger Crushing Combo, if you will! Whether we're talking whole snacking tree nuts (or peanuts) or spreads, nuts offer protein, fiber, and healthy mono- and polyunsaturated fats, along with antioxidants (e.g., selenium, vitamin E, and zinc). We also know that exposing kids regularly to peanuts and tree nut products starting immediately when they begin solids up through early childhood and beyond can help reduce the rate of nut and peanut allergy by adolescence by over 70 percent.[11] Although most schools require nut-free lunches, there are plenty of at-home opportunities to cash in on nut nutrition. Try adding nuts or nut butters to smoothies, oats, and baked goods, make homemade

nut-based energy bites or bars, use them for sweet or savory
dips and sauces, or keep it classy with nut butter toasts and
sammies.

- **Whole-Milk Dairy.** One of the reasons dairy is still lauded
  as a useful tool in infant, child, and adolescent nutrition
  is that it packs multiple key nutrients into one generally
  well-accepted package. When you throw that yogurt cup
  into your kid's lunchbox, you know they're getting a solid
  dose of protein, healthy fat, carbohydrates, calcium, vitamin
  D (when fortified), plus a cocktail of other essential nutrients
  that help build bones, support growth, and fuel activity. And
  again, remember, fat is back (and should have never been out
  of style in the first place). Updated research has found that
  whole-fat dairy is *not* associated with obesity or excess weight
  gain in kids or teens, nor is it linked to any kind of cardiometabolic risk.[12] Whole dairy generally has a more palatable texture and consistency, which reduces the need to add extra
  sugars or syrups to make it taste good to picky kids. More
  Hunger Crushing Compounds and nutrition, less added
  sugar. Of course, if your kiddo is lactose intolerant, look for
  lactose-free versions, or choose a fortified nondairy alternative with protein and no added sugar (e.g., soy- or pea-based
  milk).
- **Sweet Potatoes.** Sweet potatoes win some big awards with
  kids and parents alike, because they're the closest thing in the
  veggie family to candy, while also packing fiber, energizing
  carbs, vitamin A (from beta-carotene), vitamin C, and potassium. Cut them into strips and roast 'em at 425°F to make
  fries. Mash them with cinnamon and butter for an easy side.
  Or throw them into smoothies or muffin recipes for color,
  fiber, and natural sweetness.

## HCC Example Day for
## Kids & Adolescents

Trying to build out a family meal plan that satisfies every family member often feels like a full-time job in itself. I therefore prefer to have simple meal "building blocks" that can be assembled in different forms and portions to satisfy the whole lot. For example, a big batch of plain rice can be used as a "safe food" for fussier kiddos, and can be transformed into chicken fried rice for more adventurous children and adults. Here's just a very rudimentary example of how meals and snacks could play out for kids:

> Breakfast: Scrambled eggs with whole-grain peanut butter toast with sliced strawberries and honey
>
> Snack: Whole-grain muffins (see page 330) with 1 cup whole milk or soy milk
>
> Lunch: Chicken quesadilla with guacamole and sour cream, served with carrot sticks and ranch dip
>
> Snack: Olive oil–roasted chickpeas, mandarin orange, and a small chocolate chip cookie
>
> Dinner: Whole-grain spaghetti and meatballs with garlic bread and steamed broccoli
>
> Snack: Smoothie with Greek yogurt, whole milk, hemp hearts, banana, berries, and almond butter

## Supplements to Consider for
## Kids & Adolescents

Going from the "clean plate club" toward a low-pressure approach to feeding may bring up some real anxieties when the **what** or **how much** your child decides to eat doesn't match *your* expectations or desires. And while kids *absolutely can* meet their nutrient needs through food alone, for a lot of families, a simple supplement routine can help alleviate some anxiety to allow you to trust the long-game process. Here are some of the most commonly useful vitamins to discuss with your child's pediatrician:

- **Kids' Multivitamin.** Kids' food intake can be as unpredictable as a reality TV reunion episode. Thankfully, children's multivitamins can serve as an assurance policy for those days when even their "favorites" end up in the trash. When choosing a multivitamin, look for one with vitamins A and D, B vitamins, calcium, zinc, iron, choline, and DHA omega-3s. Always choose a vitamin brand that has been third-party tested for purity and dose consistency, and keep vitamins away from young children (many are designed to look and taste like candy, and overdosing on vitamins can cause real harm). If you're concerned about your kid's diet, it may be worth having their vitamin levels checked annually, particularly for iron and vitamin D status, since deficiency in children is so prevalent. Depending on your kid's stores, your pediatrician may prescribe a specific vitamin dosage based on their weight and unique needs.

- **Probiotics.** Supplemental probiotics certainly aren't a must-have for all kids, but specific strains may be useful in some circumstances. For example, *Lactobacillus rhamnosus* GG and *Saccharomyces boulardii* (which is technically a yeast) have been consistently shown to reduce the severity and duration of antibiotic-associated and viral diarrhea in children.[13] There is also emerging (though less conclusive) research showing potential benefits of specific strains for colic, IBS, eczema, and asthma. Speak to your dietitian or pediatrician about which probiotic strains (if any) are appropriate for your child.

## Lifestyle Considerations for
## Raising Healthy Kids

Raising healthy kids involves a lot more than peas and broccoli. It's committing to balancing that broccoli with other physical, emotional, mental, and social well-being considerations. Which means sometimes the family pizza night *will be* the healthy choice. Here are some other important considerations for supporting your kids' holistic sense of health:

- **Model a Healthy Relationship with Food.** How our kids think about and interact with food is largely dependent on what we model as parents or caregivers. Even if you're still working through your own internal challenges, make an effort to visibly model the behavior and food beliefs you want your kids to carry with them through life.

- **Encourage Physical Activity (Outdoors, If Possible).** We all know the mental madness that a cooped-up rainy day indoors can cause busy-bodied kids (*and their parents*). Kids need to move. Aim for at least sixty minutes of moderate to vigorous activity daily through a combination of aerobic, muscle-strengthening, and bone-strengthening activities. Getting outside for independent unstructured play and age-appropriate "risky play" like climbing, jumping, exploring nature, or building, can help foster risk assessment and decision-making skills, boost creativity, and build self-confidence. And don't forget about the power of social interaction! While solo bike rides and swims are amazing cardiovascular activities (and great stress release, too), engaging in sports with friends can also help teach resilience, conflict resolution, leadership, and cooperation.

- **Limit Social Media and Screen Time.** Mounting research clearly shows that social media use in childhood increases

the risk of anxiety, depression, cyberbullying, body dissatisfaction, loneliness, and eating disorders.[14] It also may dimin-
ish critical social skills and attention span, while negatively
affecting academic achievement and learning. And I'm barely
scratching the surface. Consider setting screen time limits,
monitor and restrict usage and content access, and teach kids
to critically evaluate what they see online.

- **Sleep Hygiene.** Children's physical, cognitive, and emotional health depends on them having a good night's rest.
  Most kids need between nine and twelve hours per night to
  function optimally in the day (depending on their age and
  circumstance), so establishing healthy sleep habits early on is
  key. See pages 159–161 for tips on optimal sleep hygiene.

- **Emotional Intelligence & Mental Health.** You are the
  greatest role model in your kids' lives, and while none of us is
  perfect, we can make a mindful effort to demonstrate empathy and conflict resolutions in our own relationships. Communication is also key, so remind your kids that they can
  speak to you about anything without judgment, while seeking opportunities to teach them about empathy and healthy
  coping strategies for managing frustration or stress.

- **Hygiene and Health Maintenance.** One of the best things
  my kids took out of our COVID-19 era is their unwavering
  commitment to washing their hands every single time they
  walk in the door. Teaching personal hygiene is an important
  life skill! So, build a routine of teeth brushing, handwashing,
  sleeve sneezing, bathing, and other personal and community
  health–promoting behaviors from a young age, when habits
  are easier to form. Also, do your best to stay on top of your
  child's regular medical, dental, and vision checkups to catch
  potential issues early on.

## Wrapping Up: Raising a Healthy Eater for Life

If there's one major takeaway from this chapter, let it be this: You're doing a great job. If your kids refuse to eat green things, you are doing a great job. If your kid has been classified as "overweight," you're doing a great job. If your kid rejects lunch and whines for snacks every damn day, you're doing a great job. You are taking strides to break that generational diet cycle and nurture your kids' relationship with food, simply by reading this chapter. Give yourself a huge pat on the back. Remember, raising healthy, competent eaters is far more about the *how* of feeding than the *what* they actually eat. So, if you feel that you're failing, you're probably on the right track. You got this.

# PART 3

# PUTTING IT ON YOUR PLATE

You're clear on the structure. You know the perks. You've got the cold hard science on deck.

Now . . .

We eat.

# CHAPTER 11

. . . . . . . . . . . . . . . . . . .

## Making It Easy:
## HCC Cheat Sheets

The Hunger Crushing Combo is designed to feel intuitive, so a lot of the meals you're already making probably meet these criteria nicely. But if you're just getting started, here's some extra direction.

These lists may just give you some inspiration, or an aha moment of realizing all of the expansive and exciting meal possibilities. If you have more specific wellness goals, these can help guide you to make the most efficient and effective choices. While I do explicitly share the grams of protein, fiber, and fat in this book's recipes for those with specific goals or health concerns, I don't do that in these cheat sheets. That's because I want this to become a natural and effortless process for you, where you don't need to obsessively weigh or measure things out. Instead, I've prepared the list with visual portion cues (see the following box) in the order of the most "efficient" Hunger Crushing Compound sources toward the top. This generally means that the foods at the top of the list offer more protein, fiber, and/or healthy fat for fewer calories, so you don't need to eat a massive portion (plus potentially excess calories) to meet your nutrient needs.

## Visual Portion Cues

Baseball or fist (small—average—large) = ¾ cup—1 cup—1¼ cups

Tennis ball or child's fist = ½ cup

Ping-Pong ball or ice cream scoop = ¼ cup

Small thumb = 1 tbsp

Small thumb tip = 1 tsp

Deck of cards or hand palm = 3.5 to 4 oz

Pair of dice = 1.5 to 2 oz

Try to focus most often on choosing "efficient" sources of Hunger Crushing Compounds (especially those with greater portion sizes, volume, and dual citizenship), and on combining smaller amounts of "less-efficient" foods to satisfy nutrient and calorie needs. Generally, two "snack dose" servings will yield the equivalent of one "meal dose."

## Power Proteins

There are endless ways to create satiating and satisfying meals that meet your protein needs. If your goals (or your unique body needs) depend on prioritizing protein, you generally want to aim for around **20 to 35 grams per meal**, and **8 to 20 grams per snack**. The more calories you need, the more likely you need to aim for the upper end of those ranges, and the more meals or snacks you need.

Here's a list of some simple visual cues standardized to a goal of around 25 grams of protein per meal, and 10 to 15 grams per snack.

Remember, if you have a weight-management goal, focusing on lean protein options near the top of the list (especially those with larger portions) will be advantageous. For example, you'd need to eat five times the amount of calories of quinoa instead of egg whites or shrimp to get a full 25 grams of protein, if weight management is your goal.

| PROTEIN SOURCE | MEAL DOSE | SNACK DOSE | DUAL STATUS |
|---|---|---|---|
| **ANIMAL PROTEIN** | | | |
| Egg whites | Fist or baseball 1 cup or 8 egg whites | Tennis ball or child's fist ½ cup or 4 egg whites | |
| Shrimp, cooked | 10 medium shrimp, cooked 3.5 to 4 oz | 5 medium shrimp 2 oz | |
| Lean white fish (e.g., cod, halibut, haddock), cooked | Deck of cards or hand palm 4 to 4.5 oz | Pair of large dice 2 oz | |
| Whey protein powder | Ice cream scoop or Ping-Pong ball 1 provided scoop | 2 small thumbs ½ provided scoop | |
| Lean poultry breast (e.g., chicken or turkey breast), cooked | Deck of cards or hand palm 3.5 to 4 oz | Pair of large dice 2 oz | |
| Canned fish (e.g., tuna in water) | Tennis ball or child's fist 3.5 oz cooked | Ping-Pong ball or ice cream scoop 1.75 oz cooked | Fat |
| Lean pork (e.g., tenderloin), cooked | Deck of cards or hand palm 3.5 oz cooked | Pair of large dice 2 oz cooked | Fat |
| Eggs | 4 whole eggs | 2 whole eggs | Fat |

| | | | |
|---|---|---|---|
| 2% plain Greek or Skyr yogurt | Large fist 1¼ cups | Tennis ball or child's fist ½ cup | Fat |
| 2% plain cottage cheese | Fist or baseball 1 cup | Tennis ball or child's fist ½ cup | Fat |
| Salmon fillet, cooked | Deck of cards or hand palm 3.5 to 4 oz | Pair of large dice 2 oz | Fat |
| Lean beef (e.g., tenderloin, sirloin), cooked | Deck of cards or hand palm 3 to 3.5 oz cooked | Pair of small dice 1.5 oz cooked | Fat |
| Dairy milk (1%) | 3 (8-oz) glasses 3 cups | 1½ (8-oz) glasses 1½ cups | Fat |
| Semifirm cheese (e.g., Cheddar, mozzarella) | 4 slices or small fist (shredded) 3.5 oz, or ¾ cup | 2 slices or small child's fist (shredded) 1.5 oz, or 6 tbsp | Fat |

**PLANT PROTEIN**

| | | | |
|---|---|---|---|
| Seitan (wheat gluten), cooked | Deck of cards or hand palm 3.5 to 4 oz | Pair of large dice 2 oz | |
| Vegan protein powder | Ice cream scoop or Ping-Pong ball 1 provided scoop | 2 small thumbs ½ provided scoop | |
| Soy ground round ("faux meat"), cooked and crumbled | Fist or baseball 1 cup | Tennis ball or child's fist ½ cup | Fat |
| Nutritional yeast | Small fist ¾ cup | Ice-cream scoop or Ping-Pong ball ¼ cup | Fat |
| Mycoprotein (Quorn), crumbled. Note: May cause allergic reactions and GI distress for some. | 1½ fists or baseballs 1½ cups | Small fist ¾ cup | Fiber |

| | | | |
|---|---|---|---|
| Firm tofu, cooked and cubed | Fist or baseball 1 cup | Tennis ball or child's fist ½ cup | |
| Unsweetened soy milk | 3 (8-oz) glasses 3 cups | 1½ (8-oz) glasses 1½ cups | Fat |
| Edamame, cooked and shelled | 1½ fists or baseballs 1½ cups | Small fist ¾ cup | Fat, fiber |
| Lentils, cooked | 1½ fists or baseballs 1½ cups | Small fist ¾ cup | Fiber |
| Beans (e.g., black beans, chickpeas, kidney beans), cooked | 2 small fists 1¾ cups | Small fist ¾ cup | Fiber |
| Hemp seeds (hulled)/ hemp hearts | Tennis ball or child's fist ½ cup | 3 small thumbs 3 tbsp | Fat |
| Quinoa, cooked | 3 fists or baseballs 3 cups | 1½ fists or baseballs 1½ cups | Fiber |

## Fabulous Fiber Foods

If your priority at this stage of life is fiber, I generally like to aim for 6 to 12 grams per meal and at least 3 to 6 grams per snack. Now, you're going to look at the chart and think, "*Abbey, HCC sounds great and I'm so game. But two cups of blueberries? In this economy?!*" I got you! Those numbers are there so you have awareness of the many different ways to meet these fiber goals. But in most cases, you're going to be combining multiple snack doses to yield a super-high-fiber satiating meal. For example, when building a stir-fry bowl, you might be getting mini doses of fiber from broccoli, carrots, rice, and tofu! The more the merrier, so don't limit yourself to just one source (but, hey, if the blueberries are on clearance, go wild!). For comparison, this list is standardized for a goal of around 7 grams of fiber per meal and 4 grams per snack. And remember, foods at the top of the list with larger portions will offer the best fiber returns on your calorie budget.

| FIBER SOURCE | MEAL DOSE | SNACK DOSE | DUAL STATUS |
|---|---|---|---|
| **VEGETABLES** | | | |
| Artichoke, cooked | Fist or baseball 1 cup | Child's fist or tennis ball ½ cup | |
| Collard greens, cooked | Fist or baseball 1 cup | Child's fist or tennis ball ½ cup | |
| Spinach, cooked | 1½ fists or baseballs 1½ cups | Small fist ¾ cup | |
| Cauliflower, cooked | 2½ fists or baseballs 2½ cups | Large fist 1¼ cups | |
| Broccoli, cooked | 1½ fists or baseballs 1½ cups | Small fist ¾ cup | |
| Carrots, cooked | 1½ fists or baseballs 1½ cups | Small fist ¾ cup | |
| Brussels sprouts, cooked | 1½ fists or baseballs 1½ cups | Small fist ¾ cup | |
| Kale, cooked | 2½ fists or baseballs 2½ cups | Large fist 1¼ cups | |

| Sweet potato with skin, cooked | 1 large fist<br>1 medium, or 1 cup, cubed | Tennis ball or child's fist<br>½ medium, or ½ cup, cubed |
|---|---|---|
| Corn, shucked and cooked | 1½ fists or baseballs<br>1½ cups | Small fist<br>¾ cup |
| Baked potato with skin, cooked | 1½ large fists<br>1½ large potatoes, or 1½ cups, cubed | Small fist<br>1 small potato, or ¾ cup, cubed |

**FRUITS**

| Raspberries | Fist or baseball<br>1 cup | Child's fist or tennis ball<br>½ cup |
|---|---|---|
| Blackberries | Fist or baseball<br>1 cup | Child's fist or tennis ball<br>½ cup |
| Pears, with skin | Large fist<br>2 small, or 1¼ cups diced | Small fist<br>1 small, or ¾ cup diced |
| Strawberries, sliced | 2 fists or baseballs<br>2 cups | 1 fist or baseball<br>1 cup |
| Orange segments | 1½ fists or baseballs<br>1½ cups | Small fist<br>¾ cup |
| Kiwi, with skin | Large fist<br>3 medium fruit, or 1¼ cups diced | Small fist<br>1½ kiwis, or ¾ cup diced |
| Apple, with skin | 1½ fists or baseballs<br>1½ medium fruit, or 1½ cups diced | Small fist<br>¾ medium fruit, or ¾ cup diced |

| | | | |
|---|---|---|---|
| Blueberries | 2 fists or baseballs<br>2 cups | 1 fist or baseball<br>1 cup | |
| Avocado | Small fist<br>¾ medium, or<br>¾ cup | Tennis ball or child's<br>fist<br>½ medium, or<br>½ cup | Fat |
| Banana | 2 fists or baseballs<br>2 medium bananas,<br>or 2 cups | 1 fist or baseball<br>1 medium banana, or<br>1 cup | |

**GRAINS**

| | | | |
|---|---|---|---|
| Bran cereal (e.g., bran flakes) | Fist or baseball<br>1 cup | Tennis ball or child's<br>fist<br>½ cup | Protein |
| Bulgur, cooked | Fist or baseball<br>1 cup cooked | Tennis ball or child's<br>fist<br>½ cup | Protein |
| Air-popped popcorn | 6 fists or baseballs<br>6 cups | 3 fists or baseballs<br>3 cups | Protein |
| Farro, cooked | Large fist<br>1¼ cups | Small fist<br>¾ cup | Protein |
| Barley, cooked | Large fist<br>1¼ cups | Small fist<br>⅔ cup | Protein |
| Buckwheat groats, cooked | 1½ fists or<br>baseballs<br>1½ cups | Small fist<br>¾ cup | Protein |
| Whole-grain or sourdough bread | 3½ hand palms<br>3½ slices | 2 hand palms<br>2 slices | Protein |
| Oats, dried | Small fist<br>¾ cup dried<br>(~2 cups cooked) | Tennis ball or child's<br>fist<br>½ cup (~1 cup<br>cooked) | Protein |
| Quinoa, cooked | 1½ fists or<br>baseballs<br>1½ cups | Small fist<br>¾ cup | Protein |

| Long-grain brown rice, cooked | 2 fists or baseballs 2 cups | Fist or baseball 1 cup | Protein |
| --- | --- | --- | --- |

**HIGH-FIBER LEGUMES, NUTS, AND SEEDS**

| Green peas, shelled and cooked | Fist or baseball 1 cup | Tennis ball or child's fist ½ cup | Protein |
| --- | --- | --- | --- |
| Lentils, cooked | Tennis ball or child's fist ½ cup | Ice cream scoop or Ping-Pong ball ¼ cup | Protein |
| Chia seeds | 2 small thumbs 2 tbsp | 1 small thumb 1 tbsp | Fat, protein |
| Flaxseeds | 2 small thumbs 2 tbsp | 1 small thumb 1 tbsp | Fat, protein |
| Beans (e.g., chickpeas, black beans, kidney beans), cooked | Tennis ball or child's fist ½ cup | Ice cream scoop or Ping-Pong ball ¼ cup | Protein |
| Edamame, shelled and cooked | Fist or baseball 1 cup | Tennis ball or child's fist ½ cup | Fat, protein |
| Wheat germ | Tennis ball or child's fist ½ cup | Ice cream scoop or Ping-Pong ball ¼ cup | Fat, protein |
| Nuts (e.g., almonds, pistachios) | Tennis ball or child's fist 2 oz, or ~½ cup | Ice cream scoop or Ping-Pong ball 1 oz, or ~¼ cup | Fat, protein |
| Seeds (e.g., sunflower, pumpkin) | Small fist 3 oz, or ¾ cup | Tennis ball or child's fist 2 oz, or ½ cup | Fat, protein |

## Fantastic Fat-Filled Foods

Unlike protein and fiber, we don't have as much solid data on how much fat per meal is "optimal." But there are so many benefits to including more anti-inflammatory healthy fats in our meals and snacks for overall health. To meet general guidelines without fussing, I recommend aiming for **8 to 15 grams of healthy fats per meal and 4 to 10 grams of healthy fats per snack.** For simple comparison, this list uses calories instead of absolute grams of fat (around 150 calories worth of fat-rich foods per meal and 80 calories for a snack). And this is because for fat specifically, the amount in grams is far less important in this framework than its dual-citizen status, volume (portion size), and calorie density. The greater the volume, the more fiber and protein to stretch the fat's staying power without tipping the calorie scales. This is why for the same 15 grams of healthy fats, we'd feel far more satiated eating two-thirds of a medium-size avocado vs. a tablespoon of avocado oil. Of course, I absolutely support adding mindful portions of cooking oils and fats for flavor and cooking, but with an emphasis on whole food dual citizens most often.

| FRUITS | MEAL DOSE | SNACK DOSE | DUAL STATUS |
|---|---|---|---|
| Olives (medium whole) | 1 fist or baseball 30 olives, or 1 cup | Tennis ball or child's fist 15 olives, or ½ cup | Fiber |
| Avocado | Tennis ball or child's fist ⅔ medium, or ½ cup mashed | Ice cream scoop or Ping-Pong ball ⅓ medium, or ¼ cup mashed | Fiber |
| Shredded unsweetened coconut | 3 small thumbs 3 tbsp | 1½ small thumbs 1½ tbsp | Fiber |
| **PEANUTS, TREE NUTS, AND SEEDS** | | | |
| Hummus | Small child's fist ⅓ cup | 3 small thumbs 3 tbsp | Protein, fiber |

| | | | |
|---|---|---|---|
| Ground flaxseeds | Ice cream scoop or Ping-Pong ball ¼ cup | 2 small thumbs 2 tbsp | Protein, fiber |
| Pistachios | Ice cream scoop or Ping-Pong ball ¼ cup, or 37 nuts | 2 small thumbs 2 tbsp, or 18 nuts | Protein, fiber |
| Almonds | Ice cream scoop or Ping-Pong ball ¼ cup, or 22 nuts | 2 small thumbs 2 tbsp, or 11 nuts | Protein, fiber |
| Peanuts | Ice cream scoop or Ping-Pong ball ¼ cup, or 30 peanuts | 2 small thumbs 2 tbsp, or 15 peanuts | Protein, fiber |
| Cashews | Ice cream scoop or Ping-Pong ball ¼ cup, or 18 nuts | 2 small thumbs 2 tbsp, or 6 nuts | Protein |
| Pecan halves | Ice cream scoop or Ping-Pong ball ¼ cup, or 15 nuts | 2 small thumbs 2 tbsp, or 7 nuts | Protein, fiber |
| Walnut halves | Ice cream scoop or Ping-Pong ball ¼ cup, or 11 nuts | 2 small thumbs 2 tbsp, or 6 nuts | Protein, fiber |
| Hazelnuts | 3 small thumbs 3 tbsp, or 25 nuts | 1 small thumb 1 tbsp, or 8 to 10 nuts | Protein, fiber |
| Sesame seeds | 3 small thumbs 3 tbsp | 1 small thumb 1 tbsp | Protein, fiber |
| Sunflower seeds | 3 small thumbs 3 tbsp | 1 small thumb 1 tbsp | Protein, fiber |
| Hemp seeds | 2½ small thumbs 2½ tbsp | 1 small thumb 1 tbsp | Protein |
| Pumpkin seeds | 2½ small thumbs 2½ tbsp | 1 small thumb 1 tbsp | Protein, fiber |
| Chia seeds | 2 small thumbs 2 tbsp | 1 small thumb 1 tbsp | Protein, fiber |

| Cacao nibs | 2 small thumbs<br>2 tbsp | 1 small thumb<br>1 tbsp | Protein, fiber |
| --- | --- | --- | --- |
| Macadamia nuts | 1½ small thumbs<br>1½ tsp, or 7 nuts | 2 small thumb tips<br>2 tsp, or 4 nuts | Fiber |
| Pine nuts | 1½ small thumbs<br>1½ tsp | 2 small thumb tips<br>2 tsp | Protein |
| Tahini | 1½ small thumbs<br>1½ tbsp | 1 small thumb<br>1 tbsp | Protein, fiber |
| Natural almond butter | 1½ small thumbs<br>1½ tbsp | 1 small thumb<br>1 tbsp | Protein |
| Natural peanut butter | 1½ small thumbs<br>1½ tbsp | 1 small thumb<br>1 tbsp | Protein |
| **PROTEIN FOODS** | | | |
| Edamame, cooked and shelled | Fist or baseball<br>¾ to 1 cup | Tennis ball or child's fist<br>½ cup | Protein, fiber |
| 4% plain Greek yogurt | Small fist<br>¾ cup | Ice cream scoop or Ping-Pong ball<br>¼ cup | Protein |
| 4% plain cottage cheese | Small fist<br>⅔ to ¾ cup | Ice cream scoop or Ping-Pong ball<br>¼ cup | Protein |
| Firm tofu, cooked and cubed | Small fist<br>¾ cup | Ice cream scoop or Ping-Pong ball<br>¼ cup, cubed | Protein |
| Whole egg | Tennis ball or child's fist<br>2 to 3 eggs, or ~½ cup | Ice cream scoop or Ping-Pong ball<br>1 egg, or ½ cup | Protein |
| Salmon fillet | Palm or deck of cards<br>3 oz cooked | Pair of large dice<br>1.5 oz cooked | Protein |

# Simple Hunger Crushing Combos
## to Get You Started

I'm sure you'll come up with your own favorite Hunger Crushing Combos, but here are just a few of mine. In a lot of cases, the ingredients may be dual citizens and straddle two or more HCC categories, but because I like my tables neat and tidy (#TypeA), we've placed them in their "Primary Residence." Naked carbs are optional (but obviously, they make life more fun!).

| PROTEIN | FIBER | FAT | NAKED CARB |
|---|---|---|---|
| Greek yogurt | Raspberries | Sliced almonds | Mini chocolate chips |
| Canned tuna | Chopped veggies | Olive oil mayonnaise | Crackers |
| Hard-boiled egg | Whole-grain toast | Avocado | Your choice! |
| Edamame | Mandarin oranges | Cashews | Take your pick! |
| Protein powder | Berries | Nut butter | You name it! |
| Turkey meatballs | Sautéed spinach | Parmesan cheese | Pasta |
| Protein powder | Oatmeal | Flax | Pure maple syrup |
| Eggs | Whole-grain waffle | Nut butter | Honey |
| Salmon | Sweet potatoes & green beans | Cashews | Teriyaki sauce |
| Chickpeas | Salad greens | Avocado | Croutons |
| Shrimp | Whole-grain tortilla | Guacamole | As you wish! |
| Chicken kebabs | Whole-grain pita | Hummus | Follow your heart! |
| Protein pancake | Strawberries | Peanut butter | Pure maple syrup |

| | | | |
|---|---|---|---|
| Chicken breast | Whole-grain pizza dough | Shredded cheese | You're the boss! |
| Chicken soup | Cooked vegetables | Pesto | Noodles |
| Soy milk | Whole-grain muffin | Almond butter | Mini chocolate chips |
| Egg omelet | Bell peppers and mushrooms | Cheese | Toast |
| Nutritional yeast | Popcorn | Parmesan cheese | Dealer's choice! |
| Cottage cheese | Apple | Nut butter | Your call! |
| Mini mozzarella cheese balls | Cherry tomatoes | Pesto | Rosé? Yes, please! |
| Smoked salmon | Rye bread | Cream cheese | Select away! |
| Tofu satay | Stir-fried broccoli | Peanut sauce | White rice |

## How to Turn Your Fear Foods into Balanced Meals

If you have "fear foods" that diet culture has convinced you that you cannot be around, I'm here to tell you (again) that this is a safe space for *all* foods. Even though foods will never all be nutritionally equal, we can make them morally equal, and thereby strip them of their power over us by putting them on a level playing field. And the easiest way to do that is to *quite literally* serve them on the same plate. It's not a "cheat meal" that precedes a "clean meal," it's just another collection of foods that together help satisfy both your physical and emotional needs.

Get ready to have your mind blown.

| FEAR FOOD | THE HACK | PROTEIN | FIBER | HEALTHY FATS |
|---|---|---|---|---|
| Chocolate cake | Serve it with . . . | Greek yogurt | Raspberries | Toasted almonds |
| Chocolate sandwich cookies | Make a cookie protein shake using . . . | Protein powder and soy or cow's milk | Banana | Almond butter |
| Mini Halloween chocolate bars | Serve it on top of your oatmeal using . . . | Soy milk for cooking | Cooked oats & banana | Peanut butter |
| Boxed mac and cheese | Upgrade the recipe on the box by adding . . . | Cottage cheese | Steamed broccoli and cauliflower | Cheddar cheese |
| Potato chips | Make a snack plate with . . . | Greek yogurt chip dip | Sliced veggies | Olives |
| Candy | Crush it into energy balls by combining . . . | Protein powder | Dates and oats | Nut butter and coconut |
| Juice | Make chia seed ice pops by pureeing and freezing with . . . | Skyr yogurt | Frozen fruit | Chia seeds |
| Croissant | Turn it into a meal with . . . | Sliced turkey | Apple | Brie cheese |
| Chocolate chip cookies | Make a cookie sandwich using . . . | Whipped ricotta | Smashed raspberries | Shredded coconut |
| Pizza | Load up your slice with . . . | Grilled chicken | Mixed vegetables | Olives |

| Sugary cereal | Use it to top . . . | Greek yogurt | Berries | Hemp hearts |
| --- | --- | --- | --- | --- |
| Ice cream | Make a sundae with . . . | Greek yogurt | Cherries | Peanuts |
| White bagel | Build a sandwich with . . . | Tuna salad | Sliced veggies and greens | Smashed avocado |
| White pasta | Make it a meal with . . . | Turkey meatballs | Spiralized zucchini | Olives |
| White rice | Make fried rice with . . . | Egg and tofu | Stir-fried vegetables | Sesame seeds |
| French fries | Use as a base for . . . | Veggie bean chili | Fajita sautéed bell peppers and onions | Avocado |

## My Favorite HCC Recipes

Remember "choose your own adventure" books? That's what I hope you can experience with these HCC recipes that follow. Don't eat chicken? Head on over to page 254 and swap in your favorite protein. Not a fan of green beans? There are plenty of high fiber goodies on page 257 to explore. You now have the building blocks to make a recipe work for you—not just the recipes in this book, but anything else in your repertoire or library! Let's get cooking.

# THE RECIPES

Here are thirty of my favorite satiating, delicious HCC recipes. You'll see the HCC breakdown at the end of each one, calculated for the recipe as instructed, but I welcome you to make these recipes your own or use one of my suggested swaps!

# THE BREAKFAST CLUB

## Fluffy Lemon Blueberry Protein Pancakes

*Makes 16 to 18 pancakes, or 4 servings*
*Vegetarian, Soy-Free, Gluten-Free (Option), Nut-Free (Option)*

Whether you whip 'em up on a lazy Sunday for the fam, or meal-prep a batch for breakfast on the go, these Fluffy Lemon Blueberry Protein Pancakes are a fantastic way to use the late summer's berry bounty, or lean on that frozen fruit you got on sale.

1 cup whole wheat flour
1 teaspoon baking powder
1 teaspoon baking soda
½ teaspoon salt
1 teaspoon ground cinnamon
1 cup 4% cottage cheese
2 tablespoons honey
2 teaspoons pure vanilla extract
3 large eggs, separated

½ cup whole milk, or more if
    needed
2 teaspoons lemon zest
1 tablespoon freshly squeezed
    lemon juice
1 cup frozen or fresh wild
    blueberries
Unsalted butter or avocado oil, for
    cooking

**For Serving:**
1 cup Greek or Skyr yogurt
½ cup toasted almonds

1 cup wild blueberries
Pure maple syrup or honey

Combine the flour, baking powder, baking soda, salt, and cinnamon in a medium-size bowl.

Place the cottage cheese in a food processor or blender, and process until pureed and smooth. Transfer the pureed cottage cheese to a large bowl and then add the honey, vanilla, two of the egg yolks (discard the third yolk or use in another recipe), the milk, lemon zest, and lemon juice. Mix well with a spatula.

Stir the flour mixture into the cottage cheese mixture. Add the blueberries to the bowl of pancake batter. Gently fold to combine.

Wipe out the bowl used for the flour mixture and add the three egg whites to the bowl. Using an electric beater (or a strong arm), whip the egg whites until fluffy but not stiff, then fold them into the batter.

Heat a large skillet or griddle over medium-low heat. Apply a small pat of unsalted butter or avocado oil to the hot surface and brush it around to cover.

Working in batches, using a ¼-cup measuring spoon, scoop the pancake batter onto the hot cooking surface. Allow the pancakes to cook until small bubbles form on the uncooked side, 3 to 4 minutes. Carefully flip the pancakes with a spatula and cook for an additional 3 to 4 minutes, or until they are cooked through.

Serve immediately, topped with a big dollop of Greek yogurt, toasted almonds, extra blueberries, and maple syrup.

**Make-Ahead Tips:**

To store, place the cooled pancakes, separated by parchment paper, in a container in the fridge for up to 5 days. Reheat in a microwave for 30 seconds, or in a 350°F oven for 5 minutes.

To freeze, place the pancakes, separated by parchment paper, in a freezer-safe bag or container for up to 3 months. Reheat from frozen in a microwave for 1 minute or in a 350°F oven for 10 minutes.

| The HCC Lineup | Make It Your Own |
|---|---|
| Protein 25 g<br>Cottage cheese, egg whites, milk, Greek yogurt | Use ricotta or Skyr yogurt in place of cottage cheese. |
| Fiber 7 g<br>Wheat flour, blueberries | Replace the blueberries with frozen raspberries or diced cherries! You can also make this gluten-free with a gluten-free flour. |
| Fat 12 g<br>Egg yolks, almonds | Go nut-free and top your pancakes with crumbled goat cheese or sunflower seeds. |

## Apple Pie Baked Protein French Toast

*Serves 6*
*Vegetarian, Dairy-Free (Option), Soy-Free (Option),*
*Gluten-Free (Option), Vegan (Option), Nut-Free (Option)*

Imagine maple syrup–drenched French toast and cinnamony apple pie had a baby, but it was miraculously born with a whopping 27 grams of blood sugar–balancing protein. This French toast is just what brunch dreams are made of, packed with hearty sourdough, crisp apples, and crunchy pecans.

Nonstick spray
8 slices (375 to 400 grams total) whole-grain sourdough bread, torn into pieces
4 large eggs
1½ cups cow's, soy, or pea milk
½ cup vanilla protein powder (pea or whey)
1 tablespoon pure maple syrup

1 tablespoon unsalted butter, melted
1 teaspoon ground cinnamon
⅛ teaspoon freshly grated nutmeg
¼ teaspoon salt
1 large apple
2 ounces pecan halves, plus more for serving, if desired

### For Serving (as desired):

1 cup 4% plain Greek or soy yogurt

Additional diced apple
Pure maple syrup

Lightly spray a 9 x 12–inch baking sheet with nonstick spray. Arrange the torn bread in a single layer and set aside.

Whisk together the eggs, milk, protein powder, maple syrup, butter, cinnamon, nutmeg, and salt in a medium-size bowl.

Pour the mixture over the bread and soak well. Cover and refrigerate overnight.

The next morning, preheat the oven to 350°F.

Core and dice the apple, and sprinkle the diced apple and pecan halves over the bread; press firmly down into the bread pieces. Bake for 45 to 50 minutes, or until lightly browned. Remove from the oven and allow to set for 5 minutes before serving as desired with yogurt, extra pecans, and/or maple syrup.

**Make-Ahead Tips:**

Cover the cooled, baked French toast with plastic wrap or store in an airtight container in the fridge for up to 5 days. Remove the plastic wrap and reheat in a microwave for 30 seconds, or in the oven at 350°F for 8 to 10 minutes.

To freeze, bake in a freezer-safe container, and cover with plastic wrap and foil. Remove the plastic wrap and reheat from frozen at 350°F for 20 to 25 minutes, or until browned.

| The HCC Lineup | Make It Your Own |
|---|---|
| Protein 27 g<br>Eggs, protein powder, mylk/milk, Greek yogurt, pecans | Switch up the protein powder flavor or use a cup of cartoned egg whites in place of whole eggs. Make it vegan with plant-based egg replacement, mylk, and pea-based protein powder. |
| Fiber 5 g<br>Whole-grain sourdough, apple, pecans | Use a high-fiber multigrain loaf, or try a pear in place of the apple. You can also make it gluten-free using your favorite hearty gluten-free bread (just make sure to let it get a little stale first). |
| Fat 17 g<br>Pecans, eggs | Replace the pecans with pumpkin seeds for a nut-free option. |

# Bougie British Beans on Toast

*Serves 4*
*Vegetarian, Nut-Free, Dairy-Free (Option), Vegan (Option),*
*Gluten-Free (Option), Soy-Free (Option)*

I have British ancestry and have spent a lot of time in the UK, so I'm pretty sure 90 percent of my protein intake as a child came from Heinz baked beans. And as a dietitian mom today, I'm not mad about it, but this homemade version is a significant upgrade! Prepared with humble pantry staples (and a few fresh additions for color, crunch, and luxe), this take on the British breakfast staple is a meatless Monday meal you'll want all week.

2 teaspoons extra-virgin olive oil

½ yellow onion, diced finely

2 garlic cloves, minced

1 teaspoon smoked paprika

½ teaspoon garlic powder

1 teaspoon chili powder, or more to taste

4 tablespoons tomato paste

2 tablespoons prepared yellow mustard

1½ teaspoons reduced-sodium soy sauce, tamari, or coconut aminos (for soy- or gluten-free)

4 to 5 tablespoons pure maple syrup, or to taste

3 tablespoons cider vinegar

2 (19-ounce) cans reduced-sodium navy beans, drained and rinsed

2 cups fresh spinach or kale leaves, chopped finely

Salt and freshly ground black pepper

**For Serving:**

4 large slices whole-grain sourdough or whole-grain wheat bread, toasted

2 ounces sharp aged Cheddar cheese, grated

2 cups cherry tomatoes, halved (optional)

Flat-leaf parsley, chopped, for garnish (optional)

Heat the olive oil in a large, nonstick skillet over medium heat. Add the onion and cook for 2 to 3 minutes, or until soft.

Add the minced garlic, smoked paprika, garlic powder, and chili powder, and stir until fragrant, about 1 minute. Then, add the tomato paste, yellow mustard, soy sauce, maple syrup, vinegar, and beans. Toss the beans in the sauce mixture.

Add the greens and cook until they're wilted and the sauce is thickened, 5 to 6 minutes. Season with salt and black pepper to taste.

To serve, place the toast on plates, sprinkle the cheese among the toast slices, then pile the beans on top to allow the cheese to melt. Garnish with cherry tomatoes and parsley, if desired. Enjoy hot with a fork and knife (*because she's messy!*).

**Make-Ahead Tip:**
Double or triple the bean portion and store in the fridge for up to 5 days. Serve the beans on top of quinoa, baked potatoes, or hash browns for lunches and dinners throughout the week.

| The HCC Lineup | Make It Your Own |
|---|---|
| Protein 23 g<br>Navy beans, Cheddar cheese | Replace the navy beans with cannellini beans, black-eyed peas, chickpeas, or lentils, and make it fully vegan by using plant-based Cheddar. |
| Fiber 17 g<br>Navy beans, sourdough or whole-grain bread, spinach or kale, tomatoes | Throw in some leftover minced carrots, bell peppers, or alternative greens that you have left in your fridge. You can make this gluten-free by using your favorite gluten-free bread. |
| Fat 11 g<br>Cheddar cheese, olive oil | Replace the cheese with mashed avocado or your favorite hummus spread. |

# Whipped Cheesecake Toast

*Serves 1*
*Vegetarian, Soy-Free, Gluten-Free (Option), Nut-Free (Option),*
*Vegan (Option), Dairy-Free (Option)*

Look, if I want cheesecake, only the dense full-fat real deal is gonna do. But I can't be mad about starting my day with the sweet and tangy flavors of my favorite treats! This breakfast looks wildly Instagrammable but is shockingly simple to throw together, making it a staple for busy mornings or a postworkout snack.

½ cup cottage cheese

1 tablespoon cream cheese (optional)

Scant teaspoon lemon zest (optional)

2 teaspoons strawberry preserves (low-sugar, if desired)

2 slices whole-grain sourdough bread, toasted

½ cup hulled and sliced strawberries

2 tablespoons thinly sliced almonds, toasted

Combine the cottage cheese, plus the cream cheese and lemon zest, if using, in a small blender or food processor, and process until well whipped and smooth.

Fold and swirl the preserves into the cottage cheese mixture.

Divide the cottage cheese mixture between the two pieces of toast. Top with the sliced strawberries and almonds. Enjoy immediately.

**Make-Ahead Tip:**
Prepare a big batch of the whipped cottage cheese mixture and store in the fridge for up to a week.

| The HCC Lineup | Make It Your Own! |
|---|---|
| Protein 24 g<br>Cottage cheese | Replace the cottage cheese with ricotta or Skyr, or go dairy-free with a plant-based Greek-style yogurt. |
| Fiber 7 g<br>Sourdough bread, strawberries, almonds | Switch up the preserves and fruit toppings by replacing the strawberries with blueberries, raspberries, cherries, or pear. You can also go gluten-free by using your favorite gluten-free bread. |
| Fat 18 g<br>Almonds, cream cheese | Use chia jam in place of fruit preserves, make it nut-free with hemp hearts or pumpkin seeds, or go vegan with plant-based cream cheese. |

# Taco Egg Bites

*Serves 6 (2 bites each)*
*Vegetarian, Gluten-Free, Nut-Free, Soy-Free, Dairy-Free (Option)*

Made with a mixture of protein-rich ingredients, plus all your favorite taco fixings, these bites are the perfect make-ahead morning meal. I love to serve them with a healthy dollop of guacamole and hot sauce with fresh fruit on the side, or tuck them into a whole wheat wrap for a breakfast burrito on the go.

Olive oil or avocado oil nonstick
  spray, for muffin molds
1 cup 2% to 4% cottage cheese
7 large eggs
¾ cup finely minced red bell
  pepper
1 jalapeño, minced finely

¼ teaspoon salt
¼ teaspoon freshly ground black
  pepper
¼ teaspoon chili powder
¼ teaspoon garlic powder
1 cup shredded Colby Jack cheese

### For Topping:

1 cup guacamole
Sour cream, if desired

Salsa, if desired
Hot sauce, if desired

Preheat your oven to 325°F. Lightly spray twelve silicone muffin molds with the nonstick spray.

Puree the cottage cheese in a blender or food processor until smooth. Add the eggs and pulse to combine (being careful not to overwhip). Transfer the mixture to a large bowl.

Stir in the bell pepper, jalapeño, salt, black pepper, chili powder, garlic, and ½ cup of the shredded cheese. Divide among the prepared muffin molds and sprinkle with the remaining shredded cheese.

Bake for 23 to 25 minutes, or until the centers are set.

Remove from the oven and top with guacamole, sour cream, salsa, and hot sauce, as desired.

Enjoy immediately, or store for later.

## Make-Ahead Tips:

To store in the fridge, let cool completely, then place the egg bites in an airtight container, separated by parchment paper to prevent sticking, for up to 5 days. Reheat for 30 seconds in a microwave or for 5 to 10 minutes in a 350°F oven.

To freeze, arrange the cooled egg bites in a single layer on a baking sheet lined with parchment paper. Freeze for 1 hour, then transfer to a freezer-safe container or bag and eat within 2 to 3 months. Reheat from frozen in 30-second increments in a microwave, or for 7 to 12 minutes in a 350°F oven.

| The HCC Lineup | Make It Your Own |
|---|---|
| Protein 25 g<br>Cottage cheese, eggs, cheese | Make this meal dairy-free by replacing the cottage cheese with five additional eggs, and using plant-based Jack cheese. |
| Fiber 4 g<br>Bell pepper, jalapeño, guaca-mole | Switch up the veggies (try broccoli or spinach), and serve with high-fiber toast or a whole-grain wrap. |
| Fat 24 g<br>Guacamole, eggs, cheeses | Go dairy-free with plant-based cheeses, or add olives for a salty bite! |

# Baked Chocolate Zucchini Oats

*Makes 4 servings*
*Vegetarian, Soy-Free, Gluten-Free (Option), Dairy-Free (Option),*
*Vegan (Option), Nut-Free (Option)*

My kids like to call this "oatmeal cake"; I call this one of my greatest mom inventions of all time, thanks to the time it saves me during the work week, *and* the nutrition I know I'm packing in. This oats recipe upgrades our favorite pantry staple with fruits *and* veggies, heart-healthy omega-3 fats, and chocolate to boot! Because everything is better as cake.

Olive oil or avocado oil nonstick spray, for pan

1 medium-size zucchini

1 cup quick oats (gluten-free, as needed)

¼ cup hemp hearts

1 teaspoon ground cinnamon

¼ teaspoon freshly grated nutmeg

1½ teaspoons unsweetened cocoa powder

½ teaspoon baking powder

½ teaspoon salt

2 tablespoons pure maple syrup

1 large egg

2 teaspoons avocado oil

1 teaspoon pure vanilla extract

1 medium-size ripe banana, mashed

¼ cup walnuts, minced finely

3 tablespoons mini dark chocolate chips

2 tablespoons hemp hearts

**For Serving:**

1 cup Greek yogurt

Berries, if desired

Extra walnuts, if desired

Pure maple syrup, if desired

Preheat your oven to 375°F. Spray a 9 x 9–inch baking pan with nonstick spray and set aside.

Finely grate the zucchini into a piece of cheesecloth and firmly squeeze all of the liquid out. If you don't have cheesecloth, pressing it down super hard into a fine colander will also work. Set aside.

Combine the oats, hemp hearts, cinnamon, nutmeg, cocoa powder, baking powder, and salt in a blender or food processor and pulse until almost smooth. Transfer to a large bowl.

Combine the milk, maple syrup, egg, avocado oil, vanilla, mashed banana, and zucchini in a medium-size bowl. Pour the milk mixture into the oat mixture and mix well with a spatula or spoon. Fold in the walnuts.

Pour the mixture into the prepared baking pan and sprinkle with the chocolate chips and hemp hearts.

Bake for 22 to 25 minutes, or until golden brown on the outside and firm to the touch. Remove from the oven and allow to cool before cutting into squares, then serve warm or at room temperature with yogurt, berries, maple syrup, and walnuts, as desired.

### Make-Ahead Tips:

To store for the week, cover the baked oatmeal or store in an airtight container in the fridge for up to 5 days. Reheat slices in a microwave for 30 to 60 seconds, or in a 350°F oven for 8 to 10 minutes.

To freeze, cut the baked oatmeal into portions and wrap individually in plastic wrap. Store in a freezer-safe container or bag for up to 3 to 4 months. Reheat in a microwave for 1 to 2 minutes, or in a 350°F oven for 10 to 12 minutes.

| The HCC Lineup | Make It Your Own |
|---|---|
| Protein 20 g<br>Hemp hearts, egg, yogurt | Go dairy-free with soy-based yogurt (just look for one with at least 10 grams of protein per serving), and make it vegan with a plant-based egg replacement. |
| Fiber 7 g<br>Oatmeal, hemp hearts, banana, zucchini, walnuts | Try mixing your favorite dried fruits, diced apples, and nuts into the batter before baking. |
| Fat 24 g<br>Walnuts, avocado oil, egg | Drizzle your slice with drippy nut butter before serving for an extra dose of healthy fats. You can also go fully nut-free and school-safe by using pumpkin seeds in place of the walnuts. |

# Almond Soufflé Sheet Pan Protein Pancakes

*Serves 6*
*Vegetarian, Gluten-Free, Dairy-Free (Option), Soy-Free (Option)*

With hungry kids at my feet threatening my undercaffeinated six a.m. patience, my days of leisurely weekday pancake-making are in the past. These flip-free sheet pan pancakes not only make prep and cleanup a breeze, they're also uniquely high in Hunger Crushing Compounds, are naturally gluten-free, and taste like an almond sponge cake. Because I'd much rather spend my precious morning sitting on my tuchus eating a delicious breakfast than making it.

Olive oil or avocado oil nonstick spray, for pan

4 large eggs, at room temperature

1 cup sliced ripe (lightly spotted) banana (about 2 small to medium-size)

½ cup soy, pea, or cow's milk

2 tablespoons avocado oil or melted unsalted butter

2 tablespoons pure maple syrup (can omit if your protein powder is very sweet)

2 teaspoons pure vanilla extract

1 teaspoon almond extract

1¾ cups packed blanched fine almond flour (not almond meal)

1 cup vanilla protein powder

2 teaspoons baking powder

½ teaspoon salt

**For Topping:**
1 cup chopped frozen cherries

**For Serving (Optional):**
Greek yogurt
Sliced almonds, toasted
Additional thawed cherries

Pure maple syrup (*but is syrup ever really optional?*)

Preheat your oven to 400°F and line a 12 x 19–inch baking sheet with parchment paper, and give the parchment a light spritz of nonstick spray.

Combine the eggs, banana, soy milk, avocado oil, maple syrup, vanilla, almond extract, almond flour, protein powder, baking powder, and salt in a blender. Puree until smooth and whipped.

Spread the mixture on the prepared baking sheet and top with the cherries. Bake, turning the pan around at around the 4-minute point to ensure even baking, for a total of 8 to 11 minutes, or until golden brown around the edges and springy when touched in the middle.

Slice into squares and serve topped with a drizzle of Greek yogurt, toasted almonds, thawed cherries, and maple syrup, if desired.

**Make-Ahead Tips:**

To store, slice the pancakes into squares and store between slices of parchment paper in an airtight container or bag for up to 5 days. Reheat for 10 to 20 seconds in a microwave or for 3 minutes in a 350°F oven.

To freeze, store the sliced pancakes between parchment paper in a freezer-safe airtight container, or bag for up to 3 months. Reheat from frozen for 30 seconds in a microwave, or for 5 minutes in a 350°F oven.

| The HCC Lineup | Make It Your Own |
|---|---|
| Protein 21 g<br>Protein powder, eggs, almond flour, mylk/milk | Top with ⅓ cup of Greek yogurt or Skyr for an additional 5 grams of satiating protein.<br>Protein powder tip: Choose a protein powder that has been third-party tested (e.g., Neue Theory), to ensure purity and safety. Depending on the type and texture of your protein powder, you may need to add an extra tablespoon or two of milk, to ensure the pancakes aren't dry. |
| Fiber 6 g<br>Almond flour, cherries, banana | Use sliced bananas, strawberries, or blueberries or add a spoonful of wheat germ in place of some of the almond flour. |
| Fat 23 g<br>Almond flour, eggs, avocado oil | Top with sliced almonds or hemp hearts before baking for a little extra crunch. |

## Choose Your Adventure Protein Granola

*Makes 12 (¼-cup) servings*
*Vegetarian, Soy-Free, Gluten-Free (Option), Dairy-Free (Option),*
*Vegan (Option), Nut-Free (Option)*

I've been making this granola with my vanilla bean Neue Theory pro-biotic protein powder for years now, and I just love its versatility. Pick a nut or seed for healthy fats, dried fruit for fiber, and your go-to protein powder for protein, and you'll have a nutrient-dense breakfast or snack for weeks to come!

1 large egg white
2 cups rolled oats (gluten-free, if needed)
½ cup vanilla protein powder (or flavor of choice)
¾ cup nuts and seeds (e.g., walnuts, sliced almonds, cashew pieces, pepitas, or sunflower seeds)

¼ cup dried fruits (raisins, cranberries, minced dried apricots, or dried cherries)
½ teaspoon ground cinnamon
⅓ cup honey
3 tablespoons avocado oil or melted coconut oil
1 tablespoon sesame seeds
½ teaspoon fancy salt (e.g., Maldon sea salt or fleur de sel)

### For Serving:

⅔ cup Greek yogurt or high-protein soy yogurt (per serving)

½ cup berries or fruit (per serving)
Honey, if desired

Preheat the oven to 325°F. Line a baking sheet with parchment paper and set aside.

Whip the egg white until frothy, in a bowl with a whisk or drink frother, and set aside.

Combine the oats, protein powder, nuts and seeds, dried fruit, and cin-namon in a large bowl. Then, add the whipped egg white, honey, and oil. Toss well to combine.

Spread the granola mixture evenly on the prepared baking sheet, using a spatula or wooden spoon. Bake for 15 minutes.

Remove from the oven and gently stir the granola, taking care not to break up the clusters. Return the granola to the oven and bake for an additional 10 to 15 minutes, or until golden brown. Immediately sprinkle the hot granola with the sesame seeds and flaky salt.

Allow to cool completely in the pan before transferring to a container. Serve with Greek yogurt and berries, or your preferred base and toppings.

**Make-Ahead Tip:**

To store, keep in an airtight container at room temperature for up to 4 weeks.

| The HCC Lineup | Make It Your Own |
| --- | --- |
| Protein 26 g<br>Protein powder, egg white, nuts, seeds, Greek yogurt | Enjoy a bowlful with soy or cow's milk instead of yogurt, or make it vegan, using plant-based protein powder and whipped canned chickpea liquid (aquafaba); sounds crazy but it works! |
| Fiber 4 g<br>Oats, nuts, seeds, dried fruit, berries | Add a few spoonfuls of wheat germ to the oats for an extra hit of insoluble fiber. |
| Fat 10 g<br>Nuts, seeds, avocado oil | Throw in some "supersprinkles," chia, flax, or hemp hearts for some heart-healthy omega-3s, and go fully nut-free by leaning on sunflower or pumpkin seeds. |

### Feel free to get creative, but here are some of my flavor combo ideas:

| Protein | Fiber | Healthy Fats |
| --- | --- | --- |
| Vanilla protein | Dried apples and cranberries | Pecans |
| Chocolate protein | Dried cherries | Almonds |
| Berry protein | Dried blueberries | Walnuts |

# Vegan Tofu Shakshuka

*Serves 4*
*Vegetarian, Vegan, Nut-Free, Dairy-Free, Gluten-Free (Option), Soy-Free (Option)*

While traditionally made by poaching runny eggs in a bed of spicy tomato sauce, my version of shakshuka utilizes tofu for a plant-based alternative. Vibrantly spiced with cumin, paprika, and chili powder, complimented by a hint of savory nutritional yeast and maple syrup for balance, this meal is as nourishing as it is flavorful.

1 teaspoon extra-virgin olive oil
1 small onion, diced finely
3 garlic cloves, diced finely
2 medium-size red bell peppers, diced finely
1 tablespoon tomato paste
1 teaspoon ground cumin
½ teaspoon chili powder
½ teaspoon smoked paprika
1 (28-ounce) can San Marzano tomatoes (chopped up with kitchen shears while in the can)

1 teaspoon freshly ground black pepper
1 teaspoon salt
1 tablespoon nutritional yeast
1 tablespoon dark maple syrup or dark brown sugar
1 (15-ounce) package of medium-firm tofu (leave unpressed!), cut into ½-inch slices

**For Topping and Serving:**

¼ cup pitted kalamata olives
¼ cup vegan feta cheese
3 tablespoons minced fresh parsley

8 slices whole-grain sourdough bread or pita

Heat the olive oil in a large skillet over medium-high heat. Add the onion, garlic, and bell peppers. Sauté until lightly golden, 3 to 4 minutes.

Add the tomato paste, cumin, chili powder, and smoked paprika to the pan. Coat the vegetables with the spice mixture and cook until fragrant, 1 to 2 minutes.

Stir in the tomatoes, black pepper, salt, nutritional yeast, and maple syrup. Bring the mixture to a simmer and cook, uncovered, until bubbly and slightly reduced, 8 to 10 minutes.

Add the sliced tofu to the top of the shakshuka and season liberally with salt and pepper. Lower the heat to low and simmer for an additional 15 minutes, uncovered, or until the sauce has further thickened.

Remove from the heat and top with the kalamata olives, vegan feta cheese, and fresh parsley before serving. Serve with fresh sourdough bread or pita.

### Make-Ahead Tips:

To store, transfer to an airtight container, or cover tightly with plastic wrap and refrigerate for up to 3 days. To reheat, cover with aluminum foil and bake at 350°F for 15 minutes, or microwave a portion for 90 seconds.

To double or triple the recipe when entertaining for a crowd, make a big batch of the sauce to the desired consistency, then refrigerate until game time. Before guests arrive, simply transfer it to a large cast-iron casserole dish, add enough servings of tofu for your guests, and bake at 375°F for 20 minutes.

| The HCC Lineup | Make It Your Own |
|---|---|
| Protein 20 g<br>Tofu | For a traditional soy-free shakshuka, use eggs instead of tofu. Simply create little wells in the sauce and crack an egg into each well. Cover the skillet with a lid and cook until the whites are set and the yolks remain runny, 6 to 8 minutes. |
| Fiber 8 g<br>Onions, tomatoes, bell peppers, tofu, sourdough bread | Add leftover zucchini, chopped kale, or spinach to your sauce for a slightly more vegetal base. Make it gluten-free by serving with a gluten-free bread or pita. |
| Fat 10 g<br>Olives, vegan feta cheese, olive oil | Top with sliced avocado or serve your bread smeared with olive tapenade. |

# MAIN ATTRACTIONS

# Protein Cauli Mac and Cheese

*Makes 4 servings*
*Vegetarian, Nut-Free, Soy-Free, Gluten-Free (Option)*

It's time that the words "comfort food" and "junk food" underwent some "conscious uncoupling," and that's where this dish comes into play. Whipped cottage cheese and sharp Cheddar make for a rich, thick, savory sauce, while steamed cauliflower adds fiber and volume to whole wheat pasta. It's a stick-to-your-ribs meal that proves that balanced eating is inherently one of life's greatest comforts.

8 ounces uncooked whole wheat short-cut pasta (e.g., macaroni, penne, rigatoni, farfalle, or fusilli)

3 cups cauliflower pieces (florets)

1 cup 2% to 4% cottage cheese

½ cup 2% to 4% milk

1½ tablespoons cornstarch

¼ cup nutritional yeast

1¼ cups shredded sharp Cheddar cheese

¼ teaspoon salt

¼ teaspoon freshly ground black pepper

¼ teaspoon garlic powder

¼ teaspoon paprika

Cook the pasta according to the package directions in a large pot of boiling, well-salted water. In the last 3 minutes, add the cauliflower florets to finish cooking with the pasta. Once tender, remove at least 1 cup of pasta water and set aside. Drain the pasta, and set aside.

Meanwhile, process the cottage cheese, milk, cornstarch, nutritional yeast, Cheddar cheese, salt, pepper, garlic powder, and paprika in a blender or food processor until smooth to create the cheese sauce.

Transfer the cheese sauce to a large saucepan over medium-high heat and cook until bubbly and thick, 4 to 5 minutes.

Add the cooked pasta and cauliflower to the cheese sauce. Add ¼ to ½ cup of cooking water, as needed, to thin out the sauce. Toss well to combine. Serve hot.

**Make-Ahead Tips:**

To store, let cool, then transfer to an airtight container and refrigerate
for up to 4 days. Reheat a portion in the microwave for 1 minute,
or the entire casserole (covered with aluminum foil) for 20 minutes
in a 350°F oven.

To freeze, transfer to an oven-safe disposable or silicone container, cover
tightly with plastic wrap, then a layer of aluminum foil, and freeze
for up to 3 months. Remove the plastic wrap, cover with aluminum
foil, and bake the entire casserole from frozen at 375°F for 45 to 60
minutes, or until hot and bubbling in the center.

| The HCC Lineup | Make It Your Own |
|---|---|
| Protein 27 g<br>Cottage cheese, milk, nutritional yeast, Cheddar cheese | Make it gluten-free with chickpea or lentil pasta instead of whole wheat, which adds an extra 7 grams of protein per serving. |
| Fiber 7 g<br>Whole wheat noodles, cauliflower | Replace the cauliflower with broccoli or mixed frozen veggies. |
| Fat 15 g<br>Cottage cheese, Cheddar cheese, milk | Experiment with adding chèvre or Gruyère in place of traditional Cheddar, or top with toasted pine nuts for a more sophisticated flavor profile. |

# Avocado Mango Shrimp Salad

*Makes 4 servings*
*Nut-Free, Dairy-Free, Soy-Free, Vegetarian (Option),*
*Vegan (Option), Gluten-Free (Option)*

Salads do not need to be unsatisfying bland, boring bird food that you drag yourself through to "pay" for skipping the gym. They can and *should* be colorful and flavorful, and provide your body with the fuel it deserves. This Avocado Mango Shrimp Salad will prove you *can* have it all.

### Salad:

1 teaspoon avocado oil
¾ cup dried pearl couscous
1 cup water
Generous pinch of salt
1 pound frozen cooked deveined shrimp, defrosted in fridge, then diced

1 large avocado, peeled, pitted, and diced
1 large mango, peeled, pitted, and diced
1 orange bell pepper, diced
1 cup cherry tomatoes, halved
3 tablespoons diced red onion
6 cups butter lettuce

### Lime Dressing:

4 teaspoons Tajín
1 teaspoon honey
¼ cup freshly squeezed lime juice

¼ cup avocado oil
Salt and freshly ground black pepper

### For Garnish:

¼ cup toasted unsweetened coconut chips

¼ cup fresh cilantro
Extra Tajín, if desired

Prepare the salad: Heat the avocado oil in a small saucepot over medium heat. Add the pearl couscous and stir constantly for 2 minutes, or until lightly golden and nutty in fragrance. Add the cup of water along with the pinch of salt, and bring to a boil. Cover the pot and simmer for 9 to 12 minutes, stirring occasionally, until the liquid has been absorbed. Remove the pan from the heat and let sit, covered, for 2 minutes. Fluff the couscous with a fork, then set aside to cool. The couscous can be served at room temperature, or made ahead and chilled in the fridge for at least an hour before assembling.

Meanwhile, make the dressing: Combine the Tajín, honey, lime juice, and olive oil in a small bowl and beat with a small whisk. Season with salt and pepper to taste, then set aside.

Build your salad: Add butter lettuce to each plate or a large serving platter. Top with cooked couscous, diced avocado, bell peppers, cherry tomatoes, red onion, and the diced shrimp. Drizzle with lime dressing and garnish with coconut chips, cilantro, and a generous sprinkle of Tajín for extra spice.

**Make-Ahead Tip:**
Cook the couscous up to 3 days in advance, and combine the salad components in an airtight container up to a day ahead. Add the avocado and dressing when ready to eat.

| The HCC Lineup | Make It Your Own |
|---|---|
| Protein 27 g<br>Shrimp | Replace shrimp with diced grilled chicken breast or make it vegan with extra-firm tofu, tempeh, or edamame. |
| Fiber 8 g<br>Avocado, vegetables, mango | Make it gluten-free by using quinoa instead of couscous, thereby doubling the fiber per serving. |
| Fat 27 g<br>Avocado, coconut, avocado oil | Add toasted macadamia nuts or cashews for extra crunch. |

# Open-Faced Sesame & Edamame Smash Sandwich

*Makes 2 servings*
*Vegetarian, Vegan, Nut-Free, Dairy-Free, Gluten-Free (Option)*

This sandwich takes the oh-so-trendy avo-toast to another level with nutty tahini, protein-rich edamame, and fresh herbs. Open-faced sammies too messy for your power lunch? There's no toast police saying you can't smash two slices together into a handheld meal, so you do you!

2 tablespoons tahini

4 teaspoons freshly squeezed lemon juice

1½ cups edamame, shelled

3 fresh basil leaves, torn

¼ medium-size ripe avocado, or ½ small avocado, peeled and pitted

Salt and freshly ground black pepper

### To Assemble:

4 slices seeded whole-grain bread, toasted

2 to 4 tablespoons pickled shallots

½ cup microgreens

2 teaspoons toasted black and white sesame seeds

Fancy salt like Maldon sea salt or fleur de sel

Combine the tahini, lemon juice, 1 cup of the edamame, the basil, and a pinch each of salt and pepper in a blender or food processor. Process until chunky. Pulse in the avocado (avoid adding too much air, or it may brown), then season with more salt, pepper, and lemon juice, as needed.

Smear the toast with the edamame smash mixture. Garnish with the remaining edamame, shallots, microgreens, sesame seeds, and a pinch of fancy salt, for crunch. Enjoy it open-faced or combine the two slices to make a sandwich.

### Make-Ahead Tip:

Batch-prep the spread up to 3 days in advance and store in the fridge, tightly covered to prevent browning.

| The HCC Lineup | Make It Your Own |
|---|---|
| Protein 24 g<br>Edamame, seeded whole-grain bread | Add a hard-boiled egg or an ounce of smoked salmon for an additional 6 grams of protein. |
| Fiber 14 g<br>Seeded whole-grain bread, edamame, tahini, avocado | Load up your toast with your favorite veggies: tomatoes, sautéed mushrooms, or grilled zucchini would all be fab! You can also go gluten-free with your favorite gluten-free bread. |
| Fat 20 g<br>Edamame, seeded whole-grain bread, avocado, tahini, sesame seeds | Swap out the sesame seeds for toasted cashews for extra crunch. |

# Herbed Turkey & Sweet Potato Shepherd's Pie

*Serves 4*
*Nut-Free, Vegetarian (Option), Soy-Free (Option),*
*Gluten-Free (Option)*

The big Thanksgiving meal is something I look forward to all year, but it wasn't until recently that I realized, hey, I'm a full-grown adult, I can make Thanksgiving food whenever the hell I want. This modern take on a classic British shepherd's pie tucks a hearty blend of ground turkey and time-slashing frozen veggies under a blanket of creamy whipped sweet potato. It's the perfect comfort food you can count on all year long.

## Sweet Potatoes:

6 medium-size sweet potatoes, washed and pierced with a fork

Olive oil or avocado oil cooking spray

½ cup whole-milk ricotta cheese

2 tablespoons whole milk

Salt and freshly ground black pepper

## Pie Filling:

1 tablespoon extra-virgin olive oil

1 pound lean ground turkey

1 medium-size onion, chopped finely

3 garlic cloves, minced

1 tablespoon tomato paste

1 tablespoon Worcestershire sauce (check that it's soy-free and/or gluten-free, if needed)

1 teaspoon fresh thyme leaves

2 teaspoons minced fresh rosemary

1 tablespoon cornstarch

1 cup low-sodium chicken bone broth

1 (16-ounce) package frozen mixed vegetables

¼ cup plus 2 tablespoons grated Parmesan cheese

Salt and freshly ground black pepper

Bake the sweet potatoes: Preheat the oven to 400°F.

Spritz the potatoes with olive oil spray. Then, wrap each potato in a sheet of aluminum foil. Place the potatoes directly on the center oven rack and bake until very tender, 45 to 60 minutes. Carefully unwrap and set aside to cool.

Once cool enough to handle, slice the potatoes in half and scoop out their innards into a bowl. Mash the potatoes with the ricotta cheese, milk, and a pinch each of salt and pepper, or to taste.

Meanwhile, prepare the pie filling: Heat the olive oil in a large skillet over medium-high heat. Add the ground turkey to the pan and break up the meat with a wooden spoon or spatula. Add the chopped onion and garlic to the pan. Cook, stirring occasionally, until the turkey is cooked through, 6 to 7 minutes.

Add the tomato paste, Worcestershire sauce, thyme, and rosemary to the turkey mixture in the pan and stir to coat the meat with them.

Sprinkle the cornstarch over the mixture and stir until the meat is evenly coated. Add the broth and simmer until the mixture thickens, 5 to 7 minutes.

Add the frozen vegetables and ¼ cup of Parmesan cheese to the pan and season with salt and pepper to taste. Once the vegetables are warmed through, remove from the heat and set aside.

Pour the meat mixture into a 9 x 9–inch or 7 x 11–inch casserole dish. Spread the mashed sweet potatoes on top of the meat mixture and sprinkle with 2 tablespoons of Parmesan cheese. Bake, uncovered, for 20 to 25 minutes, or until lightly browned on top. Remove from the oven and allow to cool for 5 to 10 minutes before serving.

**Meal-Prep Tips:**

To store, cover the baking dish tightly in plastic wrap and refrigerate for up to 4 days. Reheat in a 350°F oven for 20 minutes, or microwave a portion for 90 seconds.

To batch-prep and freeze, double or triple the portions (as needed), and divide the ingredients among disposable or silicone containers. Without baking, cover tightly with plastic wrap, then a layer of aluminum foil, and freeze for up to 3 months. When ready to serve, remove the plastic wrap and re-cover with aluminum foil. Bake, covered, at 400°F for 35 to 40 minutes, then remove the foil and bake for another 10 to 15 minutes.

| The HCC Lineup | Make It Your Own |
|---|---|
| Protein 36 g<br>Ground turkey, chicken bone broth, ricotta cheese, Parmesan | Swap in ground beef or chicken or use veggie ground round ("faux meat") to make it vegetarian. |
| Fiber 8 g<br>Sweet potatoes, mixed vegetables, onions | Replace the mixed veggies with leftover finely chopped cooked veggies: Brussels sprouts, mushrooms, or parsnips. |
| Fat 14 g<br>Parmesan cheese, ricotta cheese | Top with toasted pepitas or crushed pistachios before serving for a little crunch. |

# Better Big Burger Bowl

*Serves 4*
*Gluten-Free, Nut-Free, Soy-Free, Vegetarian (Option),*
*Vegan (Option), Dairy-Free (Option)*

I'm generally an "eat with my hands" kinda girl, but this burger bowl is worth pulling out a fork. It's loaded up with all the fixings you know and love from your go-to drive-through order, with a bountiful high-fiber base.

## Meat and Potatoes:

3 cups baby new potatoes

1 tablespoon extra-virgin olive oil

1 pound extra-lean ground beef

½ teaspoon onion powder

½ teaspoon garlic powder

½ teaspoon paprika

½ teaspoon freshly ground black pepper

½ teaspoon fine kosher salt

Fleur de sel

## Special Sauce:

1½ tablespoons plain 4% Greek yogurt

1½ tablespoons mayonnaise

1 tablespoon ketchup

2 tablespoons prepared yellow mustard

1 tablespoon pickle juice

1½ teaspoons roughly chopped fresh dill

## Salad:

8 cups romaine lettuce, shredded finely

2 cups cherry tomatoes

¼ cup pickled onion or finely diced fresh red onion

¼ cup sliced dill pickles

¼ cup aged Cheddar cheese, shredded

1 large avocado, peeled, pitted, and diced

Start the meat and potatoes: Place the potatoes in a large pot. Fill with water until the potatoes are covered by an inch of water, add a generous pinch of salt, and bring to a boil. Lower the heat to a simmer and cook until the potatoes are fork-tender, 10 to 18 minutes. Drain the potatoes and let cool. Once the potatoes are cool enough to handle, cut them into ½- or ¼-inch pieces, depending upon the size of the potatoes. Set aside.

Heat 1 teaspoon of the oil in a large skillet over medium-high heat. Add the meat to the pan and break it up into little pieces with a wooden spoon or spatula. Season with the onion powder, garlic powder, paprika, ¼ teaspoon of the pepper, and the kosher salt. Cook, stirring frequently, until the meat is cooked through, 7 to 9 minutes. Remove from the pan and set aside.

Heat the remaining 2 teaspoons of olive oil in the pan over medium-high heat, and add the cooked potatoes. Allow to brown for 3 to 5 minutes, and sprinkle with the remaining black pepper and salt.

Meanwhile, prepare the sauce: Stir together the yogurt, mayonnaise, ketchup, mustard, pickle juice, and fresh dill in a small bowl. Cover and place in the fridge until ready to serve.

To build your bowl, divide the romaine among four bowls. Add the potatoes, meat mixture, and other veggies. Drizzle with a couple of spoonfuls of sauce and enjoy warm.

**Make-Ahead Tips:**
Meal-prep by preparing the sauce and cooking the meat and potatoes up to 4 days in advance. Assemble the salad when you're ready to eat.
Pro Tip: Make an extra-big batch of the special sauce for throwing on sandwiches, wraps, salads, and *actual* burgers *(and no, you don't have to hollow out the bun)*.

| The HCC Lineup | Make It Your Own |
|---|---|
| Protein 34 g<br>Lean ground beef, Greek yogurt, Cheddar cheese | Replace the beef with lean ground turkey or chicken, or make it vegetarian by using lentils, coarsely grated tofu or tempeh, or veggie "meat." |
| Fiber 5.5 g<br>Potatoes, lettuce, avocado, cherry tomatoes, red onion | Use sweet potatoes in place of new potatoes and switch up the salad ingredients with bell peppers, cucumber, steamed green beans, and arugula. |
| Fat 21 g<br>Avocado, Cheddar cheese, olive oil, mayonnaise | Go for blue cheese or chèvre, or add pimiento-stuffed olives for a salty bite. You can also go dairy-free by swapping in plant-based cheese and yogurt. |

## Baked Harissa Orzo with Shrimp and Kale

*Serves 4*
*Dairy-Free, Soy-Free, Gluten-Free (Option),*
*Vegetarian (Option), Vegan (Option)*

As a busy mompreneur, I *live* for one-pot meals, and this baked orzo is giving viral recipe vibes. Between the aromatic heat of harissa paste, the sweetness of sun-dried tomatoes, and the toasty pine nuts on top, this one-pot wonder offers huge flavor ROI for a 30-minute meal.

1 tablespoon extra-virgin olive oil
1 medium-size onion, chopped finely
2 garlic cloves, minced
1 tablespoon tomato paste
3 tablespoons harissa
6 ounces uncooked whole wheat orzo
Zest and juice of 1 lemon
1 cup sun-dried tomatoes, cut into strips
1⅔ cups low-sodium vegetable stock
1½ pounds raw peeled shrimp
Salt and freshly ground black pepper
2 roasted jarred red peppers, sliced thinly
4 cups thinly sliced kale leaves
⅔ cup frozen green peas
¼ cup toasted pine nuts
1 lemon, cut into wedges

Position a rack in the center of the oven and preheat to 425°F.

Heat the oil in an ovenproof Dutch oven over medium heat. Add the onion and garlic. Sauté, stirring regularly, for 1 to 2 minutes, until the onion is soft and translucent. Then, add the tomato paste and 2 tablespoons of the harissa to the hot pan. Add the orzo, lemon zest (reserving the juice), and sun-dried tomatoes. Stir with a spatula to combine, and add the stock. Place in the oven and bake, uncovered, for 14 to 16 minutes, or until the orzo is tender and the liquid is absorbed.

Toss the shrimp in a large bowl with the remaining 1 tablespoon of harissa, along with a pinch of salt and black pepper. Remove the casserole dish from the oven and nestle the roasted red peppers, kale, peas, and shrimp in the casserole and add the reserved lemon juice. Cover and place back in the oven for an additional 7 to 9 minutes, or until the shrimp are opaque. Adjust the seasoning with salt and black pepper to taste.

Top the casserole with toasted pine nuts and serve with lemon wedges.

**Make-Ahead Tip:**

To store, let cool, then transfer to an airtight container for up to 3 days in the fridge. Reheat a portion in a microwave for 60 to 90 seconds, or reheat the entire casserole in a 350°F oven for 15 to 20 minutes.

| The HCC Lineup | Make It Your Own |
| --- | --- |
| Protein 36 g<br>Shrimp | Replace the shrimp with precooked sliced turkey sausage, or make this vegetarian by using pressed extra-firm tofu, tempeh, or edamame. |
| Fiber 9 g<br>Orzo, kale, sun-dried tomatoes, peas, roasted red peppers | Switch out the peas and kale for green beans and spinach, and go gluten-free using gluten-free orzo. |
| Fat 13 g<br>Pine nuts, olive oil | Swap in slivered almonds or cashews for the pine nuts. |

## Creamy Crème Fraîche Salmon Pasta

*Serves 4*
*Nut-Free, Soy-Free, Vegetarian (Option), Vegan (Option),*
*Dairy-Free (Option), Gluten-Free (Option)*

This pasta dish is so easy and quick to put together, it will make you feel like a multitasking master. Popping a steamer basket on top of a large pasta pot allows you to cook your fish and penne at the same time, while also cooking down your veggies and sauce. Fast never tasted so fresh!

5 ounces uncooked whole wheat penne pasta or other whole wheat short-cut pasta
1 to 1½ pounds salmon fillets
Salt and freshly ground black pepper
1 tablespoon extra-virgin olive oil
½ medium-size onion, diced
2 garlic cloves, crushed

2 medium-size zucchini, sliced on the bias
½ cup low-sodium vegetable stock
½ cup crème fraîche or sour cream
1 cup frozen peas
½ bunch dill, chopped roughly
Zest of 1 lemon
¼ cup grated Parmesan cheese

Bring salted water to a boil in a large stockpot over medium-high heat. Add the pasta. Lower the heat to medium and cook according to the package directions.

Meanwhile, place a tiered steamer or metal colander over the pot and add the salmon fillets. Season with salt and pepper. Cover with a lid and allow the fish to steam for 8 to 10 minutes while the pasta cooks. Remove the salmon from the pot. Before draining the pasta, scoop out 1 cup of the pasta water and set aside. Drain the pasta and set aside.

Carefully remove the skin from the salmon. Then, with a fork, flake the salmon into large chunks. Set aside.

Combine 1 tablespoon of the olive oil with the onion and garlic in a large skillet. Turn the heat to medium-high and cook, stirring frequently, until the onion is soft and translucent, 1 to 2 minutes. Then, add the sliced zucchini to the pan and season everything with a pinch each of salt and pepper. Cook for 5 to 7 minutes, or until golden brown.

Add the vegetable stock, crème fraîche, and peas to the pan. Allow to cook and thicken for 2 minutes, stirring occasionally. If the sauce seems too thick, add a little of the pasta water.

Remove from the heat. Fold in the cooked pasta, half of the chopped dill, and the salmon chunks and lemon zest. Season with salt and pepper to taste. Serve warm, topped with grated Parmesan cheese and the remaining chopped dill.

**Make-Ahead Tip:**
To store, let cool, then transfer to an airtight container for up to 3 days in the fridge. Reheat a portion in the microwave for 60 to 90 seconds, or warm up the whole casserole (covered with aluminum foil) in a 350°F oven for 10 to 15 minutes.

| The HCC Lineup | Make It Your Own |
| --- | --- |
| Protein 36 g<br>Salmon, Parmesan | Skip the fish and add shredded rotisserie chicken in the last step, or go vegetarian with a can of white beans. |
| Fiber 8 g<br>Whole wheat pasta, zucchini, peas | Replace the zucchini with cauliflower or sautéed greens, and go gluten-free using high-protein chickpea pasta. |
| Fat 23 g<br>Salmon, olive oil, crème fraîche, Parmesan cheese | Garnish with a handful of toasted pine nuts for extra crunch and flavor, or swap out the dairy for plant-based sour cream and cheese. |

# Coconut Chicken Tenders

*Makes 4 servings*
*Nut-Free, Soy-Free, Dairy-Free (Option), Vegetarian (Option),*
*Vegan (Option), Gluten-Free (Option)*

These air-fried coconut-crusted tenders offer the crunch you truly crave, no messy deep-frying required. With a sweet and tangy yogurt dip in tow, they're easy enough for a weeknight family dinner with the kiddos, and impressive enough to serve to guests. Just add a blended piña colada (*with one of those cute paper umbrellas on top*), and you've got a party!

Olive oil or avocado oil nonstick cooking spray

½ cup whole wheat flour

½ teaspoon salt

¼ teaspoon freshly ground black pepper

2 teaspoons Tajín seasoning

2 large eggs

2 tablespoons coconut milk

⅔ cup unsweetened fine coconut flakes

¾ cup bran cereal (e.g., All-Bran flakes), pulsed to a flour

1½ pounds chicken tenderloins, or chicken breasts, cut into strips

**Dip:**

½ cup coconut-flavored Greek yogurt

2 tablespoons sweet chili sauce

1 teaspoon lime zest

2 teaspoons freshly squeezed lime juice

2 teaspoons sriracha, or to taste

Preheat the air fryer to 400°F and spray the air fryer basket lightly with nonstick cooking spray. If using an oven, preheat to 425°F, line a baking sheet with parchment, and spritz the paper with nonstick cooking spray.

Gather three large bowls or deep plates to create your dipping station. In the first bowl, combine the flour, salt, pepper, and 1 teaspoon of the Tajín seasoning. In the second bowl, whisk together the eggs and coconut milk. In the third bowl, combine the coconut flakes, pulverized bran cereal, and remaining teaspoon of Tajín seasoning. Set aside.

Start by dipping each chicken piece into the flour mixture, then into the egg mixture, and then finally into the cereal mixture. Lay them on the baking sheet or air fryer basket with 1 to 2 inches in between.

Air-fry at 400°F for 12 to 14 minutes per side, or bake at 425°F for 15 to 20 minutes, in either case, until the chicken is 165°F, and the outside is golden and crispy.

In the meantime, prepare the dip: Stir together the Greek yogurt, chili sauce, lime zest, lime juice, and sriracha in a small bowl. Keep cold until ready to use. Serve alongside rice, noodles, or roasted sweet potatoes or plantains, plus your favorite sautéed vegetables or salad.

**Make-Ahead Tips:**

To store, transfer the cooled chicken fingers to an airtight container and separate the fingers into layers with parchment paper. Refrigerate for up to 4 days. Reheat in a 400°F air fryer for 3 to 4 minutes, or an oven for 5 to 7 minutes.

To freeze, place the cooled chicken fingers on a baking sheet for 1 hour, then transfer to a freezer-safe container or bag. Cook from frozen in a 400°F oven for 12 to 15 minutes or in an air fryer for 10 to 15 minutes.

| The HCC Lineup | Make It Your Own |
| --- | --- |
| Protein 44 g<br>Chicken, eggs, Greek yogurt | This coconut crust is equally delicious on shrimp and extra-firm tofu, for a veggie option. You can also go dairy-free and vegan using a high-protein soy-based yogurt and a vegan egg replacement. |
| Fiber 5.5 g<br>Bran cereal, whole wheat flour, coconut flakes | Make it gluten-free by replacing the whole wheat flour and bran cereal with coconut flour and oat-based cereal, and up the fiber by serving the tenders alongside wild rice and slaw. |
| Fat 19 g<br>Coconut flakes, coconut milk, eggs | Pulsed cashews or macadamia nuts can stand in for the coconut for a nuttier flavor profile. |

# Gochujang Lettuce Wraps

*Serves 4*
*Dairy-Free, Gluten-Free (Option), Vegetarian (Option),*
*Vegan (Option), Soy-Free (Option), Nut-Free (Option)*

Gochujang is a powerful Korean chili paste that supplies the perfect balance of heat, sweet, and umami to any dish, and really elevates blank-slate poultry. Served in crisp lettuce cups with probiotic-rich kimchi, a sprightly quick-pickled cucumber salad, and creamy avocado, this dish is as addictive as it is nutritious.

### Gochujang Mixture:

2 tablespoons dark brown sugar

¼ cup low-sodium tamari or soy sauce (or coconut aminos for soy-free or gluten-free)

2 teaspoons sesame oil

¼ teaspoon crushed red pepper flakes, or to taste

2 tablespoons gochujang paste (check that it's gluten-free, if desired)

4 garlic cloves, minced

1 tablespoon grated fresh ginger

1 teaspoon avocado oil

1 pound lean ground turkey or ground chicken

¼ teaspoon freshly ground black pepper

¼ teaspoon salt

### Cucumber Salad:

6 mini cucumbers, sliced thinly

1 teaspoon salt

1 tablespoon reduced-sodium tamari or soy sauce (or coconut aminos for soy-free or gluten-free)

2 garlic cloves, minced

1 tablespoon seasoned rice vinegar

1 tablespoon granulated sugar

1 teaspoon sesame oil

1 teaspoon sesame seeds

**For Serving:**

12 to 16 butter or Bibb lettuce
  cups
1 cup kimchi
1 avocado, peeled, pitted, and
  sliced

1½ cups finely shredded red
  cabbage
2 tablespoons white and black
  sesame seeds
¼ cup crushed peanuts

Begin the gochujang mixture: Whisk together the brown sugar, tamari, sesame oil, red pepper flakes, gochujang paste, garlic, and ginger in a small bowl to create a sauce. Set aside.

Heat the avocado oil in a large skillet over medium-high heat. Add the turkey to the pan, breaking it up with a wooden spoon or spatula. Add the gochujang sauce to the pan. Cook, stirring frequently, until the meat is cooked through and is coated in the thick, sticky sauce, 5 to 7 minutes.

In the meantime, make the cucumber salad: Place the cucumbers and salt in a medium-size bowl. Toss gently to coat. Allow the cucumbers to sit for 1 to 2 minutes, or until they start to release their moisture. Next, rinse the cucumbers in cold water and pat dry with a clean kitchen towel or paper towel. Meanwhile, make a dressing by combining the tamari, garlic, rice vinegar, sugar, sesame oil, and sesame seeds in a medium-size bowl, and stir with a spoon. Transfer the cucumbers to the bowl of dressing. Toss gently to mix well. The flavors only intensify as this sits, so feel free to make a big batch and eat the leftovers throughout the week.

To build a lettuce wrap, add a heaping spoonful of the gochujang meat mixture to a lettuce cup. Top with pickled cucumber salad, kimchi, avocado, cabbage, sesame seeds, and peanuts, as desired. Serve with warm rice or noodles on the side.

**Make-Ahead Tip:**

To meal-prep, store the cooked and cooled meat mixture and the cucumber salad separately for up to 4 and 3 days, respectively. Assemble when it's time to eat.

| The HCC Lineup | Make It Your Own |
|---|---|
| Protein 34 g<br>Ground turkey or chicken | Use the gochujang sauce on ground beef, pork, or shrimp, or make it vegan with crumbled tofu, "faux meat," lentils, or edamame. |
| Fiber 8 g<br>Avocado, cucumber, lettuce, cabbage, kimchi | Top your wraps with sliced bok choy, bell peppers, carrots, or snap peas, and serve with wild rice. |
| Fat 23 g<br>Avocado, sesame seeds, peanuts, avocado oil, sesame oil | Replace the peanuts with cashews, or use sunflower seeds for nut-free. |

## Butternut Squash Chickpea Coconut Curry

*Makes 4 servings*
*Vegetarian, Vegan, Gluten-Free, Dairy-Free, Soy-Free (Option), Nut-Free (Option)*

Sweet, spicy, creamy, and tangy, this curry is stick-to-your-ribs satisfying, and really warms the soul. It's also incredibly versatile and easily adaptable based on whatever you have in your fridge. Serve it with fluffy rice or warm naan for the full takeout-at-home experience.

### Tofu:

9 ounces extra-firm tofu, pressed and cubed

1 tablespoon rice flour, cornstarch, or tapioca starch

¼ teaspoon salt

¼ teaspoon freshly ground black pepper

### Curry:

1 tablespoon coconut oil

2 cups cubed and seeded fresh butternut squash

1 large carrot, sliced thinly

1 medium-size onion, diced

2 garlic cloves, minced

2 teaspoons grated fresh ginger

1 tablespoon mild curry powder

1 teaspoon ground cumin

¼ teaspoon salt

¼ teaspoon freshly ground black pepper

1 to 2 tablespoons tomato paste

1 (14-ounce) can diced tomatoes

1 (14-ounce) can lite coconut milk

1 (16-ounce) can low-sodium chickpeas, drained and rinsed well

Juice of 1 lime

3 cups fresh spinach

¼ cup chopped cashew pieces

Fresh cilantro, if desired

Prepare the tofu: Toss the cubed pressed tofu in a bowl with the flour, salt, and pepper.

Make the curry: Heat 2 teaspoons of the coconut oil in a deep sauté pan over medium-high heat. Add the tofu and sauté on all sides until golden brown, about 5 minutes total. Remove from the pan and set aside.

Add the remaining teaspoon of oil to the pan over medium-high heat and add the butternut squash, diced onion, and carrot to the pan. Cook, stirring occasionally, for 5 to 10 minutes, until the onion is soft and translucent.

Add the garlic, ginger, curry powder, cumin, salt, pepper, and tomato paste to the warm pan and coat the vegetables with the mixture. Stir frequently for 2 minutes.

Add the diced tomatoes and coconut milk, and lower the heat to low. Simmer, uncovered, for 5 to 10 minutes before adding the chickpeas and cooking for an additional 10 minutes, or until the butternut squash is *just* fork-tender.

Remove from the heat and stir in the lime juice, spinach, and tofu. Stir until the greens are wilted, and season with additional salt and pepper to taste. Top with the cashews and cilantro, if desired, and serve with rice, noodles, or naan.

**Make-Ahead Tips:**

To store, let the curry cool, then transfer to an airtight container in the refrigerator for up to 5 days. Reheat in a microwave for 60 to 90 seconds or on the stovetop over medium-low heat.

To freeze, transfer the cooled curry to freezer containers or bags, and lay them flat on a baking sheet to freeze evenly; once frozen, they will keep for up to 3 months. When ready to serve, thaw in the fridge overnight, then reheat on the stovetop or in a microwave.

| The HCC Lineup | Make It Your Own |
|---|---|
| Protein 20 g<br>Tofu, chickpeas | Make it soy-free by swapping out the tofu for shrimp or cubed chicken breast (just remember to cook them to an internal temperature of 145°F and 165°F, respectively). |

| | |
|---|---|
| Fiber 13 g<br>Chickpeas, butternut squash, spinach, carrots | Switch it up with sweet potatoes and cauliflower, and serve your curry with wild rice or quinoa. |
| Fat 20 g<br>Coconut milk, cashews, coconut oil | Make it nut-free with pumpkin or sunflower seeds in place of cashews. |

# One-Pan Pizza Chicken

*Makes 4 servings*
*Gluten-Free, Nut-Free, Soy-Free, Vegetarian (Option),*
*Vegan (Option), Dairy-Free (Option)*

This pizza isn't another disappointing diet swap, but it *is* a damn fun way to dress up basic boring chicken breasts with all the flavors of pizza you love. We're team pepperoni in my house, but feel free to throw on whatever combination of toppings you have in the fridge (*pineapple and pickles, anyone?*).

Avocado or olive oil nonstick
  cooking spray, for pan
2 pounds new potatoes
4 colorful bell peppers, sliced
  thinly
4 teaspoons extra-virgin olive oil
2 tablespoons Italian seasoning
3 tablespoons finely grated
  Parmesan cheese
½ teaspoon salt

¼ teaspoon freshly ground black
  pepper
4 skinless boneless chicken breasts
  (about 1 pound)
½ cup pizza sauce
4 ounces fresh mozzarella cheese,
  sliced
¼ cup sliced turkey pepperoni
¼ cup sliced olives

Preheat the oven to 400°F. Spray a large rimmed baking sheet with nonstick cooking spray and set aside.

Meanwhile, place the new potatoes in a pot and cover with cold salted water. Bring to a boil, then simmer for 10 to 15 minutes, or until fork-tender. Drain the potatoes and allow to cool before cutting into quarters and transferring to a large bowl along with the sliced bell peppers and 2 teaspoons of the olive oil.

Combine the Italian seasoning, Parmesan cheese, salt, and black pepper in a small bowl. Add half of this mixture to the vegetables and toss well to coat.

Spread out the potatoes and bell peppers on the prepared baking sheet.

Next, season the chicken breasts with the remaining seasoning mixture. Heat the remaining 2 teaspoons of olive oil in a large skillet over medium-high heat. Add the chicken breasts to the hot pan and cook until golden brown, 4 to 5 minutes on each side.

Transfer the cooked chicken breasts to the baking pan that contains the potatoes and bell peppers. Bake at 400°F for 15 minutes. Remove from the oven and carefully spoon the pizza sauce over the top of the chicken breasts, then top with the mozzarella cheese, pepperoni, and olives. Return the pan to the oven and bake an additional 10 minutes, or until the cheese is melty and browned, and the chicken reaches an internal temperature of 165°F. Enjoy sizzling hot!

**Make-Ahead Tip:**

To store, transfer the cooled chicken breasts, potatoes, and vegetables to an airtight container for up to 4 days. Reheat in a 350°F oven for 10 to 13 minutes, or microwave a portion for 90 seconds.

| The HCC Lineup | Make It Your Own |
|---|---|
| Protein 44 g<br>Chicken breasts, turkey pepperoni, mozzarella, Parmesan | Make it plant-based by replacing the chicken breast with extra-firm tofu or tempeh and veggie pepperoni, and using plant-based cheese and nutritional yeast. |
| Fiber 8 g<br>Potatoes, bell peppers | Serve alongside a fresh green salad or throw extra veggies onto the pan for roasting! |
| Fat 19 g<br>Mozzarella, Parmesan, olives | Swap out the mozzarella for Cheddar or Gruyère, or garnish your bowl with toasted pine nuts. |

# Sicilian Cauliflower Pasta

*Makes 6 servings*
*Vegetarian, Gluten-Free, Soy-Free, Vegan (Option),*
*Dairy-Free (Option), Nut-Free (Option)*

This recipe is *giving* date night (without the insane bill or two-hour dining time limit). Al dente chickpea rigatoni gets cozy with caramelized cauliflower and golden raisins, finished off with a snowfall of Parm and toasty pine nuts. This isn't just dinner, it's a culinary swipe right.

1 pound uncooked chickpea or other legume rigatoni pasta (or your favorite short-cut pasta)
1 tablespoon olive oil
1 large head cauliflower, cut into small pieces
1 to 2 shallots, sliced thinly
Salt and freshly ground black pepper
2 garlic cloves, sliced thinly
2 tablespoons capers

¼ cup golden raisins
¼ cup sherry vinegar or white wine balsamic vinegar
1 tablespoon honey (or pure maple syrup, for plant-based)
Leaves from 3 sprigs thyme
⅓ cup pitted kalamata olives
¼ cup toasted pine nuts
¼ cup flat-leaf parsley
¼ cup Parmesan cheese, or to taste

Bring a large pot of salted water to a boil over medium-high heat. Cook the pasta according to the package directions, 8 to 10 minutes. Using a spider drainer, remove the pasta noodles, but not the boiling water. Add the cauliflower to the boiling water and blanch for about 1 minute. Before draining, set aside 1½ cups of the cooked pasta water. Drain the cauliflower pieces and set aside.

Heat the olive oil in a large skillet over medium-high heat. Add the shallots and cauliflower to the hot pan, along with a pinch each of salt and pepper, and sauté for 2 to 3 minutes. Add the garlic and capers, and stir for another minute, or until fragrant.

Next add the raisins, vinegar, honey, thyme leaves, and ¾ cup of the reserved cooking water to the pan. Lower the heat to low and simmer until the raisins are plump, 5 to 7 minutes.

Add the cooked pasta and olives to the pan, along with a few spoonfuls of cooking water. If you need to thin it out more, you can add additional cooking water. Toss gently and adjust seasoning as needed. Serve hot topped with pine nuts, parsley, and Parmesan cheese.

**Make-Ahead Tip:**

To store, transfer the cooled pasta to an airtight container in the fridge
for up to 5 days. Rewarm a portion in a microwave or reheat the full
casserole in a 350°F oven for 10 to 12 minutes.

| The HCC Lineup | Make It Your Own |
| --- | --- |
| Protein 21 g<br>Chickpea or legume pasta, Parmesan | If you prefer regular lower-protein wheat pasta, add your favorite neutral protein source like chickpeas, chicken, tofu, or shrimp. |
| Fiber 12 g<br>Chickpea or legume pasta, cauliflower | Replace the cauliflower with sweet potatoes, sunchokes, or parsnips (just make sure to give the root veggies some extra time in the water and pan to soften up). |
| Fat 13 g<br>Olives, olive oil, pine nuts, Parmesan cheese | Swap out the pine nuts for pumpkin seeds and a sprinkle of hemp hearts for nut-free; or go vegan, using nutritional yeast in place of Parmesan. |

# SNACKS & SWEETS

# German Cake Black Bean Brownie Bites

*Makes 24 balls (nutrition per ball)*
*Vegetarian, Vegan, Gluten-Free, Dairy-Free, Soy-Free*

I know that the idea of putting beans in your brownies sounds like the most diet-y thing ever, but you will be shocked at how fudgy and dense our beloved magical fruits make these mini noms. Rich cocoa and chocolate chips get combined with toasty coconut and nutty pecans in a bite-size, bean-based brownie with big benefits. It's the ultimate staff room snack flex that you won't want to share.

3 tablespoons unsweetened cocoa powder

1 cup fine almond flour

1 (19-ounce) can low-sodium black beans, drained and rinsed well

¼ cup natural almond butter

½ cup pure maple syrup

2 teaspoons pure vanilla extract

¼ teaspoon fine salt

½ cup mini dark chocolate chips

½ cup finely shredded unsweetened coconut, toasted

¼ cup finely minced or ground pecans

Combine the cocoa powder, almond flour, black beans, almond butter, maple syrup, vanilla, and salt in a food processor. Fold in the chocolate chips. Refrigerate the bowl for an hour.

Combine the coconut and pecans on a plate or a shallow bowl.

Roll the batter into twenty-four balls, then roll each in the coconut-pecan mixture. Put them back in the fridge to set for at least 30 minutes before serving. Enjoy with a big, cold glass of soy or cow's milk.

**Make-Ahead Tips:**

To store, transfer to an airtight container in the fridge for up to 10 days.

To freeze, transfer between layers of parchment paper to a freezer-safe container or bag for up to 3 months.

| The HCC Lineup | Make It Your Own |
|---|---|
| Protein 3 g<br>Black beans, almond butter | Boost protein even more by replacing the cocoa powder with chocolate protein powder. |
| Fiber 3 g<br>Black beans, coconut, pecans, almond butter, almond flour | For an extra fiber-boost, mix in a big handful of chia or flaxseeds. |
| Fat 7 g<br>Almond flour, almond butter, coconut, pecans | Switch up the nut butter with whatever you have on hand, or add a handful of hemp hearts to the coating for a bit of omega-3 fats. |

# Pumpkin Pie Protein Shake

*Serves 1*
*Vegetarian, Vegan, Gluten-Free, Dairy-Free,*
*Soy-Free (Option), Nut-Free (Option)*

Call me basic, but the moment that first leaf turns orange, I'm making a beeline to Starbucks in my Ugg boots and oversize scarf, singing Taylor Swift's "All Too Well" (*obviously, the ten-minute version*). That first PSL sip of the season hits like a powerful key-change bridge, but I find myself getting sugared out before I can even get my caffeine fix. This shake provides your autumnal flavor fix in a satiating milkshake-like snack.

½ frozen banana (about ½ cup, sliced)

1 cup unsweetened soy milk

¼ cup pure pumpkin puree

1 tablespoon cashew butter

1 scoop vanilla protein powder (e.g., **Neue Theory**'s 2-in-1 Plant Based Probiotic Protein Powder)

0 to 3 teaspoons pure maple syrup

½ teaspoon pumpkin pie spice, or to taste

6 ice cubes

**Optional (but not really optional for me):**
1 to 2 shots espresso

**For Serving:**
2 tablespoons soy-based Greek-style yogurt

Additional pumpkin pie spice

Combine the banana, soy milk, pumpkin puree, cashew butter, vanilla protein powder, maple syrup, pumpkin pie spice, ice cubes, and espresso, if using, in a blender. Blend until supersmooth and creamy.

Top with a dollop of Greek yogurt and a sprinkle of pumpkin pie spice. Serve chilled with a wide straw.

**Make-Ahead Tip:**

Meal-prep and then store in the fridge for up to 24 hours.

Tripled your batch and got leftovers? Freeze them in ice cube molds for up to 3 months and let thaw in the fridge overnight before drinking.

| The HCC Lineup | Make It Your Own |
|---|---|
| Protein 36 g<br>Protein powder, soy milk, yogurt | Use Greek yogurt, Skyr, soy yogurt, or cottage cheese in place of the protein powder. Or make it soy-free, using pea milk and a nut-based yogurt. |
| Fiber 6 g<br>Banana, pumpkin | Add a handful of frozen cauliflower to your smoothie, or replace the banana with applesauce or ripe pear. |
| Fat 18 g<br>Cashew butter | Make it nut-free by using sunflower seed butter, or turn it into a spoonable smoothie bowl and add a handful of pumpkin seeds for crunch. |

# Cheesy Savory Muffins

*Makes 12 muffins*
*Vegetarian, Soy-Free, Gluten-Free (Option)*

These cheese and broccoli muffins are the perfect poppable stand-in for when you're feeling like "meal food," but don't have the bandwidth (or appetite) to make and eat an actual meal. They're soft and tender on the inside, and crunchy and crackly on top, with loads of cheesy flavor.

4 large eggs
1 cup whole-milk cottage cheese
⅔ cup finely grated sharp Cheddar cheese
1 cup fine almond flour
¼ cup whole wheat flour
1 teaspoon baking powder
½ teaspoon salt

½ teaspoon freshly ground black pepper
1 cup grated broccoli crown (from 1 head of broccoli)
¼ cup finely grated Parmesan cheese
1 tablespoon fresh thyme leaves
Fleur de sel or Maldon sea salt

Preheat the oven to 400°F. Line a 12-well muffin tin with paper liners or silicone baking cups, and set aside.

Whisk the eggs in a large bowl until fully combined and fluffy.

Whisk in the cottage cheese and Cheddar cheese.

Switch to a spatula and mix in the almond flour, whole wheat flour, baking powder, salt, pepper, and broccoli until well combined.

Spoon the mixture into the prepared muffin cups until they are about three-quarters of the way full. Sprinkle the Parmesan cheese, chopped fresh thyme, and a pinch of fleur de sel on top of each muffin. Bake for 25 to 28 minutes, until golden brown and set in the center. Serve warm or at room temperature.

**Make-Ahead Tip:**

Let cool completely after baking, then transfer to an airtight container in the fridge for up to 5 days. Reheat in a microwave for 20 to 30 seconds.

| The HCC Lineup | Make It Your Own |
|---|---|
| Protein 10 g<br>Cottage cheese, Cheddar, Parmesan, eggs, almond flour | Add finely diced turkey breast or chicken sausage to pump up the protein, flavor, and texture. |
| Fiber 2 g<br>Broccoli, almond flour, whole wheat flour | Ditch the broccoli in favor of mushrooms, potatoes, or sun-dried tomatoes, or add a couple of spoonfuls of ground flaxseed to the batter. You can also make them gluten-free by using gluten-free flour in place of whole wheat. |
| Fat 10 g<br>Cottage cheese, Cheddar, Parmesan, eggs, almond flour | Try folding in some sliced olives for a more sophisticated, savory flavor. |

# Cheese Plate Bites

*Makes 4 bites*
*Vegetarian, Soy-Free, Gluten-Free (Option), Nut-Free (Option)*

Tangy chèvre, crunchy pear, and toasted walnuts find their home on a not-too-sweet graham cracker base. These pretty little things make for a simple crowd-pleasing dessert, or a late-night solo hit of self-care.

¾ cup whole-milk ricotta

¼ cup chèvre

4 sheets graham crackers (gluten-free, if desired)

½ pear, cored and sliced thinly

2 ounces walnut halves, toasted and chopped roughly

4 teaspoons honey, or to taste

Puree the ricotta and chèvre together in a small blender or food processor (*or just give it a good whip with a strong arm*).

Divide the ricotta cheese among the crackers, top with sliced pear and walnuts, and drizzle with honey. Enjoy . . . *ideally with a glass of Chablis*!

**Make-Ahead Tip:**

If entertaining a crowd, batch-prep the ricotta filling and store in the fridge for up to a week. (*PS: This also makes a delicious spoonable breakfast with berries and nuts!*) Assemble the bites right before serving.

| The HCC Lineup | Make It Your Own |
|---|---|
| Protein 9 g <br> Ricotta, chèvre, walnuts | Use cottage cheese in place of ricotta for an even greater protein punch, or garnish with a few slices of prosciutto on top. |
| Fiber 2.2 g <br> Pear, walnuts | Eat seasonal and swap out the pear for raspberries, blueberries, figs, or apple. |
| Fat 18 g <br> Ricotta, chèvre, walnuts | Use pistachios, almonds, pecans, or pine nuts if walnuts aren't your jam, or go nut-free, using pumpkin seeds. |

# Honey Mustard Popcorn Party Mix

*Serves 4 (makes 2½ to 3 cups)*
*Vegetarian, Gluten-Free, Dairy-Free, Soy-Free,*
*Vegan (Option), Nut-Free (Option)*

Sweet, salty, zingy, *and* crunchy, this party mix delivers on *all* our sensory needs. So, whether you're meal-prepping snacks for the week, hosting a game night, or just looking to level up your solo Netflix marathon snacks, this mix understands the assignment.

1 (19-ounce) can low-sodium chickpeas, drained, rinsed, and patted very dry
4 teaspoons avocado oil
½ cup shelled pistachios
3 tablespoons mustard powder

3 tablespoons honey (or pure maple syrup for vegan)
10 cups air-popped popcorn
1 teaspoon fleur de sel or fine sea salt

Preheat the oven to 400°F and line a baking sheet with parchment paper.

Dump the chickpeas onto a clean kitchen towel and rub to remove the skins and any moisture. The more moisture you can remove, the crunchier the mix!

Toss with 2 teaspoons of the avocado oil, then bake them for 35 to 45 minutes, or until crispy and browned, shaking the pan every 10 to 12 minutes to cook evenly.

Mix together the mustard, honey, and remaining 2 teaspoons of avocado oil in a small bowl.

Add the roasted chickpeas and pistachios to the sauce and toss well to coat. Return the mixture to the baking sheet and spread out in an even layer. Bake for an additional 6 to 8 minutes, keeping a close eye on it to prevent burning.

Remove from the oven and allow to cool for 15 minutes, then mix with the popcorn and season generously with fleur de sel.

**Make-Ahead Tip:**

To store, transfer to an airtight container or bag and keep at room temperature, away from heat or moisture, for up to 5 days.

| The HCC Lineup | Make It Your Own |
| --- | --- |
| Protein 10 g<br>Chickpeas, pistachios | Swap in dry-roasted edamame for the chickpeas (especially if you're looking for the menopause-supporting perks). |
| Fiber 9 g<br>Popcorn, chickpeas, pistachios | Add a heaping spoonful of ground flax-seeds or wheat bran alongside the honey-mustard sauce for an extra boost of fiber. |
| Fat 17 g<br>Pistachios, avocado oil | Try peanuts or mixed nuts for a more traditional snack mix, or use sunflower or pumpkin seeds instead. |

# PB Cup Tofu Mousse

*Makes 4 servings*
*Vegan, Vegetarian, Gluten-Free, Dairy-Free, Nut-Free (Option)*

I know, I know. The word "tofu" doesn't exactly scream "serve me seconds" in the dessert department, but after trying this, you *will* be buying tofu in bulk. Silken tofu offers a neutral yet high-protein base that blends seamlessly with peanut butter and maple syrup, creating a luscious mousse that's rich on the palate but light on the tongue.

1½ cups (about 12 ounces) silken tofu

¼ cup natural peanut butter

2 tablespoons pure maple syrup, or to taste

1 teaspoon pure vanilla extract

¼ teaspoon salt

### Dark Chocolate Ganache:

1.5 ounces (1 scant cup) dark chocolate chips (dairy-free, if needed)

¼ teaspoon coconut oil

¼ cup full-fat coconut milk (shaken in the can)

### For Serving:

¼ cup chopped salted peanuts

¼ cup cacao nibs

Fleur de sel or Maldon sea salt

Combine the tofu, peanut butter, maple syrup, vanilla, and salt in a food processor or blender, and puree until smooth. Divide equally among four small cups or ramekins and set in the fridge.

Combine the dark chocolate chips and coconut oil in a microwave-safe dish. Microwave on 50% power for 45 seconds. Stir, then microwave in 20-second intervals, until the chocolate is melted and smooth. While hot, whisk in the shaken canned coconut milk.

Divide the chocolate ganache on top of the cups of mousse and let sit in the fridge for 30 minutes to set up before serving. When ready to eat, top with salted peanuts, cacao nibs, and a pinch of fleur de sel.

**Make-Ahead Tip:**

To prep ahead or store for later, cover the cups or ramekins tightly with plastic wrap and refrigerate for up to 48 hours. Garnish with the peanuts, cacao nibs, and salt when serving.

| The HCC Lineup | Make It Your Own |
|---|---|
| Protein 11 g<br>Silken tofu, peanut butter, peanuts | Replace the tofu with Greek yogurt and blend as usual for a slightly heavier mousse that's jam-packed with protein. |
| Fiber 4 g<br>Peanut butter, peanuts, cacao nibs | For a fiber boost, blend some ground chia seeds into the mousse base, or top with fresh berries. |
| Fat 24 g<br>Peanut butter, coconut milk, peanuts, cacao nibs | Go nut-free by using sunflower butter and seeds in place of the peanut products. |

# Pumpkin Chocolate Bread

*Makes 12 servings*
*Vegetarian, Nut-Free, Soy-Free, Gluten-Free (Option),*
*Dairy-Free (Option), Vegan (Option)*

Canned pumpkin is such a versatile year-round staple for adding moisture, natural sweetness, and fiber to baked goods, and we put it to work in this hearty bread. Okay, okay, so with the addition of rich, dark chocolate and salty pepitas, it really didn't have to work that hard.

Avocado or olive oil nonstick cooking spray, for pan
1½ cups canned pure pumpkin puree
1 large egg
⅓ cup plain 5% Greek yogurt
½ cup pure maple syrup
2 tablespoons avocado oil
2 teaspoons pure vanilla extract
1 teaspoon baking soda
2 teaspoons ground cinnamon
¼ teaspoon freshly grated nutmeg
¼ teaspoon ground cloves
¼ teaspoon salt
1¼ cups whole wheat flour
¼ teaspoon ground flax meal
½ cup mini dark chocolate chips
½ cup pepitas (pumpkin seeds)
2 tablespoons demerara sugar (raw cane sugar)

Preheat an oven to 325°F. Line an 8 x 4–inch loaf pan with parchment paper (leaving extra "wings" of paper on the long sides of the pan, for easy removal), spray with nonstick cooking spray, and set aside.

Combine the pumpkin puree, egg, Greek yogurt, maple syrup, avocado oil, and vanilla in a large bowl and stir with a spatula.

In another large bowl, combine the baking soda, cinnamon, nutmeg, cloves, salt, whole wheat flour, and flax meal.

Create a well in the center of the flour mixture. Pour the pumpkin mixture into the well and fold gently with a spatula until combined. Once well mixed, fold in the chocolate chips.

Pour the batter into the prepared loaf pan and sprinkle with the pepitas and demerara sugar.

Bake for 25 to 30 minutes, then tent with foil and bake for an additional 30 to 40 minutes, or until a toothpick inserted into the center comes out clean. Remove from the oven and allow to cool fully on a baking rack before slicing and serving.

**Make-Ahead Tips:**

To store, wrap tightly in plastic wrap or aluminum foil to lock in the moisture, then keep in an airtight container or storage bag at room temperature for up to 3 days, or in the fridge for up to 5 days.

To freeze, wrap the loaf in plastic wrap and then foil, then store in a freezer-safe bag for up to 3 months. Allow to thaw at room temperature for a few hours or microwave a slice for 30 seconds.

| The HCC Lineup | Make It Your Own |
| --- | --- |
| Protein 5 g<br>Greek yogurt, egg, flax meal, pepitas | Go dairy-free and vegan by replacing the Greek yogurt with soy-based yogurt and using a plant-based egg replacement. |
| Fiber 3 g<br>Pumpkin, whole wheat flour, flax meal | Replace the flax meal with wheat bran as an effective baked-good fiber booster, or go gluten-free, using your favorite gluten-free flour. |
| Fat 9 g<br>Greek yogurt, pepitas, flax meal, avocado oil | Swap out the seeds in favor of crushed pistachios or pecans, or smear your loaf with almond butter when serving. |

# Blueberry Walnut Power Muffins

*Makes 12 muffins*
*Vegetarian, Soy-Free, Dairy-Free (Option), Vegan (Option),*
*Gluten-Free (Option), Nut-Free (Option)*

These muffins aren't just a snack; they're a whole mood. Full of hunger-crushing ingredients like Greek yogurt, flax, oats, walnuts, and antioxidant-rich blueberries, they're nutrient packed, flavorful, and moist AF, giving you sustained energy to power through your day.

¾ cup 5% plain Greek yogurt
1½ cups mashed ripe bananas (2 to 3 large bananas)
3 tablespoons melted unsalted butter or coconut oil
2 to 3 tablespoons pure maple syrup
2 large eggs
2 teaspoons pure vanilla extract

1½ cups whole wheat pastry flour
½ cup old-fashioned or rolled oats
¼ cup flax meal
1½ teaspoons ground cinnamon
1 teaspoon baking soda
½ teaspoon salt
1 cup frozen wild blueberries
⅓ cup chopped walnuts

Preheat the oven to 350°F. Line a 12-well muffin tin with paper liners and set aside.

Combine the yogurt, banana, melted butter, maple syrup, eggs, and vanilla in a large bowl and beat until the eggs are well broken up and incorporated.

In another large bowl, stir together the flour, oats, flax meal, cinnamon, baking soda, and salt.

Add the banana mixture to the flour mixture, and mix until combined. Then, fold in the blueberries and walnuts.

Scoop the muffin batter into the prepared muffin tin, filling each well about two-thirds of the way full. Bake for 20 to 22 minutes, or until a toothpick inserted into the center of a muffin comes out clean.

**Make-Ahead Tips:**

To store, place in an airtight container separated by layers of paper towel and refrigerate for up to 1 week. Bring to room temperature or warm in a microwave for 15 seconds before eating.

To freeze, wrap each muffin individually in plastic wrap or foil, and place in a single layer in a freezer-safe bag or container for up to three months. Allow to thaw for 30 to 45 minutes, or microwave for 20 to 30 seconds or 2 to 3 minutes in a 350°F oven before eating.

| The HCC Lineup | Make It Your Own |
|---|---|
| Protein 5 g<br>Greek yogurt, eggs, flax meal, walnuts | Use whipped cottage cheese in place of yogurt, or go dairy-free and vegan with soy-based yogurt and egg replacement. |
| Fiber 4 g<br>Oats, whole wheat pastry flour, bananas, blueberries, flax meal, walnuts | Mix up the fruit flavor by experimenting with diced strawberries, raspberries, cherries, pears, or apples! You can also make these gluten-free by using gluten-free flour and oats. |
| Fat 9 g<br>Greek yogurt, eggs, walnuts, flax meal | Swap out the walnuts for pumpkin seeds or coconut for a school-safe nut-free snack. |

# Berry Power Crisp

*Makes 8 servings*
*Vegetarian, Soy-Free, Gluten-Free (Option),*
*Dairy-Free (Option), Vegan (Option)*

This cozy dessert builds on my family's famous crisp recipe, with the addition of almond meal and sliced almonds, for an extra hit of staying power and crunch. Serve it warm with vanilla ice cream for a more decadent weeknight treat, or load it on top of Greek yogurt for a breakfast with benefits!

### Berry Filling:

Avocado or olive oil nonstick cooking spray, for pan

5 cups frozen berries, thawed in a large bowl

1½ tablespoons cornstarch

2 tablespoons granulated sugar

½ teaspoon ground cinnamon

1 teaspoon lemon zest

2 teaspoons pure vanilla extract

### Crumble:

½ cup old-fashioned oats or rolled oats

¼ cup whole wheat flour

¼ cup almond meal

¼ cup sliced almonds

¼ cup light brown sugar

½ teaspoon ground cinnamon

¼ teaspoon salt

¼ cup melted unsalted butter

### For Serving:

3 cups 5% to 10% vanilla Greek yogurt or crème fraîche

Prepare the berry filling: Preheat the oven to 375°F. Lightly spray a 9-inch pie dish with nonstick spray and set aside.

Drain the juice from the thawed berries (*and keep that liquid gold for smoothies!*). Add the cornstarch to the bowl and toss until the berries are coated, then add the sugar, cinnamon, lemon zest, and vanilla. Toss to combine, then pour the mixture into the prepared pie dish.

In another large bowl, stir the oatmeal, flour, almond meal, almonds, brown sugar, cinnamon, and salt together. Add the melted butter and use your fingers to create little "clusters" of crumble.

Sprinkle the clusters on top of the berry filling and bake for 30 to 40 minutes, or until the berries are bubbly and thick, and the topping is golden brown. Remove from the oven and allow to cool before serving. Serve with Greek yogurt or crème fraîche.

**Make-Ahead Tips:**

To store, allow to cool completely, then cover with plastic wrap and refrigerate for up to 3 days. Reheat in a 350°F oven for 10 to 15 minutes, or in a microwave for 45 to 60 seconds.

To freeze, bake the crisp in a freezer-safe dish and, when cool, wrap tightly in plastic wrap and foil. Reheat from frozen at 350°F for 35 to 40 minutes, or until bubbly and crisp.

| The HCC Lineup | Make It Your Own |
| --- | --- |
| Protein 10 g<br>Greek yogurt, almond meal, almonds | Add a handful of hemp hearts to the crumble for extra protein, or go dairy-free and vegan by using nondairy yogurt and butter. |
| Fiber 14.5 g<br>Berries, oats, whole wheat flour, almond meal, almonds | When the weather starts to cool, swap out the berries for stewed apples or pears. You can also make this recipe gluten-free by using gluten-free oats and flour. |
| Fat 13 g<br>Almonds, almond meal, Greek yogurt, butter | Get creative with the crust by trading in the almond slices for pecans, pistachios, or walnuts. |

# ACKNOWLEDGMENTS

This book, like most things in my life, wasn't a solo venture. In addition to my ride-or-die, coffee, it took a village of brilliant minds, loving hearts, and well-timed memes to bring *The Hunger Crushing Combo Method* to life.

To my husband, thank you for doubling down on dad duty when I was drowning in citations, editing marathons, and a fridge full of cottage cheese for recipe testing. Your validation, patience, and kid wrangling heroics kept me afloat and (at least somewhat) sane.

To my sweet boys, thank you for reminding me daily of the power of joy, curiosity, and the magic of a few chocolate chips in making hemp heart protein oats disappear.

To my parents and extended family, thank you for passing on your love of learning and your gift of teaching. You laid the foundation for this work long before I had the platform (never mind the internet) to share it.

To my friends, you magical beings, thank you for the text rants, relatable video shares, and impromptu pep talks over wine and cheese boards (which, by the way, is absolutely a Hunger Crushing Combo in my books).

To my incredibly dedicated fans and followers, whether you've been with me since the beginning, are new here (welcome!), or found me somewhere along the way: This book exists because of you. You are proof that the Hunger Crushing Combo isn't just a theory, it's a powerful tool designed for 180 transformation. Your stories, your questions, your struggles, and your wins gave this work a beating heart. I am endlessly grateful for your trust and your hunger for knowledge, freedom, and a better approach to eating well.

Professionally, I need to extend my profound gratitude to my team:

**Ginger Bertrand and Michele Yeo**, my longtime managers, protectors, cheerleaders, and friends. You saw the potential in this idea from day one and never let me forget it. Thank you for building me up and standing by me through every twist of this wild ride.

**Charlotte Chan**: You *are* Abbey's Kitchen. Thank you for literally running the rest of my life (and multiple businesses) with grace, intelligence, and a killer spreadsheet while I chipped away at this beast of a book.

**Dr. Eric Williamson**, my nutrition encyclopedia and trusted thought partner. Thank you for offering critical insights, evidence-based brilliance, and sanity-saving fact checks.

**Shoshana Pritzker, Ana Reisdorf, and Lauren Panoff**: Thank you for deep-diving into the research trenches with me. Your dietitian-informed support in recipe testing, writing, and editing has helped support this book's credibility and creativity.

And finally, to my younger self: Your struggles were not in vain. Every challenge you faced, every moment of doubt, every tear shed in front of a mirror, has helped someone else heal their relationship with food and their body. I see you. I thank you. Your lived experience is the only reason I am able to write these words today.

# NOTES

· · · · · · · · · · · · · · ·

**Introduction: The Road to Abundance**

1. Marie Galmiche et al., "Prevalence of Eating Disorders over the 2000–2018 Period: A Systematic Literature Review," *American Journal of Clinical Nutrition* 109, no. 5 (2019): 1402–13, https://doi.org:10.1093/ajcn/nqy342.

2. "Survey Finds Disordered Eating Behaviors Among Three out of Four American Women," University of North Carolina at Chapel Hill, September 26, 2008, https://sph.unc.edu/cphm/carolina-public-health-magazine-accelerate-fall-2008/survey-finds-disordered-eating-behaviors-among-three-out-of-four-american-women-fall-2008/.

**Chapter 1: The Nonrestrictive, Additive Approach to Eating and Living Well**

1. Caroline E. Childs et al., "Diet and Immune Function," *Nutrients* 11, no. 8 (August 16, 2019): 1933, https://doi.org:10.3390/nu11081933.

2. Jaecheol Moon and Gwanpyo Koh, "Clinical Evidence and Mechanisms of High-Protein Diet-Induced Weight Loss," *Journal of Obesity & Metabolic Syndrome* 29, no. 3 (2020): 166–73, https://doi.org:10.7570/jomes20028.

3. Emily Arentson-Lantz et al., "Protein: A Nutrient in Focus," *Applied Physiology, Nutrition, and Metabolism (Physiologie appliquee, nutrition et metabolisme)* 40, no. 8 (2015): 755–61, https://doi.org:10.1139/apnm-2014-0530.

4. Robert MacDonell et al., "Protein/Amino-Acid Modulation of Bone Cell Function," *BoneKey Reports* 5, no. 827 (August 10, 2016), https://doi.org:10.1038/bonekey.2016.58.

5. Andrew N. Reynolds et al., "Dietary Fibre and Whole Grains in Diabetes Management: Systematic Review and Meta-analyses," *PLoS Medicine* 17, no. 3 (March 6, 2020): e1003053, https://doi.org:10.1371/journal.pmed.1003053.

6. Ghada A. Soliman, "Dietary Fiber, Atherosclerosis, and Cardiovascular Disease," *Nutrients* 11, no. 5 (May 23, 2019): 1155, https://doi.org:10.3390/nu11051155.

7. Jun Hu et al., "Use of Dietary Fibers in Reducing the Risk of Several Cancer Types: An Umbrella Review," *Nutrients* 11 (May 30, 2023): 2545, https://doi.org:10.3390/nu15112545.

8. Pablo Alonso-Coello et al., "Fiber for the Treatment of Hemorrhoids Complications: A Systematic Review and Meta-analysis," *American Journal of Gastroenterology* 101, no. 1 (2006): 181–88, https://doi.org:10.1111/j.1572-0241.2005.00359.x.

9. Jiongxing Fu et al., "Dietary Fiber Intake and Gut Microbiota in Human Health," *Microorganisms* 10, no. 12 (December 18, 2022): 2507, https://doi.org:10.3390 /microorganisms10122507.

10. W. S. Harris et al., "Blood n-3 Fatty Acid Levels and Total and Cause-Specific Mortality from 17 Prospective Studies," *Nature Communications* 12, no. 2329 (2021): 2329, https://doi.org/10.1038/s41467-021-22370-2.

11. Jacqueline K. Innes and Philip C. Calder, "Omega-6 Fatty Acids and Inflammation," *Prostaglandins, Leukotrienes, and Essential Fatty Acids* 132 (2018): 41–48, https:// doi.org:10.1016/j.plefa.2018.03.004.

12. Suh-Ching Yang et al., "High Fat Diet with a High Monounsaturated Fatty Acid and Polyunsaturated/Saturated Fatty Acid Ratio Suppresses Body Fat Accumulation and Weight Gain in Obese Hamsters," *Nutrients* 9, no. 10 (October 19, 2017): 1148, https://doi.org:10.3390/nu9101148.

13. P. Mata et al., "Effect of Dietary Monounsaturated Fatty Acids on Plasma Lipoproteins and Apolipoproteins in Women," *American Journal of Clinical Nutrition* 56, no. 1 (1992): 77–83, https://doi.org:10.1093/ajcn/56.1.77.

14. Elena M. Yubero-Serrano et al., "Insulin Resistance Determines a Differential Response to Changes in Dietary Fat Modification on Metabolic Syndrome Risk Factors: The LIPGENE Study," *American Journal of Clinical Nutrition* 102, no. 6 (2015): 1509–17, https://doi.org:10.3945/ajcn.115.111286.

15. Yubero-Serrano et al., "Insulin Resistance Determines."

16. Nina Teicholz, "A Short History of Saturated Fat: The Making and Unmaking of a Scientific Consensus," *Current Opinion in Endocrinology, Diabetes, and Obesity* 30, no. 1 (2023): 65–71, https://doi.org:10.1097/MED.0000000000000791.

17. Laura Pimpin et al., "Is Butter Back? A Systematic Review and Meta-analysis of Butter Consumption and Risk of Cardiovascular Disease, Diabetes, and Total Mortality," *PloS One* 11, no. 6 (June 29, 2016): e0158118, https://doi.org:10.1371 /journal.pone.0158118.

18. Linxi Ma et al., "Postbiotics in Human Health: A Narrative Review," *Nutrients* 15, no. 2 (January 6, 2023): 291, https://doi.org:10.3390/nu15020291.

19. Peng Zhao et al., "Significance of Gut Microbiota and Short-Chain Fatty Acids in Heart Failure," *Nutrients* 14, no. 18 (September 11, 2022): 3758, https://doi .org:10.3390/nu14183758.

20. Morvarid Noormohammadi et al., "The Effect of Probiotic and Symbiotic Supplementation on Appetite-Regulating Hormones and Desire to Eat: A Systematic Review and Meta-analysis of Clinical Trials," *Pharmacological Research* 187 (2023): 106614, https://doi.org:10.1016/j.phrs.2022.106614.

21. Marie-Pierre St-Onge and Aubrey Bosarge, "Weight-Loss Diet That Includes Consumption of Medium-Chain Triacylglycerol Oil Leads to a Greater Rate of Weight and Fat Mass Loss Than Does Olive Oil," *American Journal of Clinical Nutrition* 87, no. 3 (2008): 621–26, https://doi.org:10.1093/ajcn/87.3.621.

22. Shinji Watanabe and Shougo Tsujino, "Applications of Medium-Chain Triglycerides in Foods," *Frontiers in Nutrition* 9 (June 2, 2022): 802805, https://doi.org:10 .3389/fnut.2022.802805; Susan Hewlings, "Coconuts and Health: Different Chain Lengths of Saturated Fats Require Different Consideration," *Journal of Cardiovascular Development and Disease* 7, no. 4 (December 17, 2020): 59, https://doi .org:10.3390/jcdd7040059.

23. Lauren K. Roth, "Revocation of Uses of Partially Hydrogenated Oils in Foods," Confirmation of Effective Date (December 11, 2023), https://www.federalregister .gov/documents/2023/12/14/2023-27506/revocation-of-uses-of-partially -hydrogenated-oils-in-foods-confirmation-of-effective-date.

24. Valeria Tosti et al., "Health Benefits of the Mediterranean Diet: Metabolic and Molecular Mechanisms," *Journals of Gerontology, Series A, Biological Sciences and Medical Sciences* 73, no. 3 (2018): 318–26, https://doi.org:10.1093/gerona/glx227.

25. Yi Wan et al., "Association Between Changes in Carbohydrate Intake and Long Term Weight Changes: Prospective Cohort Study," *BMJ (Clinical Research Ed.)* 382 (September 27, 2023): e073939, https://doi.org:10.1136/bmj-2022-073939.

26. Vasanti S. Malik and Frank B. Hu, "The Role of Sugar-Sweetened Beverages in the Global Epidemics of Obesity and Chronic Diseases," *Nature Review, Endocrinology* 18, no. 4 (2022): 205–18, https://doi.org:10.1038/s41574-021-00627-6.

## Chapter 2: Goodbye, Diets; Hello, Satiety—and Your Healthiest Weight

1. Katrin Elisabeth Giel et al., "Weight Bias in Work Settings—a Qualitative Review," *Obesity Facts* 3, no. 1 (2010): 33–40, https://doi.org/10.1159/000276992.

2. John Cawley, "The Impact of Obesity on Wages," *Journal of Human Resources* 39, no. 2 (Spring 2004): 451–74, https://www.researchgate.net/profile/John-Cawley /publication/227637102_The_Impact_of_Obesity_on_Wage/links/09e415141 d137c2146000000/The-Impact-of-Obesity-on-Wage.pdf.

3. Nathalie Auger et al., "Anorexia Nervosa and the Long-Term Risk of Mortality in Women," *World Psychiatry: Official Journal of the World Psychiatric Association (WPA)* 20, no. 3 (2021): 448–49, https://doi.org:10.1002/wps.20904.

4. J. M. Nagata et al., "Prevalence and Correlates of Disordered Eating Behaviors Among Young Adults with Overweight or Obesity," *Journal of General Internal Medicine* 33 (2018): 1337–43, https://doi.org/10.1007/s11606-018-4465-z.

5. Alice A. Gibson and Amanda Sainsbury, "Strategies to Improve Adherence to Dietary Weight Loss Interventions in Research and Real-World Settings," *Behavioral Sciences* (Basel) 7, no. 3 (July 11, 2017): 44, https://doi.org:10.3390/bs7030044.

6. D. M. Thomas et al., "Can a Weight Loss of One Pound a Week Be Achieved with a 3500-kcal Deficit? Commentary on a Commonly Accepted Rule," *International Journal of Obesity* 37, no. 12 (2013): 1611–63, https://doi.org:10.1038/ijo.2013.51.

7. E. Fothergill et al., "Persistent Metabolic Adaptation 6 Years After 'The Biggest Loser' Competition," *Obesity* (Silver Spring, MD) 24, no. 8 (2016): 1612–19, https:// doi.org/10.1002/oby.21538.

8. A. Astrup et al., "Meta-analysis of Resting Metabolic Rate in Formerly Obese Subjects," *American Journal of Clinical Nutrition* 69, no. 6 (1999): 1117–22, https:// doi.org:10.1093/ajcn/69.6.1117.

9. Nana Chung et al., "Non-exercise Activity Thermogenesis (NEAT): A Component of Total Daily Energy Expenditure," *Journal of Exercise Nutrition & Biochemistry* 22, no. 2 (2018): 23–30, https://doi.org:10.20463/jenb.2018.0013.

10. Michael Rosenbaum et al., "Long-Term Persistence of Adaptive Thermogenesis in Subjects Who Have Maintained a Reduced Body Weight," *American Journal of Clinical Nutrition* 88, no. 4 (2008): 906–12, https://doi.org:10.1093/ajcn/88.4 .906.

11. Areeba N. Memon et al., "Have Our Attempts to Curb Obesity Done More Harm Than Good?," *Cureus* 12, no. 9 (September 6, 2020): e10275, https://doi.org:10.7759/cureus.10275.

12. Brian Wansink and Pierre Chandon, "Health Halos: How Nutrition Claims Influence Food Consumption for Overweight and Normal Weight People," *FASEB Journal* 20, no. 5 (March 2006): A1008, https://doi.org/10.1096/fasebj.20.5.A1008-c.

13. Heather J. Leidy et al., "Beneficial Effects of a Higher-Protein Breakfast on the Appetitive, Hormonal, and Neural Signals Controlling Energy Intake Regulation in Overweight/Obese, 'Breakfast-Skipping,' Late-Adolescent Girls," *American Journal of Clinical Nutrition* 97, no. 4 (2013): 677–88, https://doi.org:10.3945/ajcn.112.053116.

14. Anne-Marie Ravn et al., "Thermic Effect of a Meal and Appetite in Adults: An Individual Participant Data Meta-analysis of Meal-Test Trials," *Food & Nutrition Research* 57 (December 23, 2013), https://doi.org:10.3402/fnr.v57i0.19676.

15. George A. Bray et al., "Effect of Protein Overfeeding on Energy Expenditure Measured in a Metabolic Chamber," *American Journal of Clinical Nutrition* 101, no. 3 (2015): 496–505, https://doi.org:10.3945/ajcn.114.091769.

16. Herman Pontzer et al., "Daily Energy Expenditure Through the Human Life Course," *Science* (New York) 373, no. 6556 (2021): 808–12, https://doi.org:10.1126/science.abe5017.

17. F. Zurlo et al., "Skeletal Muscle Metabolism Is a Major Determinant of Resting Energy Expenditure," *Journal of Clinical Investigation* 86, no. 5 (1990): 1423–27, https://doi.org:10.1172/JCI114857.

18. Jaecheol Moon and Gwanpyo Koh, "Clinical Evidence and Mechanisms of High-Protein Diet-Induced Weight Loss," *Journal of Obesity & Metabolic Syndrome* 29, no. 3 (2020): 166–73, https://doi.org:10.7570/jomes20028.

19. M. S. Westerterp-Plantenga et al., "High Protein Intake Sustains Weight Maintenance After Body Weight Loss in Humans," *International Journal of Obesity and Related Metabolic Disorders: Journal of the International Association for the Study of Obesity* 28, no. 1 (2004): 57–64, https://doi.org:10.1038/sj.ijo.0802461.

20. Heather J. Leidy et al., "The Role of Protein in Weight Loss and Maintenance," *American Journal of Clinical Nutrition* 101, no. 6 (2015): 1320S–29S, https://doi.org:10.3945/ajcn.114.084038.

21. D. A. VanderWeele, "Insulin Is a Prandial Satiety Hormone," *Physiology & Behavior* 56, no. 3 (1994): 619–22, https://doi.org:10.1016/0031-9384(94)90310-7.

22. Yuuki Yanagisawa, "How Dietary Amino Acids and High Protein Diets Influence Insulin Secretion," *Physiological Reports* 11, no. 2 (2023): e15577, https://doi.org:10.14814/phy2.15577.

23. Manuela Lejeune et al., "Ghrelin and Glucagon-Like Peptide 1 Concentrations, 24-h Satiety, and Energy and Substrate Metabolism During a High-Protein Diet and Measured in a Respiration Chamber," *American Journal of Clinical Nutrition* 83, no. 1 (January 2006): 89–94, https://doi.org/10.1093/ajcn/83.1.89.

24. Heather J. Leidy et al., "The Influence of Higher Protein Intake and Greater Eating Frequency on Appetite Control in Overweight and Obese Men," *Obesity* (Silver Spring, MD) 18, no. 9 (2010): 1725–32, https://doi.org:10.1038/oby.2010.45.

25. Martin Friedrichsen et al., "The Effect of Semaglutide 2.4 mg Once Weekly on Energy Intake, Appetite, Control of Eating, and Gastric Emptying in Adults with Obesity," *Diabetes, Obesity & Metabolism* 23, no. 3 (2021): 754–62, https://doi.org:doi:10.1111/dom.14280.

26. Thomas A. Wadden et al., "Effect of Subcutaneous Semaglutide vs Placebo as an Adjunct to Intensive Behavioral Therapy on Body Weight in Adults with Overweight or Obesity: The STEP 3 Randomized Clinical Trial," *JAMA* 325, no. 14 (2021): 1403–13, https://doi.org:10.1001/jama.2021.1831.

27. Wendy A. M. Blom et al., "Effect of a High-Protein Breakfast on the Postprandial Ghrelin Response," *American Journal of Clinical Nutrition* 83, no. 2 (2006): 211–20, https://doi.org:10.1093/ajcn/83.2.211.

28. Heather J. Leidy et al., "The Effects of Consuming Frequent, Higher Protein Meals on Appetite and Satiety During Weight Loss in Overweight/Obese Men," *Obesity* (Silver Spring, MD) 19, no. 4 (2011): 818–24, https://doi.org:10.1038/oby.2010.203.

29. Heather J. Leidy, "Increased Dietary Protein as a Dietary Strategy to Prevent and/or Treat Obesity," *Missouri Medicine* 111, no. 1 (2014): 54–58.

30. Karla Arnotti and Mandy Bamber, "Fruit and Vegetable Consumption in Overweight or Obese Individuals: A Meta-analysis," *Western Journal of Nursing Research* 42, no. 4 (2020): 306–14, https://doi.org:10.1177/0193945919858699.

31. Monica L. Bertoia et al., "Changes in Intake of Fruits and Vegetables and Weight Change in United States Men and Women Followed for Up to 24 Years: Analysis from Three Prospective Cohort Studies," *PLoS Medicine* 12, no. 9 (September 22, 2015): e1001878, https://doi.org:10.1371/journal.pmed.1001878.

32. Maximilian Andreas Storz, "Nutrition Facts Labels: Who Is Actually Reading Them and Does It Help in Meeting Intake Recommendations for Nutrients of Public Health Concern?," *BMC Public Health* 23, no. 1 (October 7, 2023): 1947, https://doi.org:10.1186/s12889-023-16859-2.

33. Tera L. Fazzino et al., "Ad Libitum Meal Energy Intake Is Positively Influenced by Energy Density, Eating Rate and Hyper-palatable Food Across Four Dietary Patterns," *Nature Food* 4, no. 2 (January 2023): 1–4, https://doi.org/10.1038/s43016-022-00688-4.

34. Barbara J. Rolls, "The Relationship Between Dietary Energy Density and Energy Intake," *Physiology & Behavior* 97, no. 5 (2009): 609–15, https://doi.org:10.1016/j.physbeh.2009.03.011; Jenny H. Ledikwe et al., "Dietary Energy Density Is Associated with Energy Intake and Weight Status in US Adults," *American Journal of Clinical Nutrition* 83, no. 6 (2006): 1362–68, https://doi.org:10.1093/ajcn/83.6.1362/.

35. Rolls, "The Relationship Between Dietary Energy Density and Energy Intake."

36. S. H. Holt et al., "A Satiety Index of Common Foods," *European Journal of Clinical Nutrition* 49, no. 9 (1995): 675–90.

37. Mahsa Jalili et al., "Fermented Foods in the Management of Obesity: Mechanisms of Action and Future Challenges," *International Journal of Molecular Sciences* 24, no. 3 (January 31, 2023): 2665, https://doi.org:10.3390/ijms24032665.

38. Cindy D. Davis, "The Gut Microbiome and Its Role in Obesity," *Nutrition Today* 51, no. 4 (2016): 167–74, https://doi.org:10.1097/NT.0000000000000167.

39. Dimitrios A. Koutoukidis et al., "The Association of Weight Loss with Changes in the Gut Microbiota Diversity, Composition, and Intestinal Permeability: A Systematic

Review and Meta-analysis," *Gut Microbes* 14, no. 1 (2022): 2020068, https://doi.org/10.1080/19490976.2021.2020068.

40. E. A. Carnero et al., "Host-Diet-Gut Microbiome Interactions Influence Human Energy Balance: A Randomized Clinical Trial," *Nature Communications* 14, no. 3161 (2023), https://doi.org/10.1038/s41467-023-38778-x.

41. A. J. Desai et al., "Cholecystokinin-Induced Satiety, a Key Gut Servomechanism That Is Affected by the Membrane Microenvironment of This Receptor," *International Journal of Obesity Supplements* 6, no. S1 (2016): S22–S27, https://doi.org:10.1038/ijosup.2016.5.

42. Xinping Lu et al., "Postprandial Inhibition of Gastric Ghrelin Secretion by Long-Chain Fatty Acid Through GPR120 in Isolated Gastric Ghrelin Cells and Mice," *American Journal of Physiology, Gastrointestinal and Liver Physiology* 303, no. 3 (2012): G367–76, https://doi.org:10.1152/ajpgi.00541.2011.

43. Andrew Costanzo et al., "A Fatty Acid Mouth Rinse Decreases Self-Reported Hunger and Increases Self-Reported Fullness in Healthy Australian Adults: A Randomized Cross-over Trial," *Nutrients* 12, no. 3 (March 2, 2020): 678, https://doi.org:10.3390/nu12030678.

44. P. K. Nguyen et al., "A Systematic Comparison of Sugar Content in Low-Fat vs Regular Versions of Food," *Nutrition & Diabetes* 6, no. 1 (January 25, 2016): e193, https://doi.org:10.1038/nutd.2015.43.

## Chapter 3: Glucose, Insulin, and Managing Blood Sugars

1. "Statistics About Diabetes," American Diabetes Association, accessed June 12, 2025, https://diabetes.org/about-diabetes/statistics/about-diabetes.

2. Vibhu Parcha et al., "Insulin Resistance and Cardiometabolic Risk Profile Among Nondiabetic American Young Adults: Insights from NHANES," *Journal of Clinical Endocrinology and Metabolism* 107, no. 1 (2022): e25–e37, https://doi.org:10.1210/clinem/dgab645.

3. "United States Population (Live)," Worldometer, accessed June 12, 2025, https://www.worldometers.info/world-population/us-population/.

4. Leila Ismail et al., "Association of Risk Factors with Type 2 Diabetes: A Systematic Review," *Computational and Structural Biotechnology Journal* 19 (March 10, 2021): 1759–85, https://doi.org:10.1016/j.csbj.2021.03.003.

5. Omar Ali, "Genetics of Type 2 Diabetes," *World Journal of Diabetes* 4, no. 4 (2013): 114–23, https://doi.org:10.4239/wjd.v4.i4.114.

6. "Diabetes Prevention Program (DPP)," National Institute of Diabetes and Digestive and Kidney Diseases (NIDDK), accessed June 12, 2025, https://www.niddk.nih.gov/about-niddk/research-areas/diabetes/diabetes-prevention-program-dpp.

7. Ahmad Al-Mrabeh, "Pathogenesis and Remission of Type 2 Diabetes: What Has the Twin Cycle Hypothesis Taught Us?," *Cardiovascular Endocrinology & Metabolism* 9, no. 4 (May 25, 2020): 132–42, https://doi.org:10.1097/XCE.0000000000000201.

8. Dirk Vissers et al., "The Effect of Exercise on Visceral Adipose Tissue in Overweight Adults: A Systematic Review and Meta-analysis," *PLoS One* 8, no. 2 (2013): e56415, https://doi.org:10.1371/journal.pone.0056415.

9. Yüksel Altuntaş, "Postprandial Reactive Hypoglycemia," *Sisli Etfal Hastanesi tip bulteni* 53, no. 3 (August 28, 2019): 215–20, https://doi.org:10.14744/SEMB.2019.59455.

10. Haishan Huang et al., "Visceral Fat Correlates with Insulin Secretion and Sensitivity Independent of BMI and Subcutaneous Fat in Chinese with Type 2 Diabetes," *Frontiers in Endocrinology* 14 (February 27, 2023): 1144834, https://doi.org:10.3389/fendo.2023.1144834.

11. Habib Yaribeygi et al., "Pathophysiology of Physical Inactivity-Dependent Insulin Resistance: A Theoretical Mechanistic Review Emphasizing Clinical Evidence," *Journal of Diabetes Research* 2021 (October 7, 2021): 7796727, https://doi.org:10.1155/2021/7796727.

12. M. González-Ortiz et al., "Effect of Sleep Deprivation on Insulin Sensitivity and Cortisol Concentration in Healthy Subjects," *Diabetes, Nutrition & Metabolism* 13, no. 2 (2000): 80–83; Habib Yaribeygi et al., "Molecular Mechanisms Linking Stress and Insulin Resistance," *EXCLI Journal* 21 (January 24, 2022): 317–34, https://doi.org:10.17179/excli2021-4382.

13. Christopher D. Gardner et al., "Effect of Low-Fat vs Low-Carbohydrate Diet on 12-Month Weight Loss in Overweight Adults and the Association with Genotype Pattern or Insulin Secretion: The DIETFITS Randomized Clinical Trial," *JAMA* 319, no. 7 (2018): 667–79, https://doi.org:10.1001/jama.2018.0245.

14. S. W. Rizkalla et al., "Health Benefits of Low Glycaemic Index Foods, Such as Pulses, in Diabetic Patients and Healthy Individuals," *British Journal of Nutrition* 88, no. S3 (2002): S255–62, https://doi.org:10.1079/BJN2002715.

15. Sunder Mudaliar, "The Evolution of Diabetes Treatment Through the Ages: From Starvation Diets to Insulin, Incretins, SGLT2-Inhibitors and Beyond," *Journal of the Indian Institute of Science* (February 21, 2023): 1–11, https://doi.org:10.1007/s41745-023-00357-w.

16. Guenther Boden et al., "Effect of a Low-Carbohydrate Diet on Appetite, Blood Glucose Levels, and Insulin Resistance in Obese Patients with Type 2 Diabetes," *Annals of Internal Medicine* 142, no. 6 (2005): 403–11, https://doi.org:10.7326/0003-4819-142-6-200503150-00006.

17. Vienica D. Funtanilla et al., "Continuous Glucose Monitoring: A Review of Available Systems," *P & T: A Peer-Reviewed Journal for Formulary Management* 44, no. 9 (2019): 550–53.

18. Melanie A. Jackson et al., "Type 2 Diabetes and the Use of Real-Time Continuous Glucose Monitoring," *Diabetes Technology & Therapeutics* 23, no. S1 (2021): S27–S34, https://doi.org:10.1089/dia.2021.0007; Nicole Ehrhardt and Enas Al Zaghal, "Behavior Modification in Prediabetes and Diabetes: Potential Use of Real-Time Continuous Glucose Monitoring," *Journal of Diabetes Science and Technology* 13, no. 2 (2019): 271–75, https://doi.org:10.1177/1932296818790994.

19. Ping-Yu Wang et al., "Higher Intake of Fruits, Vegetables or Their Fiber Reduces the Risk of Type 2 Diabetes: A Meta-analysis," *Journal of Diabetes Investigation* 7, no. 1 (2016): 56–69, https://doi.org:10.1111/jdi.12376; Mehran Nouri et al., "The Relationship Between Intake of Fruits, Vegetables and Dairy Products with Overweight and Obesity in a Large Sample in Iran: Findings of STEPS 2016," *Frontiers in Nutrition* 9 (January 17, 2023): 1082976, https://doi.org:10.3389/fnu.2022.1082976.

20. Viral N. Shah et al., "Continuous Glucose Monitoring Profiles in Healthy Nondiabetic Participants: A Multicenter Prospective Study," *Journal of Clinical Endocrinology and Metabolism* 104, no. 10 (2019): 4356–64, https://doi.org:10.1210/jc.2018-02763.

21. Anders Gummesson et al., "Effect of Weight Reduction on Glycated Haemoglobin in Weight Loss Trials in Patients with Type 2 Diabetes," *Diabetes, Obesity and Metabolism* 19, no. 9 (2017): 1295–1305, https://doi.org/10.1111/dom.12971.

22. Mary C. Gannon and Frank Q. Nuttall, "Control of Blood Glucose in Type 2 Diabetes Without Weight Loss by Modification of Diet Composition," *Nutrition & Metabolism* 3, no. 16 (March 23, 2006), https://doi.org:10.1186/1743-7075-3-16.

23. Sheri R. Colberg et al., "Physical Activity/Exercise and Diabetes: A Position Statement of the American Diabetes Association," *Diabetes Care* 39, no. 11 (2016): 2065–79, https://doi.org:10.2337/dc16-1728.

24. Paddy C. Dempsey et al., "Benefits for Type 2 Diabetes of Interrupting Prolonged Sitting with Brief Bouts of Light Walking or Simple Resistance Activities," *Diabetes Care* 39, no. 6 (2016): 964–72, https://doi.org:10.2337/dc15-2336.

25. Francisco B. Ortega et al., "The Intriguing Metabolically Healthy but Obese Phenotype: Cardiovascular Prognosis and Role of Fitness," *European Heart Journal* 34, no. 5 (February 1, 2013): 389–97, https://doi.org/10.1093/eurheartj/ehs174.

26. Mathieu Nollet et al., "Sleep Deprivation and Stress: A Reciprocal Relationship," *Interface Focus* 10, no. 3 (2020): 20190092, https://doi.org/10.1098/rsfs.2019.0092; Ali Darraj, "The Link Between Sleeping and Type 2 Diabetes: A Systematic Review," *Cureus* 15, no. 11 (November 3, 2023): e48228, https://doi.org:10.7759/cureus.48228.

27. Ranjit Tiwari et al., "Effects of Sleep Intervention on Glucose Control: A Narrative Review of Clinical Evidence," *Primary Care Diabetes* 15, no. 4 (2021): 635–41, https://doi.org:10.1016/j.pcd.2021.04.003; Sang Dol Kim, "Effects of Yogic Exercises on Life Stress and Blood Glucose Levels in Nursing Students," *Journal of Physical Therapy Science* 26, no. 12 (2014): 2003–6, https://doi.org:10.1589/jpts.26.2003.

28. R. Hackett and A. Steptoe, "Type 2 Diabetes Mellitus and Psychological Stress—a Modifiable Risk Factor," *National Review of Endocrinology* 13 (2017): 547–60, https://doi.org/10.1038/nrendo.2017.64.

29. Kacper Witek et al., "A High-Sugar Diet Consumption, Metabolism and Health Impacts with a Focus on the Development of Substance Use Disorder: A Narrative Review," *Nutrients* 14, no. 14 (July 18, 2022): 2940, https://doi.org:10.3390/nu14142940.

30. Lu Zhang et al., "Association Between Dietary Sugar Intake and Depression in US Adults: A Cross-sectional Study Using Data from the National Health and Nutrition Examination Survey 2011–2018," *BMC Psychiatry* 24, no. 1 (February 8, 2024): 110, https://doi.org:10.1186/s12888-024-05531-7.

31. Shane Bilsborough and Neil Mann, "A Review of Issues of Dietary Protein Intake in Humans," *International Journal of Sport Nutrition and Exercise Metabolism* 16, no. 2 (2006): 129–52, https://doi.org:10.1123/ijsnem.16.2.129.

32. Jose Antonio et al., "Casein Protein Supplementation in Trained Men and Women: Morning Versus Evening," *International Journal of Exercise Science* 10, no. 3 (May 1, 2017): 479–86, https://doi.org:10.70252/QWHA8703.

33. Berrak Basturk et al., "Evaluation of the Effect of Macronutrients Combination on Blood Sugar Levels in Healthy Individuals," *Iranian Journal of Public Health* 50, no. 2 (2021): 280–87, https://doi.org:10.18502/ijph.v50i2.5340.

34. A. Meloni et al., "GLP-1 Receptor Activated Insulin Secretion from Pancreatic β-Cells: Mechanism and Glucose Dependence," *Diabetes, Obesity & Metabolism* 15, no. 1 (2013): 15–27, https://doi.org:10.1111/j.1463-1326.2012.01663.x; Tohru Hira

et al., "Improvement of Glucose Tolerance by Food Factors Having Glucagon-Like Peptide-1 Releasing Activity," *International Journal of Molecular Sciences* 22, no. 12 (June 21, 2021): 6623, https://doi.org:10.3390/ijms22126623.

35.   B. L. Petersen et al., "A Whey Protein Supplement Decreases Post-prandial Glycemia," *Nutrition Journal* 8, no. 47 (2009), https://doi.org/10.1186/1475-2891-8-47.

36.   Stine Smedegaard et al., "Whey Protein Premeal Lowers Postprandial Glucose Concentrations in Adults Compared with Water—the Effect of Timing, Dose, and Metabolic Status: A Systematic Review and Meta-analysis," *American Journal of Clinical Nutrition* 118, no. 2 (2023): 391–405.

37.   Heather J. Leidy et al., "The Effects of Consuming Frequent, Higher Protein Meals on Appetite and Satiety During Weight Loss in Overweight/Obese Men," *Obesity* (Silver Spring, MD) 19, no. 4 (2011): 818–24, https://doi.org:10.1038/oby.2010.203.

38.   Karla E. Merz and Debbie C Thurmond, "Role of Skeletal Muscle in Insulin Resistance and Glucose Uptake," *Comprehensive Physiology* 10, no. 3 (July 8, 2020): 785–809, https://doi.org:10.1002/cphy.c190029.

39.   Merz and Thurmond, "Role of Skeletal Muscle."

40.   F. J. DiMenna and A. D. Arad, "Exercise as 'Precision Medicine' for Insulin Resistance and Its Progression to Type 2 Diabetes: A Research Review," *BMC Sport Science, Medicine and Rehabilitation* 10, no. 21 (2018), https://doi.org/10.1186/s13102-018-0110-8.

41.   R. Havenaar et al., "Inulin: Fermentation and Microbial Ecology in the Intestinal Tract," *Food Reviews International* 15, no. 1 (1999): 109–20, https://doi.org:10.1080/87559129909541179.

42.   Long Wang et al., "Inulin-Type Fructans Supplementation Improves Glycemic Control for the Prediabetes and Type 2 Diabetes Populations: Results from a GRADE-Assessed Systematic Review and Dose-Response Meta-analysis of 33 Randomized Controlled Trials," *Journal of Translational Medicine* 17, no. 1 (December 5, 2019): 410, https://doi.org:10.1186/s12967-019-02159-0.

43.   Di Zhu et al., "Can Functional Oligosaccharides Reduce the Risk of Diabetes Mellitus?," *FASEB Journal: Official Publication of the Federation of American Societies for Experimental Biology* 33, no. 11 (2019): 11655–67, https://doi.org:10.1096/fj.201802802RRR; Muhammad Akmal et al., "Alpha Glucosidase Inhibitors," last updated February 28, 2024, in *StatPearls* (Treasure Island, FL: StatPearls Publishing, 2025), https://www.ncbi.nlm.nih.gov/books/NBK557848/.

44.   Nélida Pascale et al., "The Potential of Pectins to Modulate the Human Gut Microbiota Evaluated by In Vitro Fermentation: A Systematic Review," *Nutrients* 14, no. 17 (September 2, 2022): 3629, https://doi.org:10.3390/nu14173629; D. J. Jenkins et al., "Unabsorbable Carbohydrates and Diabetes: Decreased Post-prandial Hyperglycaemia," *Lancet* (London) 2, 7978 (1976): 172–24, https://doi.org:10.1016/s0140-6736(76)92346-1.

45.   American Chemical Society, "New Low-Calorie Way to Cook Rice Could Help Cut Rising Obesity Rates," *ScienceDaily*, March 23, 2015, https://www.sciencedaily.com/releases/2015/03/150323075233.htm.

46.   Brian K. Ferguson and Patrick B. Wilson, "Ordered Eating and Its Effects on Various Postprandial Health Markers: A Systematic Review," *Journal of the American Nutrition Association* 42, no. 8 (2023): 746–57, https://doi.org:10.1080/27697061.2022.2161664.

47. Lijuan Sun et al., "Postprandial Glucose, Insulin and Incretin Responses Differ by Test Meal Macronutrient Ingestion Sequence (PATTERN Study)," *Clinical Nutrition* (Edinburgh) 39, no. 3 (2020): 950–57, https://doi.org:10.1016/j .clnu.2019.04.001; Alpana P. Shukla et al., "Food Order Has a Significant Impact on Postprandial Glucose and Insulin Levels," *Diabetes Care* 38, no. 7 (2015): e98– e99, https://doi.org:10.2337/dc15-0429; Sodai Kubota et al., "A Review of Recent Findings on Meal Sequence: An Attractive Dietary Approach to Prevention and Management of Type 2 Diabetes," *Nutrients* 12, no. 9 (August 19, 2020): 2502, https://doi.org:10.3390/nu12092502.

48. Eleanor Noss Whitney and Linda Kelly DeBruyne, *An Introduction to Nutrition*, LibreTexts, last modified October 18, 2023, https://med.libretexts.org/Bookshelves /Nutrition/An_Introduction_to_Nutrition_(Zimmerman)/05%3A_Lipids/5.04 %3A_Digestion_and_Absorption_of_Lipids.

49. Daniel K. Jass, "721-P: Fat Added to High-Glycemic-Index Foods Reduces Both Glycemic and Insulinemic Response to Moderate-Size Meals," *Diabetes* 69, no. S1 (June 1, 2020): 721-P, https://doi.org/10.2337/db20-721-P.

50. Chiara Garonzi et al., "Impact of Fat Intake on Blood Glucose Control and Cardiovascular Risk Factors in Children and Adolescents with Type 1 Diabetes," *Nutrients* 13, no. 8 (July 29, 2021): 2625, https://doi.org:10.3390/nu13082625.

51. One study followed 3,300 adults for over 4½ years and found that those who consumed higher amounts of saturated fats and animal fats were twice as likely to develop type 2 diabetes than those who consumed a lower amount; https://www .sciencedirect.com/science/article/pii/S0002916522048080?via%3Dihub.

52. One small study found that when men drank water with palm oil containing as much saturated fat as a cheeseburger and fries, they experienced a reduction in insulin sensitivity, an increase in fatty deposits in the liver, and changes in glucose metabolism similar to what's seen in type 2 diabetes; https://pubmed.ncbi.nlm.nih .gov/28112681/.

53. Esther Winters–van Eekelen et al., "Effects of Dietary Macronutrients on Liver Fat Content in Adults: A Systematic Review and Meta-analysis of Randomized Controlled Trials," *European Journal of Clinical Nutrition* 75, no. 4 (2021): 588–601, https://doi.org:10.1038/s41430-020-00778-1.

54. X. Chen et al., "High Dietary Intake of Unsaturated Fatty Acids Is Associated with Improved Insulin Resistance—a Cross-sectional Study Based on the NHANES Database," *Lipids in Health and Disease* 22, no. 216 (2023), https://doi.org/10.1186 /s12944-023-01982-1.

55. Meghana D. Gadgil et al., "The Effects of Carbohydrate, Unsaturated Fat, and Protein Intake on Measures of Insulin Sensitivity: Results from the OmniHeart Trial," *Diabetes Care* 36, no. 5 (May 2013): 1132–37, https://doi.org/10.2337 /dc12-0869.

56. Abhimanyu Garg, "High-Monounsaturated-Fat Diets for Patients with Diabetes Mellitus: A Meta-analysis," *American Journal of Clinical Nutrition* 67, no. 3 (1998): 577S–82S, https://doi.org/10.1093/ajcn/67.3.577S; Susmita Sinha et al., "The Effect of Omega-3 Fatty Acids on Insulin Resistance," *Life* 13, no. 6 (2023): 1322, https:// doi.org/10.3390/life13061322.

57. Jiyoung S. Kim et al., "Effect of Nutrient Composition in a Mixed Meal on the Postprandial Glycemic Response in Healthy People: A Preliminary Study,"

*Nutrition Research and Practice* 13, no. 2 (2019): 126–33, https://doi.org:10.4162/nrp.2019.13.2.126.

58. Lijuan Sun et al., "Effect of Chicken, Fat and Vegetable on Glycaemia and Insulinaemia to a White Rice–Based Meal in Healthy Adults," *European Journal of Nutrition* 53, no. 8 (2014): 1719–26, https://doi.org:10.1007/s00394-014-0678-z.

**Chapter 4: Effortless Nutrition for Vitality and Immunity**

1. Carol Boushey et al., *Dietary Patterns and All-Cause Mortality: A Systematic Review* (Alexandria, VA: USDA Nutrition Evidence Systematic Review, 2020), https://www.ncbi.nlm.nih.gov/books/NBK578477/, https://doi.org/10.52570/NESR.DGAC2020.SR0108.

2. K. Miyamoto et al., "Dietary Diversity and Healthy Life Expectancy—an International Comparative Study," *European Journal of Clinical Nutrition* 73 (2019): 395–400, https://doi.org/10.1038/s41430-018-0270-3.

3. Sun Ce et al., "Quantity and Variety in Fruit and Vegetable Consumption and Mortality in Older Chinese: A 15-Year Follow-Up of a Prospective Cohort Study," *Journal of Nutrition* 153, no. 7 (2023): 2061–72.

4. Karin B. Michels and Alicja Wolk, "A Prospective Study of Variety of Healthy Foods and Mortality in Women," *International Journal of Epidemiology* 31, no. 4 (2002): 847–54, https://doi.org:10.1093/ije/31.4.847.

5. Laura L. Wilkinson and Jeffrey M. Brunstrom, "Sensory Specific Satiety: More Than 'Just' Habituation?," *Appetite* 103 (2016): 221–28, https://doi.org:10.1016/j.appet.2016.04.019.

6. Roseane B. de Miranda et al., "Effects of Hydrolyzed Collagen Supplementation on Skin Aging: A Systematic Review and Meta-analysis," *International Journal of Dermatology* 60, no. 12 (2021): 1449–61, https://doi.org:10.1111/ijd.15518.

7. Luana Dias Campos et al., "Collagen Supplementation in Skin and Orthopedic Diseases: A Review of the Literature," *Heliyon* 9, no. 4 (2023): e14961, https://doi.org/10.1016/j.heliyon.2023.e14961; Daniel Martínez-Puig et al., "Collagen Supplementation for Joint Health: The Link Between Composition and Scientific Knowledge," *Nutrients* 15, no. 6 (March 8, 2023): 1332, https://doi.org:10.3390/nu15061332.

8. Alexander K. C. Leung et al., "Iron Deficiency Anemia: An Updated Review," *Current Pediatric Reviews* 20, no. 3 (2024): 339–56, https://doi.org:10.2174/1573396320666230727102042.

9. Amira Kassis et al., "Nutritional and Lifestyle Management of the Aging Journey: A Narrative Review," *Frontiers in Nutrition* 9, no. 1087505 (2023), https://doi.org:10.3389/fnut.2022.1087505; Gianluca Rizzo et al., "Vitamin B$_{12}$ Among Vegetarians: Status, Assessment and Supplementation," *Nutrients* 8, no. 12 (2016): 767, https://doi.org:10.3390/nu8120767.

10. Vikas Menon et al., "Vitamin D and Depression: A Critical Appraisal of the Evidence and Future Directions," *Indian Journal of Psychological Medicine* 42, 1 (2020): 11–21, https://doi.org:10.4103/IJPSYM.IJPSYM_160_19; F. J. Amaro-Gahete et al., "Low Vitamin D Levels Are Linked with Increased Cardiovascular Disease Risk in Young Adults: A Sub-study and Secondary Analyses from the ACTIBATE Randomized Controlled Trial," *Journal of Endocrinological Investigation* 47, no. 7 (2024): 1645–56, https://doi.org:10.1007/s40618-023-02272-4; Maheen Siddiqui

et al., "Immune Modulatory Effects of Vitamin D on Viral Infections," *Nutrients* 12, no. 9 (2020): 2879, https://doi.org:10.3390/nu12092879; Gerbenn Seraphin et al., "The Impact of Vitamin D on Cancer: A Mini Review," *Journal of Steroid Biochemistry and Molecular Biology* 231 (2023): 106308, https://doi.org:10.1016/j.jsbmb.2023.106308; Josephine Yu et al., "Vitamin D and Beta Cells in Type 1 Diabetes: A Systematic Review," *International Journal of Molecular Sciences* 23, no. 22 (2022): 14434, https://doi.org:10.3390/ijms232214434; Julia Feige et al., "Vitamin D Supplementation in Multiple Sclerosis: A Critical Analysis of Potentials and Threats," *Nutrients* 12, no. 3 (2020): 783, https://doi.org:10.3390/nu12030783; Behzad Heidari et al., "Vitamin D Deficiency and Rheumatoid Arthritis: Epidemiological, Immunological, Clinical and Therapeutic Aspects," *Mediterranean Journal of Rheumatology* 30, no. 2 (2019): 94–102, https://doi.org:10.31138/mjr.30.2.94; Jae H. Kang et al., "Effect of Vitamin D on Cognitive Decline: Results from Two Ancillary Studies of the VITAL Randomized Trial," *Scientific Reports* 11, no. 1 (2021): 23253, https://doi.org:10 /541598-021-02485-8.

11.  Gianluca Rizzo et al., "Vitamin $B_{12}$ Among Vegetarians: Status, Assessment and Supplementation," *Nutrients* 8, no. 12 (2016): 767, https://doi.org:10.3390/nu8120767.

12.  Sina Naghshi et al., "Dietary Intake of Total, Animal, and Plant Proteins and Risk of All Cause, Cardiovascular, and Cancer Mortality: Systematic Review and Dose-Response Meta-analysis of Prospective Cohort Studies," *BMJ (Clinical Research Edition)* 370 (2020): m2412, https://doi.org:10.1136/bmj.m2412.

13.  Jiaqi Huang et al., "Association Between Plant and Animal Protein Intake and Overall and Cause-Specific Mortality," *JAMA Internal Medicine* 180, no. 9 (2020): 1173–84, https://doi.org:10.1001/jamainternmed.2020.2790.

14.  Henry J. Thompson, "The Dietary Guidelines for Americans (2020–2025): Pulses, Dietary Fiber, and Chronic Disease Risk—a Call for Clarity and Action," *Nutrients* 13, no. 11 (2021): 4034, https://doi.org:10.3390/nu13114034.

15.  Abed Ghavami et al., "Soluble Fiber Supplementation and Serum Lipid Profile: A Systematic Review and Dose-Response Meta-analysis of Randomized Controlled Trials," *Advances in Nutrition* (Bethesda, MD) 14, no. 3 (2023): 465–74, https://doi.org:10.1016/j.advnut.2023.01.005.

16.  Dagfinn Aune et al., "Dietary Fibre, Whole Grains, and Risk of Colorectal Cancer: Systematic Review and Dose-Response Meta-analysis of Prospective Studies," *BMJ (Clinical research ed.)* 343 (2011): d6617, https://doi.org:10.1136/bmj.d6617.

17.  Ruo-Gu Xiong et al., "Health Benefits and Side Effects of Short-Chain Fatty Acids," *Foods* (Basel) 11, no. 18 (2022): 2863, https://doi.org:10.3390/foods11182863; María Daniella Carretta et al., "Participation of Short-Chain Fatty Acids and Their Receptors in Gut Inflammation and Colon Cancer," *Frontiers in Physiology*, no. 12 (2021): 662739, https://doi.org:10.3389/fphys.2021.662739.

18.  Jiongxing Fu et al., "Dietary Fiber Intake and Gut Microbiota in Human Health," *Microorganisms* 10, no. 12 (2022): 507, https://doi.org:10.3390/microorganisms 10122507.

19.  Dagfinn Aune et al., "Fruit and Vegetable Intake and the Risk of Cardiovascular Disease, Total Cancer and All-Cause Mortality: A Systematic Review and Dose-Response Meta-analysis of Prospective Studies," *International Journal of Epidemiology* 46, no. 3 (2017): 1029–56, https://doi.org:10.1093/ije/dyw319;

Dong D. Wang et al., "Fruit and Vegetable Intake and Mortality: Results from 2 Prospective Cohort Studies of US Men and Women and a Meta-analysis of 26 Cohort Studies," *Circulation* 143, no. 17 (2021): 1642–54, https://doi.org:10.1161 /CIRCULATIONAHA.120.048996.

20. Sabina Janciauskiene, "The Beneficial Effects of Antioxidants in Health and Diseases," *Chronic Obstructive Pulmonary Diseases* (Miami) 7, no. 3 (2020): 182–202, https://doi.org:10.15326/jcopdf.7.3.2019.0152.

21. Melanie Ziegler et al., "Cardiovascular and Metabolic Protection by Vitamin E: A Matter of Treatment Strategy?," *Antioxidants* (Basel) 9, no. 10 (2020): 935, https:// doi.org:10.3390/antiox9100935; Genea Edwards et al., "Molecular Mechanisms Underlying the Therapeutic Role of Vitamin E in Age-Related Macular Degeneration," *Frontiers in Neuroscience* 16 (2022): 890021, https://doi.org:10.3389 /fnins.2022.890021; O. Asbaghi et al., "The Effect of Vitamin E Supplementation on Selected Inflammatory Biomarkers in Adults: A Systematic Review and Meta-analysis of Randomized Clinical Trials," *Scientific Reports* 10 (2020): 17234, https://doi.org/10.1038/s41598-020-73741-6.

22. Nikolina Vrdoljak, "Carotenoids and Carcinogenesis: Exploring the Antioxidant and Cell Signaling Roles of Carotenoids in the Prevention of Cancer," *Critical Reviews in Oncogenesis* 27, no. 3 (2022): 1–13, https://doi.org:10.1615/CritRevOncog.20220 45331.

23. Shan-Shan Li et al., "Efficacy of Different Nutrients in Age-Related Macular Degeneration: A Systematic Review and Network Meta-analysis," *Seminars in Ophthalmology* 37, no. 4 (2022): 515–23, https://doi.org:10.1080/08820538.2021 .2022165.

24. Wolfgang Köpcke and Jean Krutmann, "Protection from Sunburn with Beta-carotene—a Meta-analysis," *Photochemistry and Photobiology* 84, no. 2 (2008): 284–88, https://doi.org:10.1111/j.1751-1097.2007.00253.x.

25. Xinrui Yi et al., "Flavonoids Improve Type 2 Diabetes Mellitus and Its Complications: A Review," *Frontiers in Nutrition* 10 (2023): 1192131, https://doi.org:10 .3389/fnut.2023.1192131.

26. Nancy R. Cook et al., "Joint Effects of Sodium and Potassium Intake on Subsequent Cardiovascular Disease: The Trials of Hypertension Prevention Follow-Up Study," *Archives of Internal Medicine* 169, no. 1 (2009): 32–40, https://doi.org:10.1001 /archinternmed.2008.523.

27. Rick L. Sharp, "Role of Whole Foods in Promoting Hydration After Exercise in Humans," *Journal of the American College of Nutrition* 26, no. S5 (2007): 592S–96S, https://doi.org:10.1080/07315724.2007.10719664.

28. Z. S. NattoYaghmoor et al., "Omega-3 Fatty Acids Effects on Inflammatory Biomarkers and Lipid Profiles Among Diabetic and Cardiovascular Disease Patients: A Systematic Review and Meta-analysis," *Scientific Reports* 9 (2019): 18867, https:// doi.org/10.1038/s41598-019-54535-x.

29. H. Gerster, "Can Adults Adequately Convert Alpha-Linolenic Acid (18:3n-3) to Eicosapentaenoic Acid (20:5n-3) and Docosahexaenoic Acid (22:6n-3)?," *International Journal for Vitamin and Nutrition Research* 68, no. 3 (1998): 159–73.

30. Ann C. Skulas-Ray et al., "Omega-3 Fatty Acids for the Management of Hypertriglyceridemia: A Science Advisory from the American Heart Association," *Circulation* 140, no. 12 (2019): e673–e691, https://doi.org:10.1161/CIR.0000000000000709;

Stefania Lamon-Fava et al., "Clinical Response to EPA Supplementation in Patients with Major Depressive Disorder Is Associated with Higher Plasma Concentrations of Pro-resolving Lipid Mediators," *Neuropsychopharmacology: Official Publication of the American College of Neuropsychopharmacology* 48, no. 6 (2023): 929–35, https://doi.org:10.1038/s41386-022-01527-7.

31. "Omega-3 Fatty Acids," National Institutes of Health, Office of Dietary Supplements, accessed June 17, 2025, https://ods.od.nih.gov/factsheets/Omega3FattyAcids-HealthProfessional/.

32. Esther Granot et al., "DHA Supplementation During Pregnancy and Lactation Affects Infants' Cellular but Not Humoral Immune Response," *Mediators of Inflammation* 2011 (2011): Article ID 493925, https://doi.org/10.1155/2011/493925; Emily K. K. Tai et al., "An Update on Adding Docosahexaenoic Acid (DHA) and Arachidonic Acid (AA) to Baby Formula," *Food & Function* 4, no. 12 (2013): 1767–75, https://doi.org:10.1039/c3fo60298b.

33. Cristina Augood et al., "Oily Fish Consumption, Dietary Docosahexaenoic Acid and Eicosapentaenoic Acid Intakes, and Associations with Neovascular Age-Related Macular Degeneration," *American Journal of Clinical Nutrition* 88, no. 2 (2008): 398–406, https://doi.org:10.1093/ajcn/88.2.398.

34. Ann C. Skulas-Ray et al., "Omega-3 Fatty Acids for the Management of Hypertriglyceridemia: A Science Advisory from the American Heart Association," *Circulation* 140, no. 12 (2019): e673–e691, https://doi.org:10.1161/CIR.0000000000000709.

35. "Omega-3 Fatty Acids," National Institutes of Health, Office of Dietary Supplements, accessed June 17, 2025, https://ods.od.nih.gov/factsheets/Omega3FattyAcids-HealthProfessional/.

36. Linda M. Arterburn et al., "Algal-Oil Capsules and Cooked Salmon: Nutritionally Equivalent Sources of Docosahexaenoic Acid," *Journal of the American Dietetic Association* 108, no. 7 (2008): 1204–09, https://doi.org:10.1016/j.jada.2008.04.020.

37. "EPA & DHA Intake Recommendations," Global Organization for EPA and DHA Omega-3s [GOED], 2017, https://goedomega3.com/storage/app/media/GOED%20Intake%20Recommendations.pdf; "Omega-3 Fatty Acids: Fact Sheet for Consumers," National Institutes of Health, Office of Dietary Supplements, 2024, https://ods.od.nih.gov/pdf/factsheets/Omega3FattyAcids-Consumer.pdf.

38. Brian S. Rett and Jay Whelan, "Increasing Dietary Linoleic Acid Does Not Increase Tissue Arachidonic Acid Content in Adults Consuming Western-Type Diets: A Systematic Review," *Nutrition & Metabolism* 8, no. 36 (2011), https://doi.org:10.1186/1743-7075-8-36.

39. Hang Su et al., "Dietary Linoleic Acid Intake and Blood Inflammatory Markers: A Systematic Review and Meta-analysis of Randomized Controlled Trials," *Food & Function* 8, no. 9 (2017): 3091–103, https://doi.org:10.1039/c7fo00433h; Guy H. Johnson et al, "Effect of Dietary Linoleic Acid on Markers of Inflammation in Healthy Persons: A Systematic Review of Randomized Controlled Trials," *Journal of the Academy of Nutrition and Dietetics* 112, no. 7 (2012): 1029–41, https://doi.org:10.1080/09637486.2018.1504009.

40. Maryam S. Farvid et al., "Dietary Linoleic Acid and Risk of Coronary Heart Disease: A Systematic Review and Meta-analysis of Prospective Cohort Studies," *Circulation* 130, no. 18 (2014): 1568–78, https://doi.org:10.1161/CIRCULATIONAHA.114.010236.

41. William S. Harris, "The Omega-6:Omega-3 Ratio: A Critical Appraisal and Possible Successor, *Prostaglandins, Leukotrienes, and Essential Fatty Acids* 132 (2018): 34–40, https://doi.org:10.1016/j.plefa.2018.03.003.

42. Lukas Schwingshackl and Georg Hoffmann, "Monounsaturated Fatty Acids, Olive Oil and Health Status: A Systematic Review and Meta-analysis of Cohort Studies," *Lipids in Health and Disease* 13, no. 154 (2014), https://doi.org:10 .1186/1476-511X-13-154.

43. L. S. Piers et al., "Substitution of Saturated with Monounsaturated Fat in a 4-Week Diet Affects Body Weight and Composition of Overweight and Obese Men," *British Journal of Nutrition* 90, no. 3 (2003): 717–27, https://doi.org:10.1079/bjn2003948.

44. Lijuan Sun et al., "Differential Effects of Monounsaturated and Polyunsaturated Fats on Satiety and Gut Hormone Responses in Healthy Subjects," *Foods* (Basel) 8, no. 12 (2019): 634, https://doi.org:10.3390/foods8120634; Theresia Sarabhai et al., "Monounsaturated Fat Rapidly Induces Hepatic Gluconeogenesis and Whole-Body Insulin Resistance," *JCI Insight* 5, no. 10 (2020): e134520, https://doi .org:10.1172/jci.insight.134520; Shatha S. Hammad et al., "Common Variants in Lipid Metabolism-Related Genes Associate with Fat Mass Changes in Response to Dietary Monounsaturated Fatty Acids in Adults with Abdominal Obesity," *Journal of Nutrition* 149, no. 10 (2019): 1749–56, https://doi.org:10.1093/jn/nxz136.

45. Martha Clare Morris and Christine C. Tangney, "Dietary Fat Composition and Dementia Risk," *Neurobiology of Aging* 35, no. S2 (2014): S59–S64, https://do i.org:10.1016/j.neurobiolaging.2014.03.038.

## Chapter 5: Healing Your Relationship with Food

1. Jake Linardon et al., "Intuitive Eating and Its Psychological Correlates: A Meta-analysis," *International Journal of Eating Disorders* 54, no. 7 (2021): 1073–98, https://doi.org:10.1002/eat.23509.

2. "10 Principles of Intuitive Eating," Intuitive Eating, accessed June 18, 2025, https:// www.intuitiveeating.org/about-us/10-principles-of-intuitive-eating/.

3. Linardon et al., "Intuitive Eating and Its Psychological Correlates."

4. Janet M. Warren et al., "A Structured Literature Review on the Role of Mindfulness, Mindful Eating and Intuitive Eating in Changing Eating Behaviours: Effectiveness and Associated Potential Mechanisms," *Nutrition Research Reviews* 30, no. 2 (2017): 272–83, https://doi.org/10.1017/S0954422417000154; K. Leahy et al., "The Relationship Between Intuitive Eating and Postpartum Weight Loss," *Maternal and Child Health Journal* 21, no. 8 (2017): 1591–97, https://doi.org/10.1007/s10995-017-2281-4.

## Chapter 6: Not Another Diet: HCC for Weight-Loss Goals

1. Shilpa Joshi and Viswanathan Mohan, "Pros & Cons of Some Popular Extreme Weight-Loss Diets," *Indian Journal of Medical Research* 148, no. 5 (2018): 642–47, https://doi.org:10.4103/ijmr.IJMR_1793_18.

2. Ling Chen et al., "The Effects of Weight Loss–Related Amenorrhea on Women's Health and the Therapeutic Approaches: A Narrative Review," *Annals of Translational Medicine* 11, no. 2 (2023): 132, https://doi.org:10.21037/atm-22-6366.

3. Jenna C. Gibbs et al., "Low Bone Density Risk Is Higher in Exercising Women with Multiple Triad Risk Factors," *Medicine and Science in Sports and Exercise* 46, no. 1 (2014): 167–76, https://doi.org:10.1249/MSS.0b013e3182a03b8b.

4.  E. C. Lloyd et al., "How Extreme Dieting Becomes Compulsive: A Novel Hypothesis for the Role of Anxiety in the Development and Maintenance of Anorexia Nervosa," *Medical Hypotheses* 108 (2017): 144–50, https://doi.org:10.1016/j.mehy.2017.09.001.

5.  Erin Fothergill et al., "Persistent Metabolic Adaptation 6 Years After 'The Biggest Loser' Competition," *Obesity* (Silver Spring, MD) 24, no. 8 (2016): 1612–19, https://doi.org:10.1002/oby.21538.

6.  W. H. M. Saris, "Very-Low-Calorie Diets and Sustained Weight Loss," *Obesity Research* 9, S11 (2001): 295S–301S, https://doi.org/10.1038/oby.2001.134.

7.  David B. Sarwer et al., "Behavior Therapy for Obesity: Where Are We Now?," *Current Opinion in Endocrinology, Diabetes, and Obesity* 16, no. 5 (2009): 347–52, https://doi:10.1097/MED.0b013e32832f5a79.

8.  Eun-Jung Rhee, "Weight Cycling and Its Cardiometabolic Impact," *Journal of Obesity & Metabolic Syndrome* 26, no. 4 (2017): 237–42, https://doi.org:10.7570/jomes.2017.26.4.237.

9.  Jamy Ard et al., "Weight Loss and Maintenance Related to the Mechanism of Action of Glucagon-Like Peptide 1 Receptor Agonists," *Advances in Therapy* 38, no. 6 (2021): 2821–39, https://doi.org:10.1007/s12325-021-01710-0.

10. Michael E. J. Lean et al., "5-Year Follow-Up of the Randomised Diabetes Remission Clinical Trial (DiRECT) of Continued Support for Weight Loss Maintenance in the UK: An Extension Study," *Lancet Diabetes & Endocrinology* 12, no. 4 (2024): 233–46.

11. Shijie Yang et al., "Effect of Weight Loss on Blood Pressure Changes in Overweight Patients: A Systematic Review and Meta-analysis," *Journal of Clinical Hypertension* (Greenwich, CT) 25, no. 5 (2023): 404–15, https://doi.org:10.1111/jch.14661.

12. Konstantinos I. Avgerinos et al., "Obesity and Cancer Risk: Emerging Biological Mechanisms and Perspectives," *Metabolism: Clinical and Experimental* 92 (2019): 121–35, https://doi.org:10.1016/j.metabol.2018.11.001; Rosemarie E. Schmandt et al., "Understanding Obesity and Endometrial Cancer Risk: Opportunities for Prevention," *American Journal of Obstetrics and Gynecology* 205, no. 6 (2011): 518–25, https://doi.org:10.1016/j.ajog.2011.05.042.

13. Yuan Z. Lim et al., "Recommendations for Weight Management in Osteoarthritis: A Systematic Review of Clinical Practice Guidelines," *Osteoarthritis and Cartilage Open* 4, no. 4 (August 5, 2022): 100298, https://doi.org:10.1016/j.ocarto.2022.100298.

14. Anne E. Dixon and Ubong Peters, "The Effect of Obesity on Lung Function," *Expert Review of Respiratory Medicine* 12, no. 9 (2018): 755–67, https://doi.org:10.1080/17476348.2018.1506331.

15. Sara Emerenziani et al., "Role of Overweight and Obesity in Gastrointestinal Disease," *Nutrients* 12 (December 31, 2019): 111, https://doi.org:10.3390/nu12010111; Dimitrios A. Koutoukidis et al., "The Association of Weight-Loss with Changes in the Gut Microbiota Diversity, Composition, and Intestinal Permeability: A Systematic Review and Meta-analysis," *Gut Microbes* 14, no. 1 (2022): 2020068, https://doi.org:10.1080/19490976.2021.2020068.

16. Fátima Pérez de Heredia et al., "Obesity, Inflammation and the Immune System," *Proceedings of the Nutrition Society* 71, no. 2 (2012): 332–38, https://doi.org:10.1017/S0029665112000092.

17. Evangelia Papatriantafyllou et al., "Sleep Deprivation: Effects on Weight Loss and Weight Loss Maintenance," *Nutrients* 14, no. 8 (April 8, 2022): 1549, https://doi.org:10.3390/nu14081549.

18. N. Lasikiewicz et al., "Psychological Benefits of Weight Loss Following Behavioural and/or Dietary Weight Loss Interventions: A Systematic Research Review," *Appetite* 72 (2014): 123–37, https://doi.org:10.1016/j.appet.2013.09.017.

19. Luigi Fontana and Frank B. Hu, "Optimal Body Weight for Health and Longevity: Bridging Basic, Clinical, and Population Research," *Aging Cell* 13, no. 3 (2014): 391–400, https://doi.org:10.1111/acel.12207; J. Stephenson et al., "The Association Between Obesity and Quality of Life: A Retrospective Analysis of a Large-Scale Population-Based Cohort Study," *BMC Public Health* 21, no. 1 (November 3, 2021): 1990, https://doi.org:10.1186/s12889-021-12009-8.

20. I. Ismail et al., "A Systematic Review and Meta-analysis of the Effect of Aerobic vs Resistance Exercise Training on Visceral Fat," *Obesity Reviews: An Official Journal of the International Association for the Study of Obesity* 13, no. 1 (2012): 68–91, https://doi.org:10.1111/j.1467-789X.2011.00931.x.

21. Pedro J. Benito et al., "A Systematic Review with Meta-analysis of the Effect of Resistance Training on Whole-Body Muscle Growth in Healthy Adult Males," *International Journal of Environmental Research and Public Health* 17, no. 4 (February 17, 2020): 1285, https://doi.org:10.3390/ijerph17041285.

22. Hui-Jing Bai et al., "Age-Related Decline in Skeletal Muscle Mass and Function Among Elderly Men and Women in Shanghai, China: A Cross Sectional Study," *Asia Pacific Journal of Clinical Nutrition* 25, no. 2 (2016): 326–32, https://doi.org:10.6133/apjcn.2016.25.2.14.

23. D. J. Wilkinson et al., "The Age-Related Loss of Skeletal Muscle Mass and Function: Measurement and Physiology of Muscle Fibre Atrophy and Muscle Fibre Loss in Humans," *Ageing Research Reviews* 47 (2018): 123–32, https://doi.org:10.1016/j.arr.2018.07.005.

24. J. J. Cunningham, "Body Composition as a Determinant of Energy Expenditure: A Synthetic Review and a Proposed General Prediction Equation," *American Journal of Clinical Nutrition* 54, no. 6 (1991): 963–69, https://doi.org:10.1093/ajcn/54.6.963.

25. Karla E. Merz and Debbie C. Thurmond, "Role of Skeletal Muscle in Insulin Resistance and Glucose Uptake," *Comprehensive Physiology* 10, no. 3 (July 8, 2020): 785–809, https://doi.org:10.1002/cphy.c190029.

26. Louisa Gnatiuc Friedrichs et al., "Body Composition and Risk of Vascular-Metabolic Mortality Risk in 113,000 Mexican Men and Women Without Prior Chronic Disease," *Journal of the American Heart Association* 12, no. 3 (2023): e028263, https://doi.org:10.1161/JAHA.122.028263.

27. Nazli Namazi et al., "The Effects of Supplementation with Conjugated Linoleic Acid on Anthropometric Indices and Body Composition in Overweight and Obese Subjects: A Systematic Review and Meta-analysis," *Critical Reviews in Food Science and Nutrition* 59, no. 17 (2019): 2720–33, https://doi.org:10.1080/10408398.2018.1466107; Lin-Huang Huang et al., "Effects of Green Tea Extract on Overweight and Obese Women with High Levels of Low Density-Lipoprotein-Cholesterol (LDL-C): A Randomised, Double-Blind, and Cross-over Placebo-Controlled Clinical Trial," *BMC Complementary and Alternative Medicine* 18, no. 1 (November 6, 2018): 294, https://doi.org:10.1186/s12906-018-2355-x.

28. Edda Cava et al., "Preserving Healthy Muscle During Weight Loss," *Advances in Nutrition* (Bethesda, MD) 8, no. 3 (May 15, 2017): 511–19, https://doi.org:10.3945/an.116.014506.

29. Rebecca T. McLay-Cooke et al., "Prediction Equations Overestimate the Energy Requirements More for Obesity-Susceptible Individuals," *Nutrients* 9, no. 9 (September 13, 2017): 1012, https://doi.org:10.3390/nu9091012.

30. Nana Chung et al., "Non-Exercise Activity Thermogenesis (NEAT): A Component of Total Daily Energy Expenditure," *Journal of Exercise Nutrition & Biochemistry* 22, no. 2 (2018): 23–30, https://doi.org:10.20463/jenb.2018.0013.

31. "Clinical Guidelines on the Identification, Evaluation, and Treatment of Overweight and Obesity in Adults—the Evidence Report," National Institutes of Health, *Obesity Research* 6, no. S2 (1998): 51S–209S.

32. Cava et al., "Preserving Healthy Muscle During Weight Loss."

33. Robert R. Wolfe et al., "Optimizing Protein Intake in Adults: Interpretation and Application of the Recommended Dietary Allowance Compared with the Acceptable Macronutrient Distribution Range," *Advances in Nutrition* (Bethesda, MD) 8, no. 2 (March 15, 2017): 266–75, https://doi.org:10.3945/an.116.013821.

34. Thomas P. Wycherley et al., "Effects of Energy-Restricted High-Protein, Low-Fat Compared with Standard-Protein, Low-Fat Diets: A Meta-analysis of Randomized Controlled Trials," *American Journal of Clinical Nutrition* 96, no. 6 (2012): 1281–98, https://doi.org:10.3945/ajcn.112.044321; P. M. Clifton et al., "Long Term Weight Maintenance After Advice to Consume Low Carbohydrate, Higher Protein Diets—a Systematic Review and Meta-analysis," *Nutrition, Metabolism, and Cardiovascular Diseases: NMCD* 3 (2014): 224–35, https://doi.org:10.1016/j.numecd.2013.11.006.

35. David S. Weigle et al., "A High-Protein Diet Induces Sustained Reductions in Appetite, Ad Libitum Caloric Intake, and Body Weight Despite Compensatory Changes in Diurnal Plasma Leptin and Ghrelin Concentrations," *American Journal of Clinical Nutrition* 82, no. 1 (2005): 41–48, https://doi.org:10.1093/ajcn.82.1.41.

36. Stuart M. Phillips and Luc J. C. Van Loon, "Dietary Protein for Athletes: From Requirements to Optimum Adaptation," *Journal of Sports Sciences* 29, no. S1 (2011): S29–S38, https://doi.org:10.1080/02640414.2011.619204.

37. Derek C. Miketinas et al., "Fiber Intake Predicts Weight Loss and Dietary Adherence in Adults Consuming Calorie-Restricted Diets: The POUNDS Lost (Preventing Overweight Using Novel Dietary Strategies) Study," *Journal of Nutrition* 149, no. 10 (2019): 1742–48, https://doi.org:10.1093/jn/nxz117.

38. Ghada A. Soliman, "Dietary Fiber, Atherosclerosis, and Cardiovascular Disease," *Nutrients* 11, no. 5 (May 23, 2019): 1155, https://doi.org:10.3390/nu11051155.

39. Diane Quagliani and Patricia Felt-Gunderson, "Closing America's Fiber Intake Gap: Communication Strategies from a Food and Fiber Summit," *American Journal of Lifestyle Medicine* 11, no. 1 (July 7, 2016): 80–85, https://doi.org:10.1177/1559827615588079.

40. Tonya F. Turner et al., "Dietary Adherence and Satisfaction with a Bean-Based High-Fiber Weight Loss Diet: A Pilot Study," *ISRN Obesity* 2013 (October 29, 2013): 915415, https://doi.org:10.1155/2013/915415.

41. John Blundell et al., "Effects of Once-Weekly Semaglutide on Appetite, Energy Intake, Control of Eating, Food Preference and Body Weight in Subjects with Obesity," *Diabetes, Obesity & Metabolism* 19, no. 9 (2017): 1242–51, https://doi.org:10.1111/dom.12932.

42. Elissa Driggin and Parag Goya, "Malnutrition and Sarcopenia as Reasons for Caution with GLP-1 Receptor Agonist Use in HFpEF," *Journal of Cardiac Failure* 30, no. 4 (2024): 610–12, https://doi.org:10.1016/j.cardfail.2024.01.005.

43. Roberto Roklicer et al., "The Effects of Rapid Weight Loss on Skeletal Muscle in Judo Athletes," *Journal of Translational Medicine* 18, no. 1 (March 30, 2020): 142, https://doi.org:10.1186/s12967-020-02315-x.

44. John P. H. Wilding et al., "Once-Weekly Semaglutide in Adults with Overweight or Obesity," *New England Journal of Medicine* 384, no. 11 (2021): 989–1002, https://doi.org:10.1056/NEJMoa2032183.

45. Angelo Tremblay et al., "Impact of Yogurt on Appetite Control, Energy Balance, and Body Composition," *Nutrition Reviews* 73, no. S1 (2015): 23–27, https://doi.org: 10.1093/nutrit/nuv015.

46. Haitao Jiang et al., "The Anti-obesogenic Effects of Dietary Berry Fruits: A Review," *Food Research International* (Ottawa), no. 147 (2021): 110539, https://doi.org:10.1016 /j.foodres.2021.110539.

47. Mehdi Karimi et al., "Effects of Chia Seed (*Salvia hispanica L.*) Supplementation on Cardiometabolic Health in Overweight Subjects: A Systematic Review and Meta-analysis of RCTs," *Nutrition & Metabolism* 21, no. 1 (September 16, 2024): 74, https://doi.org:10.1186/s12986-024-00847-3.

48. Sako Mizutani et al., "Vitamin D Activates Various Gene Expressions, Including Lipid Metabolism, in C2C12 Cells," *Journal of Nutritional Science and Vitaminology* 68, no. 1 (2022): 65–72, https://doi.org:10.3177/jnsv.68.65; Xingxing Lei et al., "Serum and Supplemental Vitamin D Levels and Insulin Resistance in T2DM Populations: A Meta-analysis and Systematic Review," *Scientific Reports* 13, no. 1 (July 31, 2023): 12343, https://doi.org:10.1038/s41598-023-39469-9.

49. Yukio Kadooka et al., "Effect of *Lactobacillus gasseri* SBT2055 in Fermented Milk on Abdominal Adiposity in Adults in a Randomised Controlled Trial," *British Journal of Nutrition* 110, no. 9 (2013): 1696–703, https://doi.org:10.1017 /S0007114513001037.

50. David J. Johns et al., "Diet or Exercise Interventions vs Combined Behavioral Weight Management Programs: A Systematic Review and Meta-analysis of Direct Comparisons," *Journal of the Academy of Nutrition and Dietetics* 114, no. 10 (2014): 1557–68, https://doi.org:10.1016/j.jand.2014.07.005.

51. Catarina Paixão et al., "Successful Weight Loss Maintenance: A Systematic Review of Weight Control Registries," *Obesity Reviews: An Official Journal of the International Association for the Study of Obesity* 21, no. 5 (2020): e13003, https://doi.org:10.1111 /obr.13003.

52. M. Fogelholm and K. Kukkonen-Harjula, "Does Physical Activity Prevent Weight Gain—a Systematic Review," *Obesity Reviews: An Official Journal of the International Association for the Study of Obesity* 1, no. 2 (2000): 95–111, https://doi .org:10.1046/j.1467-789x.2000.00016.x; Deborah F. Tate et al., "Long-Term Weight Losses Associated with Prescription of Higher Physical Activity Goals. Are Higher Levels of Physical Activity Protective Against Weight Regain?," *American Journal of Clinical Nutrition* 85, no. 4 (2007): 954–59, https://doi.org:10.1093/ajcn/85.4 .954.

53. Yun Jun Yang, "An Overview of Current Physical Activity Recommendations in Primary Care," *Korean Journal of Family Medicine* 40, no. 3 (2019): 135–42, https:// doi.org:10.4082/kjfm.19.0038.

54. Ozlem Celik and Bülent O. Yildiz, "Obesity and Physical Exercise," *Minerva Endocrinology* 46, no. 2 (2021): 131–44, https://doi.org:10.23736/S2724-6507.20.03361-1.

55. J. T. Lemmer et al., "Effect of Strength Training on Resting Metabolic Rate and Physical Activity: Age and Gender Comparisons," *Medicine and Science in Sports and Exercise* 33, no. 4 (2001): 532–41, https://doi.org:10.1097/00005768-200104000-00005.

56. Beau Kjerulf Greer et al., "EPOC Comparison Between Isocaloric Bouts of Steady-State Aerobic, Intermittent Aerobic, and Resistance Training," *Research Quarterly for Exercise and Sport* 86, no. 2 (2015): 190–95, https://doi.org:10.1080 /02701367.2014.999190; J. F. Phelain et al., "Postexercise Energy Expenditure and Substrate Oxidation in Young Women Resulting from Exercise Bouts of Different Intensity," *Journal of the American College of Nutrition* 16, no 2 (1997): 140–46, https://doi.org:10.1080/07315724.1997.10718664.

57. Leslie H. Willis et al., "Effects of Aerobic and/or Resistance Training on Body Mass and Fat Mass in Overweight or Obese Adults," *Journal of Applied Physiology* (Bethesda, MD) 113, no. 12 (2012): 1831–27, https://doi.org:10.1152/japplphysio l.01370.2011.

58. Sebastian M. Schmid et al., "A Single Night of Sleep Deprivation Increases Ghrelin Levels and Feelings of Hunger in Normal-Weight Healthy Men," *Journal of Sleep Research* 17, no. 3 (2008): 331–34, https://doi.org:10.1111/j.1365 -2869.2008.00662.x.

59. Evangelia Papatriantafyllou et al., "Sleep Deprivation: Effects on Weight Loss and Weight Loss Maintenance," *Nutrients* 14, no. 8 (April 8, 2022): 1549, https:// doi.org:10.3390/nu14081549; Stephanie M. Greer et al., "The Impact of Sleep Deprivation on Food Desire in the Human Brain," *Nature Communications* 4 (2013): 2259, https://doi.org:10.1038/ncomms3259.

60. Jean-Philippe Chaput et al., "The Association Between Sleep Duration and Weight Gain in Adults: A 6-Year Prospective Study from the Quebec Family Study," *Sleep* 31, no. 4 (2008): 517–23, https://doi.org:10.1093/sleep/31.4.517; Jean-Philippe Chaput et al., "Change in Sleep Duration and Visceral Fat Accumulation over 6 Years in Adults," *Obesity* (Silver Spring, MD) 22, no. 5 (2014): E9–E12, https://doi .org:10.1002/oby.20701.

61. Leena Tähkämö et al., "Systematic Review of Light Exposure Impact on Human Circadian Rhythm," *Chronobiology International* 36, no. 2 (2019): 151–70, https:// doi.org:10.1080/07420528.2018.1527773.

62. Kazue Okamoto-Mizuno and Koh Mizuno, "Effects of Thermal Environment on Sleep and Circadian Rhythm," *Journal of Physiological Anthropology* 31, no. 1 (May 31, 2012): 14, https://doi.org:10.1186/1880-6805-31-14.

63. J. S. Samra et al., "Effects of Physiological Hypercortisolemia on the Regulation of Lipolysis in Subcutaneous Adipose Tissue," *Journal of Clinical Endocrinology and Metabolism* 83, no. 2 (1998): 626–31, https://doi.org:10.1210/jcem.83.2.4547; J. Uddén et al., "Effects of Glucocorticoids on Leptin Levels and Eating Behaviour in Women," *Journal of Internal Medicine* 253, no. 2 (2003): 225–31, https://doi .org:10.1046/j.1365-2796.2003.01099.x.

64. Nicola Di Polito et al., "Real-World Intake of Dietary Sugars Is Associated with Reduced Cortisol Reactivity Following an Acute Physiological Stressor," *Nutrients* 15, no. 1, (January 1, 2023): 209, https://doi.org:10.3390/nu15010209; Debra A. Zellner et al., "Food Selection Changes Under Stress," *Physiology & Behavior* 87, no. 4 (2006): 789–93, https://doi.org:10.1016/j.physbeh.2006.01.014.

65.  Yuko Nakamura et al., "Systematic Review and Meta-analysis Reveals Acutely Elevated Plasma Cortisol Following Fasting but Not Less Severe Calorie Restriction," *Stress* (Amsterdam) 19, no. 2 (2016): 151–57, https://doi.org:10.3109/10253890 .2015.1121984.

66.  Nakamura, "Systematic Review and Meta-analysis Reveals."

67.  Simon N. Thornton, "Increased Hydration Can Be Associated with Weight Loss," *Frontiers in Nutrition* 18 (June 10, 2016): https://doi.org:10.3389/fnut.2016.00018.

68.  Jennifer L. Steiner and Charles H. Lang, "Alcohol, Adipose Tissue and Lipid Dysregulation," *Biomolecules* 1, no. 16 (February 16, 2017), https://doi.org:10.3390 /biom7010016.

69.  Laurel S. Morris et al., "Stress, Motivation, and the Gut-Brain Axis: A Focus on the Ghrelin System and Alcohol Use Disorder," *Alcoholism, Clinical and Experimental Research* (May 24, 2018): 10.1111/acer.13781, https://doi.org:10.1111/acer.13781; S. Röjdmark et al., "Alcohol Ingestion Decreases Both Diurnal and Nocturnal Secretion of Leptin in Healthy Individuals," *Clinical Endocrinology* 55, no. 5 (2001): 639–47, https://doi.org:10.1046/j.1365-2265.2001.01401.x.

70.  Gabor Egervari et al., "Alcohol and the Brain: From Genes to Circuits," *Trends in Neurosciences* 44, no. 12 (2021): 1004–15, https://doi.org:10.1016/j .tins.2021.09.006; Thomas Gough et al., "The Effect of Alcohol on Food-Related Attentional Bias, Food Reward and Intake: Two Experimental Studies," *Appetite* 162 (2021): 105173, https://doi.org:10.1016/j.appet.2021.105173.

71.  "Limiting Alcohol to Manage High Blood Pressure," American Heart Association, last modified April 20, 2023, https://www.heart.org/en/health-topics/high-blood -pressure/changes-you-can-make-to-manage-high-blood-pressure/limiting-alcohol -to-manage-high-blood-pressure.

72.  "Canada's Guidance on Alcohol and Health," Canadian Centre on Substance Use and Addiction (CCSA), accessed June 23, 2025, https://www.ccsa.ca/en /guidance-tools-resources/substance-use-and-addiction/alcohol/canadas-guidance -alcohol-and-health.

## Chapter 7: Flattening the Curve: HCC for Insulin Resistance, Diabetes & PCOS Management Goals

1.  C. D. Gardner et al., "Effect of a Ketogenic Diet Versus Mediterranean Diet on Glycated Hemoglobin in Individuals with Prediabetes and Type 2 Diabetes Mellitus: The Interventional Keto-Med Randomized Crossover Trial," *American Journal of Clinical Nutrition* 116, no. 3 (2022): 640–52, https://doi.org:10.1093/ajcn/nqac279.

2.  Alpana P. Shukla et al., "The Impact of Food Order on Postprandial Glycaemic Excursions in Prediabetes," *Diabetes, Obesity & Metabolism* 21, no. 2 (2019): 377–81, https://doi.org:10.1111/dom.13503.

3.  Chunye Chen et al., "Therapeutic Effects of Soluble Dietary Fiber Consumption on Type 2 Diabetes Mellitus," *Experimental and Therapeutic Medicine* 12, no. 2 (2016): 1232–42, https://doi.org:10.3892/etm.2016.3377.

4.  Rine Elise Halvorsen et al., "Fruit and Vegetable Consumption and the Risk of Type 2 Diabetes: A Systematic Review and Dose-Response Meta-analysis of Prospective Studies," *BMJ Nutrition, Prevention & Health* 4, no. 2 (July 2, 2021): 519–31, https://doi.org:10.1136/bmjnph-2020-000218.

5. Huaidong Du et al., "Fresh Fruit Consumption in Relation to Incident Diabetes and Diabetic Vascular Complications: A 7-Year Prospective Study of 0.5 Million Chinese Adults," *PLoS Medicine* 14, no. 4 (April 11, 2017): e1002279, https://doi.org:10.1371/journal.pmed.1002279.

6. Effie Viguiliouk et al., "Effect of Replacing Animal Protein with Plant Protein on Glycemic Control in Diabetes: A Systematic Review and Meta-analysis of Randomized Controlled Trials," *Nutrients* 7, no. 12 (December 1, 2015): 9804–24, https://doi.org:10.3390/nu7125509.

7. Mengying Fan et al., "Dietary Protein Consumption and the Risk of Type 2 Diabetes: A Dose-Response Meta-analysis of Prospective Studies," *Nutrients* 11, no. 11 (November 15, 2019): 2783, https://doi.org:10.3390/nu11112783.

8. Sina Naghshi et al., "Dietary Intake of Total, Animal, and Plant Proteins and Risk of All Cause, Cardiovascular, and Cancer Mortality: Systematic Review and Dose-Response Meta-analysis of Prospective Cohort Studies," *BMJ (Clinical Research Ed.)* 370 (July 22, 2020): m2412, https://doi.org:10.1136/bmj.m2412.

9. Makoto Funaki, "Saturated Fatty Acids and Insulin Resistance," *Journal of Medical Investigation: JMI* 56, no. 3–4 (2009): 88–92, https://doi.org:10.2152/jmi.56.88; Panu K. Luukkonen et al., "Saturated Fat Is More Metabolically Harmful for the Human Liver Than Unsaturated Fat or Simple Sugars," *Diabetes Care* 41, no. 8 (2018): 1732–39, https://doi.org:10.2337/dc18-0071.

10. Mohammad Idreesh Khan et al., "Advanced Glycation End Product Signaling and Metabolic Complications: Dietary Approach," *World Journal of Diabetes* 14, no. 7 (2023): 995–1012, https://doi.org:10.4239/wjd.v14.i7.995.

11. Mu-Yuan Ma et al., "Omega-3 Index and Type 2 Diabetes: Systematic Review and Meta-analysis," *Prostaglandins, Leukotrienes, and Essential Fatty Acids* 174 (2021): 102361, https://doi.org:10.1016/j.plefa.2021.102361.

12. A. Garg, "High-Monounsaturated-Fat Diets for Patients with Diabetes Mellitus: A Meta-analysis," *American Journal of Clinical Nutrition* 67, no. S3 (1998): 577S–82S, https://doi.org:10.1093/ajcn/67.3.577S; Xiaoran Liu et al., "Changes in Types of Dietary Fats Influence Long-Term Weight Change in US Women and Men," *Journal of Nutrition* 148, no. 11 (2018): 1821–29, https://doi.org:10.1093/jn/nxy183.

13. "Fats and Fatty Acids in Human Nutrition. Report of an Expert Consultation," *FAO Food and Nutrition Paper* 91 (2010): 1–166.

14. Tanja Kongerslev Thorning et al., "Whole Dairy Matrix or Single Nutrients in Assessment of Health Effects: Current Evidence and Knowledge Gaps," *American Journal of Clinical Nutrition* 105, no. 5 (2017): 1033–45, https://doi.org:10.3945/ajcn.116.151548.

15. Ronan Lordan et al., "Dairy Fats and Cardiovascular Disease: Do We Really Need to Be Concerned?," *Foods* (Basel) 7, no. 3 (March 1, 2018): 29, https://doi.org:10.3390/foods7030029.

16. Ritu Deswal et al., "The Prevalence of Polycystic Ovary Syndrome: A Brief Systematic Review," *Journal of Human Reproductive Sciences* 13, no. 4 (2020): 261–71, https://doi.org:10.4103/jhrs.JHRS_95_18.

17. Yan Sun et al., "Gut Microbiota Dysbiosis in Polycystic Ovary Syndrome: Mechanisms of Progression and Clinical Applications," *Frontiers in Cellular and Infection Microbiology* 13 (2023): 1142041, https://doi.org:10.3389/fcimb.2023.1142041.

18. "Polycystic Ovary Syndrome (PCOS)," Centers for Disease Control and Prevention, last reviewed February 27, 2023, https://www.cdc.gov/diabetes/risk-factors/pcos -polycystic-ovary-syndrome.html.

19. Fang Wang et al., "Effects of High-Protein Diets on the Cardiometabolic Factors and Reproductive Hormones of Women with Polycystic Ovary Syndrome: A Systematic Review and Meta-analysis," *Nutrition & Diabetes* 14, no. 1 (February 29, 2024): 6, https://doi.org:10.1038/s41387-024-00263-9; Lone B. Sørensen et al., "Effects of Increased Dietary Protein-to-Carbohydrate Ratios in Women with Polycystic Ovary Syndrome," *American Journal of Clinical Nutrition* 95, no. 1 (2012): 39–48, https:// doi.org:10.3945/ajcn.111.020693.

20. Gamze Yurtdaş and Yasemin Akdevelioğlu, "A New Approach to Polycystic Ovary Syndrome: The Gut Microbiota," *Journal of the American College of Nutrition* 39, no. 4 (2020): 371–82, https://doi.org:10.1080/07315724.2019.1657515.

21. G. Oner and I. I. Muderris, "Efficacy of Omega-3 in the Treatment of Polycystic Ovary Syndrome," *Journal of Obstetrics and Gynaecology: The Journal of the Institute of Obstetrics and Gynaecology* 33, no. 3 (2013): 289–91, https://doi.org:10.3109 /01443615.2012.751365.

22. Michael J. Davies et al., "Intergenerational Associations of Chronic Disease and Polycystic Ovary Syndrome," *PloS One* 6, no. 10 (2011): e25947, https://doi.org:10 .1371/journal.pone.0025947.

23. Kailin Yang et al., "Effectiveness of Omega-3 Fatty Acid for Polycystic Ovary Syndrome: A Systematic Review and Meta-analysis," *Reproductive Biology and Endocrinology: RB&E* 16, no. 1 (March 27, 2018): 27, https://doi.org:10.1186/s12958-018-0346-x.

24. J. E. Chavarro et al., "A Prospective Study of Dairy Foods Intake and Anovulatory Infertility," *Human Reproduction* (Oxford, UK) 22, no. 5 (2007): 1340–47, https:// doi.org:10.1093/humrep/dem019; Christian R. Juhl et al., "Dairy Intake and Acne Vulgaris: A Systematic Review and Meta-Analysis of 78,529 Children, Adolescents, and Young Adults," *Nutrients* 10, no. 8 (August 9, 2018): 1049, https://doi.org:10 .3390/nu10081049.

25. Guo-Chong Chen et al., "Association of Oily and Nonoily Fish Consumption and Fish Oil Supplements with Incident Type 2 Diabetes: A Large Population-Based Prospective Study," *Diabetes Care* 44, no. 3 (2021): 672–80, https://doi.org:10.2337 /dc20-2328.

26. "Fish and Omega-3 Fatty Acids," American Heart Association, last reviewed May 3, 2023, https://www.heart.org/en/healthy-living/healthy-eating/eat-smart/fats /fish-and-omega-3-fatty-acids.

27. Qingtao Hou et al., "The Metabolic Effects of Oats Intake in Patients with Type 2 Diabetes: A Systematic Review and Meta-analysis," *Nutrients* 7, no. 12 (December 10, 2015): 10369-87, https://doi.org:10.3390/nu7125536.

28. Tan Shot Yen et al., "Increased Vegetable Intake Improves Glycaemic Control in Adults with Type 2 Diabetes Mellitus: A Clustered Randomised Clinical Trial Among Indonesian White-Collar Workers," *Journal of Nutritional Science* 11 (June 21, 2022): e40, https://doi.org:10.1017/jns.2022.41.

29. Yen et al., "Increased Vegetable Intake."

30. Yoona Kim et al., "Benefits of Nut Consumption on Insulin Resistance and Cardiovascular Risk Factors: Multiple Potential Mechanisms of Actions," *Nutrients*

9, no. 11 (November 22, 2017): 1271, https://doi.org:10.3390/nu9111271; Andrea J. Glenn et al., "Nuts and Cardiovascular Disease Outcomes: A Review of the Evidence and Future Directions," *Nutrients* 15, no. 4 (February 11, 2023): 911, https://doi .org:10.3390/nu15040911.

31.   Lauren Houston et al., "Tree Nut and Peanut Consumption and Risk of Cardiovascular Disease: A Systematic Review and Meta-analysis of Randomized Controlled Trials," *Advances in Nutrition* (Bethesda, MD) 14, no. 5 (2023): 1029–49, https:// doi.org:10.1016/j.advnut.2023.05.004.

32.   Heitor O. Santos et al., "Vinegar (Acetic Acid) Intake on Glucose Metabolism: A Narrative Review," *Clinical Nutrition ESPEN* 32 (2019): 1–7, https://doi .org:10.1016/j.clnesp.2019.05.008; Panayota Mitrou et al., "Vinegar Consumption Increases Insulin-Stimulated Glucose Uptake by the Forearm Muscle in Humans with Type 2 Diabetes," *Journal of Diabetes Research* 2015 (2015): 175204, https://doi .org:10.1155/2015/175204; Farideh Shishehbor et al., "Vinegar Consumption Can Attenuate Postprandial Glucose and Insulin Responses: A Systematic Review and Meta-analysis of Clinical Trials," *Diabetes Research and Clinical Practice* 127 (2017): 1–9, https://doi.org:10.1016/j.diabres.2017.01.021.

33.   Wenting Xie et al., "Glucose-Lowering Effect of Berberine on Type 2 Diabetes: A Systematic Review and Meta-analysis," *Frontiers in Pharmacology* 13 (November 16, 2022): 1015045, https://doi.org:10.3389/fphar.2022.1015045.

34.   Hong Ma et al., "Efficacy and Safety of GLP-1 Receptor Agonists Versus SGLT-2 Inhibitors in Overweight/Obese Patients with or Without Diabetes Mellitus: A Systematic Review and Network Meta-analysis," *BMJ Open* 13, no. 3 (March 7, 2023): e061807, https://doi.org:10.1136/bmjopen-2022-061807.

35.   James J. DiNicolantonio and James H. O'Keefe, "Myo-inositol for Insulin Resistance, Metabolic Syndrome, Polycystic Ovary Syndrome and Gestational Diabetes," *Open Heart* 9, no. 1 (2022): e001989, https://doi.org:10.1136/openhrt-2022-001989.

36.   Scott Roseff and Marta Montenegro, "Inositol Treatment for PCOS Should Be Science-Based and Not Arbitrary," *International Journal of Endocrinology* 2020 (March 27, 2020): 6461254, https://doi.org:10.1155/2020/6461254.

37.   Hammad Ali Fadlalmola et al., "Efficacy of Resveratrol in Women with Polycystic Ovary Syndrome: A Systematic Review and Meta-analysis of Randomized Clinical Trials," *Pan African Medical Journal* 44, no. 134 (March 16, 2023), https://doi .org:10.11604/pamj.2023.44.134.32404.

38.   Felipe Mendes Delpino et al., "Omega-3 Supplementation and Diabetes: A Systematic Review and Meta-analysis," *Critical Reviews in Food Science and Nutrition* 62, no. 16 (2022): 4435–48, https://doi.org:10.1080/10408398.2021.1875977.

39.   Yang et al., "Effectiveness of Omega-3 Fatty Acid for Polycystic Ovary Syndrome."

40.   Diane Fatkin et al., "Fishing for Links Between Omega-3 Fatty Acids and Atrial Fibrillation," *Circulation* 145, no. 14 (2022): 1037–39, https://doi.org:10.1161 /CIRCULATIONAHA.121.058596.

41.   Andreea Zurbau et al., "The Effect of Oat β-glucan on Postprandial Blood Glucose and Insulin Responses: A Systematic Review and Meta-analysis," *European Journal of Clinical Nutrition* 75, no. 11 (2021): 1540–54, https://doi.org:10.1038 /s41430-021-00875-9; Soltanian Noureddin et al., "Effects of Psyllium vs. Placebo on Constipation, Weight, Glycemia, and Lipids: A Randomized Trial in Patients

with Type 2 Diabetes and Chronic Constipation," *Complementary Therapies in Medicine* 40 (2018): 1–7, https://doi.org:10.1016/j.ctim.2018.07.004.

42. Hye In Jeong et al., "*Morus alba*. L for Blood Sugar Management: A Systematic Review and Meta-Analysis," *Evidence-Based Complementary and Alternative Medicine: eCAM* 2022 (May 23, 2022): 9282154, https://doi.org:10.1155/2022/9282154; Mark Lown et al., "Mulberry-Extract Improves Glucose Tolerance and Decreases Insulin Concentrations in Normoglycaemic Adults: Results of a Randomised Double-Blind Placebo-Controlled Study," *PloS One* 12 no. 2 (February 22, 2017): e0172239, https://doi.org:10.1371/journal.pone.0172239.

43. Alessio Bellini et al., "Effects of Different Exercise Strategies to Improve Postprandial Glycemia in Healthy Individuals," *Medicine and Science in Sports and Exercise* 53, no. 7 (2021): 1334–44, https://doi.org:10.1249/MSS.0000000000002607.

44. Sandra Bonuccelli et al., "Improved Tolerance to Sequential Glucose Loading (Staub-Traugott Effect): Size and Mechanisms," *American Journal of Physiology, Endocrinology and Metabolism* 297, no. 2 (2009): E532–37, https://doi.org:10.1152/ajpendo.00127.2009.

45. Kristen L. Knutson, "Impact of Sleep and Sleep Loss on Glucose Homeostasis and Appetite Regulation," *Sleep Medicine Clinics* 2, no. 2 (2007): 187–97, https://doi.org:10.1016/j.jsmc.2007.03.004.

46. Michael A. Grandner et al., "Sleep Duration and Diabetes Risk: Population Trends and Potential Mechanisms," *Current Diabetes Reports* 16, no. 11 (2016): 106, https://doi.org:10.1007/s11892-016-0805-8; Raphael Vallat et al., "Coordinated Human Sleeping Brainwaves Map Peripheral Body Glucose Homeostasis," *Cell Reports Medicine* 4, no. 7 (2023): 101100, https://doi.org:10.1016/j.xcrm.2023.101100.

47. Jean-Philippe Chaput et al., "Sleep Duration and Health in Adults: An Overview of Systematic Reviews," *Applied Physiology, Nutrition, and Metabolism (Physiologie appliquee, nutrition et metabolisme)* 45, no. 10 (S2) (2020): S218–S231, https://doi.org:10.1139/apnm-2020-0034.

48. Habib Yaribeygi et al., "Molecular Mechanisms Linking Stress and Insulin Resistance," *EXCL Journal* 21 (January 24, 2022): 317–34, https://doi.org:10.17179/excli2021-4382.

49. Fatimata Sanogo et al., "Mind- and Body-Based Interventions Improve Glycemic Control in Patients with Type 2 Diabetes: A Systematic Review and Meta-analysis," *Journal of Integrative and Complementary Medicine* 29, no. 2 (2023): 69–79, https://doi.org:10.1089/jicm.2022.0586.

50. Meng Wang et al., "Association Between Sugar-Sweetened Beverages and Type 2 Diabetes: A Meta-analysis," *Journal of Diabetes Investigation* 6, no. 3 (2015): 360–66, https://doi.org:10.1111/jdi.12309.

51. Jean-Philippe Drouin-Chartier et al., "Changes in Consumption of Sugary Beverages and Artificially Sweetened Beverages and Subsequent Risk of Type 2 Diabetes: Results from Three Large Prospective U.S. Cohorts of Women and Men," *Diabetes Care* 42, no. 12 (2019): 2181–89, https://doi.org:10.2337/dc19-0734.

52. M. Yanina Pepino et al., "Sucralose Affects Glycemic and Hormonal Responses to an Oral Glucose Load," *Diabetes Care* 36, no. 9 (2013): 2530–35, https://doi.org:10.2337/dc12-2221; Francisco Javier Ruiz-Ojeda et al., "Effects of Sweeteners on the Gut Microbiota: A Review of Experimental Studies and Clinical Trials,"

*Advances in Nutrition* (Bethesda, MD) 10, no. S1 (2019): S31–S48, https://doi
.org:10.1093/advances/nmy037.

53. Matcha Angelin et al., "Artificial Sweeteners and Their Implications In Diabetes: A Review," *Frontiers in Nutrition* 11 (June 25, 2024): 1411560, https://doi
.org:10.3389/fnut.2024.1411560; Ingrid Toews et al., "Association Between Intake
of Non-sugar Sweeteners and Health Outcomes: Systematic Review and Meta-
analyses of Randomised and Non-randomised Controlled Trials and Observational
Studies," *BMJ* 364 (January 2, 2019): k4718, https://doi.org/10.1136/bmj.k4718.

54. Emilio González-Reimers et al., "Alcoholism: A Systemic Proinflammatory
Condition," *World Journal of Gastroenterology* 20, no. 40 (2014): 14660-71, https://
doi.org:10.3748/wjg.v20.i40.14660.

55. James D. Lane et al., "Caffeine Impairs Glucose Metabolism in Type 2 Diabetes,"
*Diabetes Care* 27, no. 8 (2004): 2047–8, https://doi.org:10.2337/diacare.27.8.2047;
Rob M. van Dam and Frank B. Hu, "Coffee Consumption and Risk of Type 2
Diabetes: A Systematic Review," *JAMA* 294, no. 1 (2005): 97–104, https://doi.org:
10.1001/jama.294.1.97.

56. Daniele Wikoff et al., "Systematic Review of the Potential Adverse Effects of Caffeine Consumption in Healthy Adults, Pregnant Women, Adolescents, and Children," *Food and Chemical Toxicology: An International Journal Published for the
British Industrial Biological Research Association* 109, pt. 1 (2017): 585–648, https://
doi.org:10.1016/j.fct.2017.04.002.

## Chapter 8: Strength and Endurance: HCC for Sports & Fitness Nutrition

1. Amy J. Hector et al., "Pronounced Energy Restriction with Elevated Protein Intake
Results in No Change in Proteolysis and Reductions in Skeletal Muscle Protein
Synthesis That Are Mitigated by Resistance Exercise," *FASEB Journal: Official
Publication of the Federation of American Societies for Experimental Biology* 32, no. 1
(2018): 265–75, https://doi.org:10.1096/fj.201700158RR.

2. Juan Mielgo-Ayuso and Diego Fernández-Lázaro, "Nutrition and Muscle Recovery,"
*Nutrients* 13, no. 2 (January 20, 2021): 294, https://doi.org:10.3390/nu13020294.

3. Robert W. Morton et al., "A Systematic Review, Meta-analysis and Meta-regression
of the Effect of Protein Supplementation on Resistance Training-Induced Gains in
Muscle Mass and Strength in Healthy Adults," *British Journal of Sports Medicine* 52,
no. 6 (2018): 376–84, https://doi.org:10.1136/bjsports-2017-097608.

4. Brad Jon Schoenfeld et al., "Pre- Versus Post-Exercise Protein Intake Has Similar
Effects on Muscular Adaptations," *PeerJ* 5 (January 3, 2017): e2825, https://doi
.org:10.7717/peerj.2825; Brad Jon Schoenfeld et al., "The Effect of Protein Timing on Muscle Strength and Hypertrophy: A Meta-analysis," *Journal of the International Society of Sports Nutrition* 10, no. 1 (December 3, 2013): 53, https://doi
.org:10.1186/1550-2783-10-53; Shawn M. Arent et al., "Nutrient Timing: A Garage
Door of Opportunity?," *Nutrients* 12, no. 7 (June 3, 2020): 1948, https://doi.org:
10.3390/nu12071948.

5. Brad Jon Schoenfeld and Alan Albert Aragon, "How Much Protein Can the
Body Use in a Single Meal for Muscle-Building? Implications for Daily Protein
Distribution," *Journal of the International Society of Sports Nutrition* 15, no. 10
(February 27, 2018), https://doi.org:10.1186/s12970-018-0215-1.

6. Daniel R. Moore, "Maximizing Post-exercise Anabolism: The Case for Relative Protein Intakes," *Frontiers in Nutrition* 6, no. 147 (September 10, 2019), https://doi.org:10.3389/fnut.2019.00147.

7. Nicholas A. Burd et al., "Dietary Protein Quantity, Quality, and Exercise Are Key to Healthy Living: A Muscle-Centric Perspective Across the Lifespan," *Frontiers in Nutrition* 6 (June 6, 2019): 83, https://doi.org:10.3389/fnut.2019.00083.

8. Jorn Trommelen et al., "The Anabolic Response to Protein Ingestion During Recovery from Exercise Has No Upper Limit in Magnitude and Duration in Vivo in Humans," *Cell Reports Medicine* 4, no. 12 (2023): 101324, https://doi.org:10.1016/j.xcrm.2023.101324.

9. Michaela C. Devries et al., "Changes in Kidney Function Do Not Differ Between Healthy Adults Consuming Higher- Compared with Lower- or Normal-Protein Diets: A Systematic Review and Meta-analysis," *Journal of Nutrition* 148, no. 11 (2018): 1760–75, https://doi.org:10.1093/jn/nxy197; Jose Antonio et al., "A High Protein Diet (3.4 g/kg/d) Combined with a Heavy Resistance Training Program Improves Body Composition in Healthy Trained Men and Women—a Follow-Up Investigation," *Journal of the International Society of Sports Nutrition* 12, no. 39 (October 20, 2015), https://doi.org:10.1186/s12970-015-0100-0.

10. Alistair J. Monteyne et al., "Vegan and Omnivorous High Protein Diets Support Comparable Daily Myofibrillar Protein Synthesis Rates and Skeletal Muscle Hypertrophy in Young Adults," *Journal of Nutrition* 153, no. 6 (2023): 1680–95, https://doi.org:10.1016/j.tjnut.2023.02.023; Alistair J. Monteyne et al., "A Mycoprotein-Based High-Protein Vegan Diet Supports Equivalent Daily Myofibrillar Protein Synthesis Rates Compared with an Isonitrogenous Omnivorous Diet in Older Adults: A Randomised Controlled Trial," *British Journal of Nutrition* 126, no. 5 (2021): 674–84, https://doi.org:10.1017/S0007114520004481.

11. Charles P. Lambert et al., "Macronutrient Considerations for the Sport of Bodybuilding," *Sports Medicine* (Auckland, NZ) 34, no. 5 (2004): 317–27, https://doi.org:10.2165/00007256-200434050-00004.

12. Menno Henselmans et al., "The Effect of Carbohydrate Intake on Strength and Resistance Training Performance: A Systematic Review," *Nutrients* 14, no. 4 (February 18, 2022): 856, https://doi.org:10.3390/nu14040856.

13. Lambert et al., "Macronutrient Considerations."

14. Alfonso J. Cruz-Jentoft et al., "Nutritional Strategies for Maintaining Muscle Mass and Strength from Middle Age to Later Life: A Narrative Review," *Maturitas* 132 (2020): 57–64, https://doi.org:10.1016/j.maturitas.2019.11.007.

15. D. Travis Thomas et al., "Position of the Academy of Nutrition and Dietetics, Dietitians of Canada, and the American College of Sports Medicine: Nutrition and Athletic Performance," *Journal of the Academy of Nutrition and Dietetics* 116, no. 3 (2016): 501–28, https://doi.org:10.1016/j.jand.2015.12.006; L. M. Burke et al., "Guidelines for Daily Carbohydrate Intake: Do Athletes Achieve Them?," *Sports Medicine* (Auckland, NZ) 31, no. 4 (2001): 267–99, https://doi.org:10.2165/00007256-200131040-00003.

16. Asker Jeukendrup, "A Step Towards Personalized Sports Nutrition: Carbohydrate Intake During Exercise," *Sports Medicine* (Auckland, NZ) 44, no. S1 (2014): S25–S33, https://doi.org:10.1007/s40279-014-0148-z.

17. Chad M. Kerksick et al., "International Society of Sports Nutrition Position Stand: Nutrient Timing," *Journal of the International Society of Sports Nutrition* 14, no. 33 (August 29, 2017), https://doi.org:10.1186/s12970-017-0189-4.

18. Javier Díaz-Lara et al., "Delaying Post-exercise Carbohydrate Intake Impairs Next-Day Exercise Capacity but Not Muscle Glycogen or Molecular Responses," *Acta Physiologica* (Oxford, UK) 240, no. 10 (2024): e14215, https://doi.org:10.1111/apha.14215.

19. Kenneth Vitale and Andrew Getzin, "Nutrition and Supplement Update for the Endurance Athlete: Review and Recommendations," *Nutrients* 11, no. 6 (June 7, 2019): 1289, https://doi.org:10.3390/nu11061289; Daniel R. Moore et al., "Beyond Muscle Hypertrophy: Why Dietary Protein Is Important for Endurance Athletes," *Applied Physiology, Nutrition, and Metabolism (Physiologie appliquee, nutrition et metabolisme)* 39, no. 9 (2014): 987–97, https://doi.org:10.1139/apnm-2013-0591.

20. M. J. Schuster et al., "A Comprehensive Review of Raisins and Raisin Components and Their Relationship to Human Health," *Journal of Nutrition and Health* 50, no. 3 (June 2017): 203–16, https://doi.org/10.4163/jnh.2017.50.3.203.

21. Mark Kern et al., "Metabolic and Performance Effects of Raisins Versus Sports Gel as Pre-exercise Feedings in Cyclists," *Journal of Strength and Conditioning Research* 21, no. 4 (2007): 1204–7, https://doi.org:10.1519/R-21226.1.

22. Atsushi Kanda et al., "Effects of Whey, Caseinate, or Milk Protein Ingestion on Muscle Protein Synthesis After Exercise," *Nutrients* 8, no. 6 (2016): 339, https://doi.org:10.3390/nu8060339.

23. Aaron Bridge et al., "Greek Yogurt and 12 Weeks of Exercise Training on Strength, Muscle Thickness and Body Composition in Lean, Untrained, University-Aged Males," *Frontiers in Nutrition* 6, no. 55 (April 30, 2019), https://doi.org:10.3389/fnut.2019.00055.

24. Tim Snijders et al., "The Impact of Pre-sleep Protein Ingestion on the Skeletal Muscle Adaptive Response to Exercise in Humans: An Update," *Frontiers in Nutrition* 6, no. 17 (March 6, 2019), https://doi.org:10.3389/fnut.2019.00017.

25. Nicolas Babault et al., "Pea Proteins Oral Supplementation Promotes Muscle Thickness Gains During Resistance Training: A Double-Blind, Randomized, Placebo-Controlled Clinical Trial vs. Whey Protein," *Journal of the International Society of Sports Nutrition* 12, no. 1 (January 21, 2015): 3, https://doi.org:10.1186/s12970-014-0064-5; Luiz Lannes Loureiro et al., "Comparison of the Effects of Pea Protein and Whey Protein on the Metabolic Profile of Soccer Athletes: A Randomized, Double-Blind, Crossover Trial," *Frontiers in Nutrition* 10 (September 22, 2023): 1210215, https://doi.org:10.3389/fnut.2023.1210215.

26. M. Negro et al., "Branched-Chain Amino Acid Supplementation Does Not Enhance Athletic Performance but Affects Muscle Recovery and the Immune System," *Journal of Sports Medicine and Physical Fitness* 48, no. 3 (2008): 347–51.

27. Abbie E. Smith-Ryan et al., "Creatine Supplementation in Women's Health: A Lifespan Perspective," *Nutrients* 13, no. 3 (March 8, 2021): 877, https://doi.org:10.3390/nu13030877; J. R. Poortmans and M. Francaux, "Long-Term Oral Creatine Supplementation Does Not Impair Renal Function in Healthy Athletes," *Medicine and Science in Sports and Exercise* 31 no. 8 (1999): 1108–10, https://doi.org:10.1097/00005768-199908000-00005; K. Vannas-Sulonen et al., "Gyrate

Atrophy of the Choroid and Retina: A Five-Year Follow-Up of Creatine Supplementation," *Ophthalmology* 92, no. 12 (1985): 1719–27, https://doi.org:10.1016/s0161-6420(85)34098-8.

28. Richard B. Kreider et al., "International Society of Sports Nutrition Position Stand: Safety and Efficacy of Creatine Supplementation in Exercise, Sport, and Medicine," *Journal of the International Society of Sports Nutrition* 14, no. 18 (June 13, 2017), https://doi.org:10.1186/s12970-017-0173-z.

29. Maria Alessandra Gammone et al., "Omega-3 Polyunsaturated Fatty Acids: Benefits and Endpoints in Sport," *Nutrients* 11, no. 1 (December 27, 2018): 46, https://doi.org:10.3390/nu11010046.

30. Frank Thielecke and Andrew Blannin, "Omega-3 Fatty Acids for Sport Performance—Are They Equally Beneficial for Athletes and Amateurs? A Narrative Review," *Nutrients* 12, no. 12 (November 30, 2020): 3712, https://doi.org:10.3390/nu12123712.

31. "Scientific Opinion on the Substantiation of Health Claims Related to Soy Isoflavones and Maintenance of Bone Mineral Density (ID 1655) and Reduction of Vasomotor Symptoms Associated with Menopause (ID 1654, 1704, 2140, 3093, 3154, 3590) (Further Assessment) Pursuant to Article 13(1) of Regulation (EC) No 1924/2006," European Food Safety Authority, *EFSA Journal* 10, no. 7 (2012): 2811, https://doi.org/10.2903/j.efsa.2012.2811.

32. Slaheddine Delleli et al., "Does Beetroot Supplementation Improve Performance in Combat Sports Athletes? A Systematic Review of Randomized Controlled Trials," *Nutrients* 15, no. 2 (January 12, 2023): 398, https://doi.org:10.3390/nu15020398; Raúl Domínguez et al., "Effects of Beetroot Juice Supplementation on Intermittent High-Intensity Exercise Efforts," *Journal of the International Society of Sports Nutrition* 15, no. 2 (January 5, 2018), https://doi.org:10.1186/s12970-017-0204-9.

33. Hamid Arazi and Ehsan Eghbali, "Possible Effects of Beetroot Supplementation on Physical Performance Through Metabolic, Neuroendocrine, and Antioxidant Mechanisms: A Narrative Review of the Literature," *Frontiers in Nutrition* 8 (May 13, 2021): 660150, https://doi.org:10.3389/fnut.2021.660150.

34. Sergio L. Jiménez et al., "Caffeinated Drinks and Physical Performance in Sport: A Systematic Review," *Nutrients* 13, no. 9 (August 25, 2021): 2944, https://doi.org:10.3390/nu13092944.

35. Nanci S. Guest et al., "International Society of Sports Nutrition Position Stand: Caffeine and Exercise Performance," *Journal of the International Society of Sports Nutrition* 18, no. 1 (January 2, 2021): 1, https://doi.org:10.1186/s12970-020-00383-4.

36. Eric T. Trexler et al., "International Society of Sports Nutrition Position Stand: Beta-alanine," *Journal of the International Society of Sports Nutrition* 12, no. 30 (July 15, 2015), https://doi.org:10.1186/s12970-015-0090-y.

37. A. Jeukendrup et al., "Carbohydrate-Electrolyte Feedings Improve 1 H Time Trial Cycling Performance," *International Journal of Sports Medicine* 18, no. 2 (1997): 125–29, https://doi.org:10.1055/s-2007-972607; Danielle McCartney et al., "The Effect of Different Post-exercise Beverages with Food on Ad Libitum Fluid Recovery, Nutrient Provision, and Subsequent Athletic Performance," *Physiology & Behavior* 201 (2019): 22–30, https://doi.org:10.1016/j.physbeh.2018.12.013.

38. Lawrence E. Armstrong, "Rehydration During Endurance Exercise: Challenges, Research, Options, Methods," *Nutrients* 13, no. 3 (March 9, 2021): 887, https://doi .org:10.3390/nu13030887.

39. Jonathan Charest and Michael A. Grandner, "Sleep and Athletic Performance: Impacts on Physical Performance, Mental Performance, Injury Risk and Recovery, and Mental Health," *Sleep Medicine Clinics* 15, no. 1 (2020): 41–57, https://doi .org:10.1016/j.jsmc.2019.11.005; Neil P. Walsh et al., "Sleep and the Athlete: Narrative Review and 2021 Expert Consensus Recommendations," *British Journal of Sports Medicine* (November 3, 2020): bjsports-2020-102025, https://doi.org:10 .1136/bjsports-2020-102025.

40. Lúcio A. Cunha et al., "The Impact of Sleep Interventions on Athletic Performance: A Systematic Review," *Sports Medicine—Open* 9, no. 1 (July 18, 2023): 58, https:// doi.org:10.1186/s40798-023-00599-z.

## Chapter 9: Healthy Aging: HCC for Perimenopause, Menopause, and Beyond

1. Priscilla Rayanne E. Silva Noll et al., "Life Habits of Postmenopausal Women: Association of Menopause Symptom Intensity and Food Consumption by Degree of Food Processing," *Maturitas* 156 (2022): 1–11, https://doi.org:10.1016/j.maturitas .2021.10.015.

2. Carla Gonçalves et al., "Systematic Review of Mediterranean Diet Interventions in Menopausal Women," *AIMS Public Health* 11, no. 1 (January 10, 2024): 110-129, https://doi.org:10.3934/publichealth.2024005; Antonio Cano et al., "The Mediterranean Diet and Menopausal Health: An EMAS Position Statement," *Maturitas* 139 (2020): 90–97, https://doi.org:10.1016/j.maturitas.2020.07.001.

3. Herman Pontzer et al., "Daily Energy Expenditure Through the Human Life Course," *Science* (New York) 373, no. 6556 (2021): 808–12, https://doi.org:10.1126 /science.abe5017.

4. Thais R. Silva et al., "Nutrition in Menopausal Women: A Narrative Review," *Nutrients* 13, no. 7 (June 23, 2021): 2149, https://doi.org:10.3390/nu13072149.

5. T. T. Fung et al., "Protein Intake and Risk of Hip Fractures in Postmenopausal Women and Men Age 50 and Older," *Osteoporosis International: A Journal Established as Result of Cooperation Between the European Foundation for Osteoporosis and the National Osteoporosis Foundation of the USA* 28, no. 4 (2017): 1401–11, https://doi.org:10.1007/s00198-016-3898-7.

6. Sijia Tang et al., "Effects of Soy Foods in Postmenopausal Women: A Focus on Osteosarcopenia and Obesity," *Journal of Obesity & Metabolic Syndrome* 29, no. 3 (2020): 180–87, https://doi.org:10.7570/jomes20006.

7. Oscar Franco et al., "Use of Plant-Based Therapies and Menopausal Symptoms," *JAMA* 315, no. 23 (2016): 2554–63, https://doi.org: 10.1001/jama.2016.8012.

8. Prasanth Surampudi et al., "Lipid Lowering with Soluble Dietary Fiber," *Current Atherosclerosis Reports* 18, no. 12 (2016): 75, https://doi.org:10.1007/s11883-016 -0624-z.

9. Sharon Dormire and Chularat Howharn, "The Effect of Dietary Intake on Hot Flashes in Menopausal Women," *Journal of Obstetric, Gynecologic, and Neonatal Nursing: JOGNN* 36, no. 3 (2007): 255–62, https://doi.org:10.1111/j.1552-6909 .2007.00142.x.

10.  Zhao-Min Liu et al., "Whole Plant Foods Intake Is Associated with Fewer Meno-pausal Symptoms in Chinese Postmenopausal Women with Prehypertension or Untreated Hypertension," *Menopause* (New York) 22, no. 5 (2015): 496–504, https://doi.org:10.1097/GME.0000000000000349; Maryam Safabakhsh et al., "Higher Intakes of Fruits and Vegetables Are Related to Fewer Menopausal Symp-toms: A Cross-sectional Study," *Menopause* (New York) 27, no. 5 (2020): 593–604, https://doi.org:10.1097/GME.0000000000001511.

11.  Claudia Vetrani et al., "Mediterranean Diet: What Are the Consequences for Menopause?," *Frontiers in Endocrinology* 13 (April 25, 2022): 886824, https://doi.org:10.3389/fendo.2022.886824.

12.  Asghar Z. Naqvi et al., "Monounsaturated, Trans, and Saturated Fatty Acids and Cognitive Decline in Women," *Journal of the American Geriatrics Society* 59, no. 5 (2011): 837–43, https://doi.org:10.1111/j.1532-5415.2011.03402.x.

13.  Ioannis Boutas et al., "Soy Isoflavones and Breast Cancer Risk: A Meta-analysis," *In Vivo* (Athens, Greece) 36, no. 2 (2022): 556–62, https://doi.org:10.21873/invivo.12737.

14.  Sijia Tang et al., "Effects of Soy Foods in Postmenopausal Women: A Focus on Osteosarcopenia and Obesity," *Journal of Obesity & Metabolic Syndrome* 29, no. 3 (2020): 180–87, https://doi.org:10.7570/jomes20006; Annette J. Thomas et al., "Effects of Isoflavones and Amino Acid Therapies for Hot Flashes and Co-occurring Symptoms During the Menopausal Transition and Early Postmenopause: A Sys-tematic Review," *Maturitas* 78, no. 4 (2014): 263–76, https://doi.org:10.1016/j.maturitas.2014.05.007; Abolfazl Fattah, "Effect of Phytoestrogen on Depres-sion and Anxiety in Menopausal Women: A Systematic Review," *Journal of Meno-pausal Medicine* 23, no. 3 (2017): 160–65, https://doi.org:10.6118/jmm.2017.23.3160.

15.  Mark Messina, "Soy and Health Update: Evaluation of the Clinical and Epidemiologic Literature," *Nutrients* 8, no. 12 (November 24, 2016): 754, https://doi.org:10.3390/nu8120754.

16.  Sarah J. O. Nomura et al., "Dietary Intake of Soy and Cruciferous Vegetables and Treatment-Related Symptoms in Chinese-American and Non-Hispanic White Breast Cancer Survivors," *Breast Cancer Research and Treatment* 168, no. 2 (2018): 467–79, https://doi.org:10.1007/s10549-017-4578-9.

17.  Carroll A. Reider et al., "Inadequacy of Immune Health Nutrients: Intakes in US Adults, the 2005–2016 NHANES," *Nutrients* 12, no. 6. (June 10, 2020): 1735, https://doi.org:10.3390/nu12061735; M. Ouzir, Nutritional and Health-Beneficial Values of Almond Nuts Consumption," *Nutrire* 48, no. 53 (2023), https://doi.org/10.1186/s41110-023-00239-2.

18.  David J. Baer et al., "Nuts, Energy Balance and Body Weight," *Nutrients* 15, no. 5 (February 25, 2023): 1162, https://doi.org:10.3390/nu15051162.

19.  Celia Bauset et al., "Nuts and Metabolic Syndrome: Reducing the Burden of Metabolic Syndrome in Menopause," *Nutrients* 14, no. 8 (April 18, 2022): 1677, https://doi.org:10.3390/nu14081677.

20.  Nuray Egelioglu Cetisli et al., "The Effects of Flaxseed on Menopausal Symptoms and Quality of Life," *Holistic Nursing Practice* 29, no. 3 (2015): 151–57, https://doi.org:10.1097/HNP.0000000000000085; Márcia Constantino Colli et al., "Evaluation of the Efficacy of Flaxseed Meal and Flaxseed Extract in Reducing

Menopausal Symptoms," *Journal of Medicinal Food* 15, no. 9 (2012): 840–45, https://doi.org:10.1089/jmf.2011.0228.

21. Andrea R. Josse et al., "Increased Consumption of Dairy Foods and Protein During Diet- and Exercise-Induced Weight Loss Promotes Fat Mass Loss and Lean Mass Gain in Overweight and Obese Premenopausal Women," *Journal of Nutrition* 141, no. 9 (2011): 1626–34, https://doi.org:10.3945/jn.111.141028.

22. Maryam Safabakhsh et al., "Higher Intakes of Fruits and Vegetables Are Related to Fewer Menopausal Symptoms: A Cross-sectional Study," *Menopause* (New York) 27, no. 5 (2020): 593–604, https://doi.org:10.1097/GME.0000000000001511.

23. Jong Min Baek et al., "Caffeine Intake Is Associated with Urinary Incontinence in Korean Postmenopausal Women: Results from the Korean National Health and Nutrition Examination Survey," *PloS One* 11, no. 2 (February 22, 2016): e0149311, https://doi.org:10.1371/journal.pone.0149311; Paru S. David et al., "Vasomotor Symptoms in Women Over 60: Results from the Data Registry on Experiences of Aging, Menopause, and Sexuality (DREAMS)," *Menopause* (New York) 25, no. 10 (2018): 1105–9, https://doi.org:10.1097/GME.0000000000001126; Andrew W. McHill et al., "Effects of Caffeine on Skin and Core Temperatures, Alertness, and Recovery Sleep During Circadian Misalignment," *Journal of Biological Rhythms* 29, no. 2 (2014): 131–43, https://doi.org:10.1177/0748730414523078.

24. Ramandeep Bansal and Neelam Aggarwal, "Menopausal Hot Flashes: A Concise Review," *Journal of Mid-life Health* 10, no. 1 (2019): 6–13, https://doi.org:10.4103/jmh.JMH_7_19.

25. Sharon Dormire and Chularat Howharn, "The Effect of Dietary Intake on Hot Flashes in Menopausal Women," *Journal of Obstetric, Gynecologic, and Neonatal Nursing: JOGNN* 36, no. 3 (2007): 255–62, https://doi.org:10.1111/j.1552-6909.2007.00142.x.

26. Mina Mohammady et al., "Effect of Omega-3 Supplements on Vasomotor Symptoms in Menopausal Women: A Systematic Review and Meta-analysis," *European Journal of Obstetrics, Gynecology, and Reproductive Biology* 228 (2018): 295–302, https://doi.org:10.1016/j.ejogrb.2018.07.008.

27. Ayesha Zafar Iqbal et al., "Effects of Omega-3 Polyunsaturated Fatty Acids Intake on Vasomotor Symptoms, Sleep Quality and Depression in Postmenopausal Women: A Systematic Review," *Nutrients* 15, no. 19 (September 30, 2023): 4231, https://doi.org:10.3390/nu15194231.

28. Abbie E. Smith-Ryan et al., "Creatine Supplementation in Women's Health: A Life-span Perspective," *Nutrients* 13, no. 3 (March 8, 2021): 877, https://doi.org:10.3390/nu13030877.

29. Darren G. Candow et al., "Effectiveness of Creatine Supplementation on Aging Muscle and Bone: Focus on Falls Prevention and Inflammation," *Journal of Clinical Medicine* 8, no. 4 (April 11, 2019): 488, https://doi.org:10.3390/jcm8040488.

30. Alexandra C. Purdue-Smithe et al., "Vitamin D and Calcium Intake and Risk of Early Menopause," *American Journal of Clinical Nutrition* 105, no. 6 (2017): 1493–1501, https://doi.org:10.3945/ajcn.116.145607.

31. Jia-Guo Zhao et al., "Association Between Calcium or Vitamin D Supplementation and Fracture Incidence in Community-Dwelling Older Adults: A Systematic Review and Meta-analysis," *JAMA* 318, no. 24 (2017): 2466–82, https://doi.org:10.1001/jama.2017.19344.

32. Seung-Kwon Myung et al., "Calcium Supplements and Risk of Cardiovascular Disease: A Meta-analysis of Clinical Trials," *Nutrients* 13, no. 2 (January 26, 2021): 368, https://doi.org:10.3390/nu13020368.

33. Blerina Shkembi and Thom Huppertz, "Calcium Absorption from Food Products: Food Matrix Effects," *Nutrients* 14, no. 1 (December 30, 2021): 180, https://doi.org:10.3390/nu14010180.

34. Aliz Erdélyi et al., "The Importance of Nutrition in Menopause and Perimenopause—a Review," *Nutrients* 16, no. 1 (December 21, 2023): 27, https://doi.org:10.3390/nu16010027.

35. Tae Won Kim et al., "The Impact of Sleep and Circadian Disturbance on Hormones and Metabolism," *International Journal of Endocrinology* 2015 (2015): 591729, https://doi.org:10.1155/2015/591729.

36. T. Liu et al., "Effects of Exercise on Vasomotor Symptoms in Menopausal Women: A Systematic Review and Meta-analysis," *Climacteric: The Journal of the International Menopause Society* 25, no. 6 (2022): 552–61, https://doi.org:10.1080/13697137.2022.2097865; Barbara Sternfeld et al., "Efficacy of Exercise for Menopausal Symptoms: A Randomized Controlled Trial," *Menopause* (New York) 21, no. 4 (2014): 330–38, https://doi.org:10.1097/GME.0b013e31829e4089.

37. Debra J. Anderson et al., "Obesity, Smoking, and Risk of Vasomotor Menopausal Symptoms: A Pooled Analysis of Eight Cohort Studies," *American Journal of Obstetrics and Gynecology* 222, no. 5 (2020): 478.e1–478.e17, https://doi.org:10.1016/j.ajog.2019.10.103.

38. Seo Yeon Choi et al., "Effects of Inhalation of Essential Oil of *Citrus aurantium* L. var. amara on Menopausal Symptoms, Stress, and Estrogen in Postmenopausal Women: A Randomized Controlled Trial," *Evidence-Based Complementary and Alternative Medicine: eCAM*, 2014 (2014): 796518, https://doi.org:10.1155/2014/796518.

39. Zahra Abbaspoor et al., "The Effect of *Citrus aurantium* Aroma on the Sleep Quality in Postmenopausal Women: A Randomized Controlled Trial," *International Journal of Community Based Nursing and Midwifery* 10, no. 2 (2022): 86–95, https://doi.org:10.30476/IJCBNM.2021.90322.1693.

**Chapter 10: Raising Healthy Happy Eaters: HCC for Kids**

1. Lori A. Francis and Leann L. Birch, "Maternal Influences on Daughters' Restrained Eating Behavior," *Health Psychology: Official Journal of the Division of Health Psychology, American Psychological Association* 24, no. 6 (2005): 548–54, https://doi.org:10.1037/0278-6133.24.6.548.

2. Katherine N. Balantekin, "The Influence of Parental Dieting Behavior on Child Dieting Behavior and Weight Status," *Current Obesity Reports* 8, no. 2 (2019): 137–44, https://doi.org:10.1007/s13679-019-00338-0.

3. "The Division of Responsibility in Feeding," Ellyn Satter Institute, accessed June 24, 2025, https://www.ellynsatterinstitute.org/how-to-feed/the-division-of-responsibility-in-feeding/.

4. Rafaella Dusi et al., "Division of Responsibility in Child Feeding and Eating Competence Among Brazilian Caregivers," *Nutrients* 15, no. 9 (May 8 2023): 2225, https://doi.org:10.3390/nu15092225.

5. Jerica M. Berge et al., "Cumulative Encouragement to Diet from Adolescence to Adulthood: Longitudinal Associations with Health, Psychosocial Well-Being, and

Romantic Relationships," *Journal of Adolescent Health: Official Publication of the Society for Adolescent Medicine* 65, no. 5 (2019): 690–97, https://doi.org:10.1016/j .jadohealth.2019.06.002.

6. Elizabeth A. O'Connor et al., "Screening for Obesity and Intervention for Weight Management in Children and Adolescents: Evidence Report and Systematic Review for the US Preventive Services Task Force," *JAMA* 317, no. 23 (2017): 2427–44, https://doi.org:10.1001/jama.2017.0332.

7. Giovanni Savarino et al., "Macronutrient Balance and Micronutrient Amounts Through Growth and Development," *Italian Journal of Pediatrics* 47, no. 1 (May 8, 2021): 109, https://doi.org:10.1186/s13052-021-01061-0.

8. Leann L. Birch et al., "Learning to Overeat: Maternal Use of Restrictive Feeding Practices Promotes Girls' Eating in the Absence of Hunger," *American Journal of Clinical Nutrition* 78, no. 2 (2003): 215–20, https://doi.org:10.1093/ajcn/78.2.215.

9. Chia-Yu Chang et al., "Essential Fatty Acids and Human Brain," *Acta neurologica Taiwanica* 18, no. 4 (2009): 231–41.

10. Maureen Spill et al., "Repeated Exposure to Foods and Early Food Acceptance: A Systematic Review," *USDA Nutrition Evidence Systematic Review* (April 2019), https://doi.org:10.52570/NESR.PB242018.SR0401.

11. George Du Toit et al., "Follow-Up to Adolescence After Early Peanut Introduction for Allergy Prevention," *NEJM Evidence* 3, no. 6 (2024): EVIDoa2300311, https:// doi.org:10.1056/EVIDoa2300311.

12. Therese A. O'Sullivan et al., "Whole-Fat or Reduced-Fat Dairy Product Intake, Adiposity, and Cardiometabolic Health in Children: A Systematic Review," *Advances in Nutrition* (Bethesda, MD) 11, no. 4 (2020): 928–50, https://doi.org:10 .1093/advances/nmaa011.

13. Ya-Ting Li et al., "Efficacy of *Lactobacillus rhamnosus* GG in Treatment of Acute Pediatric Diarrhea: A Systematic Review with Meta-analysis," *World Journal of Gastroenterology* 25, no. 33 (2019): 4999–5016, https://doi.org:10.3748/wjg.v25 .i33.4999.

14. Gwenn Schurgin O'Keeffe et al., "The Impact of Social Media on Children, Adolescents, and Families," *Pediatrics* 127, no. 4 (2011): 800–04, https://doi.org:10.1542 /peds.2011-0054; Yvonne Kelly et al., "Social Media Use and Adolescent Mental Health: Findings from the UK Millennium Cohort Study," *eClinicalMedicine* 6 (January 4, 2019): 59–68, https://doi.org:10.1016/j.eclinm.2018.12.005.

# RECIPE INDEX

· · · · · · · · · · · · · · · · · · · · · · · · · ·

# INDEX